DRUG USE
IN PREGNANCY

to my son, Peter

DRUG USE
IN PREGNANCY

JENNIFER R. NIEBYL, M.D.

Associate Professor,
Gynecology, Obstetrics, and Pediatrics,
Director, Division of Maternal-Fetal Medicine
Johns Hopkins University School of Medicine
Baltimore, Maryland

Second Edition

LEA & FEBIGER *Philadelphia*

1988

Lea & Febiger
600 Washington Square
Philadelphia, PA   19106-4198
U.S.A.
(215) 922-1330

First Edition, 1982

Library of Congress Cataloging-in-Publication Data

Drug use in pregnancy.

   Includes bibliographies and index.
   1. Obstetrical pharmacology. 2. Fetus—
Effect of drugs on. I. Niebyl, Jennifer R.
[DNLM: 1. Drug Therapy—adverse effects. 2. Drug
Therapy—in pregnancy. 3. Substance Abuse—in
pregnancy. WQ 240 D793]
RG528.D78   1988   618.2′061   87-17270
ISBN 0-8121-1119-2

PRINTED IN THE UNITED STATES OF AMERICA

Print number: 5   4   3   2   1

PREFACE

Caution has always been warranted about drug administration in pregnancy. With increasing emphasis on fetal health and well being, pregnant women often question the advisability of drug ingestion. In many medical situations, drug therapy is indicated.

This book addresses the use of drug groups for various clinical indications. In general, non-pharmacologic remedies are recommended if these will suffice before drug therapy is instituted. Known adverse effects of drugs are documented and caution is advised because of the many unknowns about long-term effects of drug exposure to the developing fetus.

This second edition has been expanded considerably to include coverage of drugs used for the common cold, antituberculosis agents, antihypertensives, anticonvulsants, and marijuana and cocaine exposure. Also, several new authors have contributed to chapters on the topics covered in the first edition. It is hoped that this book will be a useful resource for physicians who care for pregnant women.

I would like to thank Ms. Diane Wheeler who provided excellent secretarial assistance in the typing of several of the manuscripts.

Baltimore, Maryland   Jennifer R. Niebyl

CONTRIBUTORS

Ernest L. Abel, Ph.D.
Professor, Department of Obstetrics and Gynecology
Wayne State University School of Medicine
Division of Research
C.S. Mott Center for Human Growth and Development
Detroit, Michigan 48226

Gertrud S. Berkowitz, Ph.D.
Assistant Professor, Departments of Obstetrics, Gynecology and Reproductive Science and Community Medicine
Mount Sinai School of Medicine
New York, New York 10029

Richard E. Besinger, M.D.
Instructor, Department of Gynecology and Obstetrics
The John Hopkins University School of Medicine
Baltimore, Maryland 21205

David A. Blake, Ph.D.
Associate Professor, Gynecology and Obstetrics
Associate Dean for Research
The Johns Hopkins University School of Medicine
Baltimore, Maryland 21205

John Buscema, M.D.
Instructor, Gynecology and Obstetrics
The Johns Hopkins Hospital
Baltimore, Maryland 21205

Loretta P. Finnegan, M.D.
Director of Family Center Program
Professor of Pediatrics, and Psychiatry and Human Behavior
Jefferson Medical College of Thomas Jefferson University
Philadelphia, Pennsylvania 19107

Edward Goldberg, M.D.
Assistant Professor, Department of Gynecology and Obstetrics
The Johns Hopkins University School of Medicine
Baltimore, Maryland 21205

Kamal A. Hamod, M.D., M.P.H.
Assistant Professor, Department of Gynecology and Obstetrics
The Johns Hopkins University School of Medicine
Baltimore, Maryland 21205

John W.C. Johnson, M.D.
Professor and Acting Chairman, Department of Obstetrics and Gynecology
University of Florida College of Medicine
Gainesville, Florida 32611

Timothy R.B. Johnson, M.D.
Assistant Professor, Department of Gynecology and Obstetrics
Divsion of Maternal-Fetal Medicine
The Johns Hopkins University School of Medicine
Baltimore, Maryland 21205

Victor A. Khouzami, M.D.
Assistant Professor, Department of Gynecology and Obstetrics
The Johns Hopkins University School of Medicine
Baltimore, Maryland 21205

Paul S. Lietman, M.D.
Wellcome Professor, Clinical Pharmacology
The Johns Hopkins University School of Medicine
Baltimore, Maryland 21205

Charles Lockwood, M.D.
Fellow in Maternal-Fetal Medicine
Department of Obstetrics and Gynecology
Yale University School of Medicine
New Haven, Connecticut 06510–8063

Keith D. Maxwell, M.D.*
Instructor, Department of Gynecology and Obstetrics
The Johns Hopkins University School of Medicine
Baltimore, Maryland 21205

Jennifer R. Niebyl, M.D.
Associate Professor, Department of Gynecology and Obstetrics and Pediatrics
Director, Division of Maternal-Fetal Medicine
The Johns Hopkins University School of Medicine
Baltimore, Maryland 21205

---

*Deceased

Roberto Romero, M.D.
Associate Professor, Department of Obstetrics and
Gynecology
Section of Maternal-Fetal Medicine
Director, Perinatal Research
Yale University School of Medicine
New Haven, Connecticut   06510–8063

Anthony R. Scialli, M.D.
Director, Reproductive Toxicology Center
Columbia Hospital for Women
Washington, D.C.   20037

Robert J. Sokol, M.D.
Professor, Chairman, and Chief of Gynecology
and Obstetrics
Wayne State University School of Medicine
Hutzel Hospital
Detroit, Michigan   48201

Jeffrey L. Stern, M.D.
Assistant Professor, Obstetrics and Gynecology
University of California, San Francisco
San Francisco, California   94123

Ronald L. Thomas, M.D.
Instructor, Department of Gynecology and Ob-
stetrics
The Johns Hopkins University School of Medicine
Baltimore, Maryland   21205

Ronald J. Wapner, M.D.
Associate Professor, Obstetrics and Gynecology
Division of Maternal-Fetal Medicine
Jefferson Medical College of Thomas Jefferson
University
Philadelphia, Pennsylvania   19107

Frank R. Witter, M.D.
Assistant Professor, Department of Gynecology
and Obstetrics
Division of Maternal-Fetal Medicine
The Johns Hopkins University School of Medicine
Baltimore, Maryland   21205

CONTENTS

Chapter 1

Requirements and Limitations in Reproductive and Teratogenic Risk Assessment

David A. Blake and Jennifer R. Niebyl

Prompted by the thalidomide incident of the early 1960s, regulatory agencies initiated requirements for animal testing of therapeutic drugs to detect teratogenic potential prior to their widespread distribution. The experience of two subsequent decades of extensive testing has failed to demonstrate the reliability of animal studies in the prediction of human teratogenic potential. There are so many examples of inconsistency between results of animal teratologic studies and the human experience that a credibility gap has developed. Epidemiologic studies have shown that numerous drugs have insignificant human teratogenic potential,[1] and yet many of these drugs have produced positive results in multiple laboratory animal species.[2] This chapter will outline the current procedures for in vivo teratogenicity testing in animals, discuss probable reasons for their limitations, and provide a preliminary critical evaluation of the degree of predictability.

Teratogenicity means the capacity to induce congenital monsters. Historically the focus has been on major overt morphologic abnormalities. There is, however, a growing tendency to broaden the definition of teratogenicity beyond major dysmorphogenesis by including minor and latent (covert) structural abnormalities. Furthermore, it is recognized that functional behavioral abnormalities should also be considered. Unfortunately, the majority of teratologic testing has focused only on the state of anatomic development at the end of pregnancy.

HUMAN CORRELATIONS

Developmental defects in humans may be from genetic or environmental causes, or from interactions between both of these. Drug exposure accounts for only 2 to 3% of birth defects. In approximately 25% of the defects, the etiology is genetic. Thus, the vast majority of anomalies are of unknown causes.

The incidence of major malformations in the general population is approximately 2 to 3%. A major malformation is defined as one that is incompatible with survival such as anenecephaly, or one which requires major surgery for correction such as cleft palate or congenital heart disease. If all minor malformations are also included such as ear tags or extra digits, the rate may be high as 7 to 10% The risk of malformation after exposure to a drug must be compared with this background rate.

1

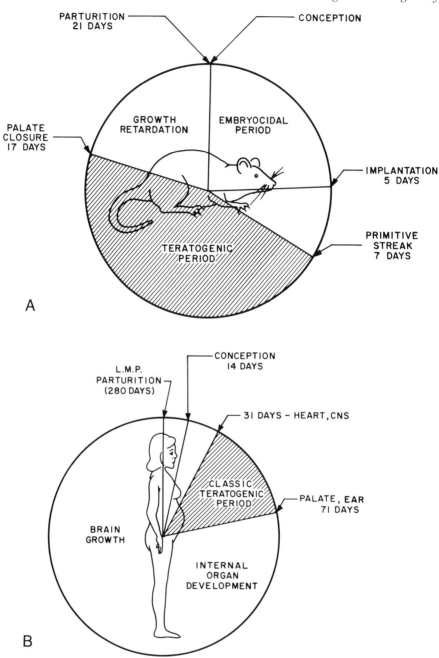

Fig. 1–1. A. This diagram indicates the approximate gestational days encompassing the teratogenic period in the rat. This period coincides with the period of organogenesis and is the time of greatest sensitivity to dysmorphic abnormalities. B. The classic teratogenic period in the human comprises a smaller proportion of pregnancy than in the rat. Exposure to teratogens during this period results in overt defects usually recognizable at birth. Other organ development continues in the second and third trimester, and effects of exposure to drugs at this time may not be recognized until later in life.

The classic teratogenic period in the human is a critical 6 weeks, but a smaller percentage of the total pregnancy than in the rat (Fig. 1–1). It lasts from approximately 31 days after the last menstrual period (a few days after the missed period) through 10 weeks from the last menstrual period. The effect of any known teratogen is dependent on the timing of exposure as well as the nature of the teratogen. Early in the teratogenic period when the heart and central nervous system are forming, exposure to a known teratogen will result in an anomaly such as congenital heart disease or neural tube defect. Nearer the end of the classic teratogenic period, malformations of the palate or ear may occur. As the heart is already formed by 10 weeks from the last menstrual period, exposure at that time cannot cause congenital heart disease.

There is a great deal of species specificity. Thalidomide was tested in rats and mice and was not teratogenic, but it was subsequently noted to be a significant human teratogen. Alternately, although certain strains of mice are extremely sensitive to corticosteroids in producing cleft lip, there is no evidence to date suggesting that corticosteroids used for human diseases in therapeutic doses cause any increased risk of congenital defects in the offspring.

Prior to the time of the classic teratogenic period, exposure to a teratogen has an all or none effect. Thus, an exposure around the time of conception or implantation may kill the conceptus and the patient may not realize that she is pregnant, but if the pregnancy continues, there is no increased risk of congenital anomalies if the exposure is before organogenesis. At this early time, the cells are totipotential. In fact, the conceptus can split in half and form identical twins, both of which are normal. Careful evaluation of time of exposure is therefore important in counselling for risk of birth defects.

Although it is commonly stated that once the teratogenic period is passed the risk of congenital anomalies is gone, it is becoming increasingly clear that important other development continues throughout pregnancy. Some of the exposures to diethylstilbestrol were as late as 20 weeks of gestation causing anomalies in the internal organs which were not recognized in the offspring until puberty or later. Another example of continued organ growth and development during pregnancy is that of the brain. Because it is recognized that chronic exposure to psychoactive medications such as alcohol may cause mental retardation, one should be cautious about chronic prescription of any psychoactive drugs even in the second and third trimester of pregnancy at the time when the brain is continuing to grow. A new field of "behavioral teratology" is developing, looking at later behavioral effects of in utero exposures. Thus, although the defects produced in the classic teratogenic period are overt at birth, other developing organs may be affected and their abnormalities not recognized until years later.

The Food and Drug Administration lists five categories of labeling for drug use in pregnancy:

A. Controlled studies in women fail to demonstrate a risk to the fetus in the first trimester, and the possibility of fetal harm appears remote.

B. Animal studies do not indicate a risk to the fetus and there are no controlled human studies, or animal studies to show an adverse effect on the fetus but well-controlled studies in pregnant women have failed to demonstrate a risk to the fetus.

C. Studies have shown the drug to have animal teratogenic or embryocidal effects, but there are no controlled studies in women, or no studies are available in either animals or women.

D.   Positive evidence of human fetal risk exists, but benefits in certain situations (e.g., life-threatening situations or serious diseases for which safer drugs cannot be used or are ineffective) may make use of the drug acceptable despite its risks.

E.   Studies in animals or humans have demonstrated fetal abnormalities or there is evidence of fetal risk based on human experience, or both, and the risk clearly outweighs any possible benefit.

Patients should be educated about avenues other than the use of drugs to cope with various disorders during pregnancy. The risk-benefit ratio should justify the use of a particular drug and the minimum effective dose should be employed. As long term effects of drug exposure in utero may not be revealed for many years, caution is warranted with regard to the use of any drug in pregnancy.

Animal Procedures

Pregnant animals are treated during the period of embryonic development (organogenesis) (Fig. 1–1) and fetuses are removed from killed mothers a few days prior to parturition. It is observed that mothers will cannibalize abnormal or dead offspring if allowed to deliver spontaneously. The usual periods of treatment (in days of gestation with day zero being the day of conception) are: mice and rats—6 to 15 days; rabbits—6 to 18 days. Treatments are avoided before and after these periods to minimize the chance that the teratogenic potential of a chemical might be obscured by its lethal effect on the conceptus. In addition, there is some evidence that initiating treatment substantially before the critical period of gestation will provide an opportunity for induction of detoxification enzyme activity resulting in reduced fetal exposure to the agent. Potential embryo lethality is evaluated by decreased litter size or disparity between ovarian corpora lutea and implantations.

It is common practice to evaluate gross abnormalties initially and then to group living fetuses for examination of visceral anomalies or skeletal anomalies. Results are separately tabulated as: litter size (number of implantations), lethal effect (number of resorbed embryos and dead fetuses), teratogenic effect (number of malformed live fetuses), and fetal growth retardation (reduced body weight of live fetuses). The practice of separate categorization of offspring hampers statistical analysis for dose-related effects since an embryopathic chemical often causes primarily deaths at high levels resulting in decreased apparent malformation rates. In studies with thalidomide in rabbits, Schumacher et al.[3] demonstrated a linear relationship between the log of dose and total "abnormalities" when dead or malformed fetuses were considered to be abnormal. Such a categorization seems reasonable unless fetal death and fetal malformation can be shown to be mutually exclusive events. A linear dose-response curve provides the opportunity for statistical determination of the 50% embryopathic effect level which can be compared to the maternal LD_{50} for evaluation of direct embryotoxicity. Using this approach to evaluate animal teratogenicity data from the literature, Jusko[4] has demonstrated that drugs can be classified into two categories: those that have a dose threshold for teratogenic effect and those that do not. The former group (including aspirin) has 50% embryopathic doses that are close to the maternal lethal doses, whereas the latter group (including thalido-mide) has greater direct embryopathic potential. Presumably, there is greater teratogenic risk with a compound that has no apparent threshold to its effect and causes malformations at a dose level considerably below that causing ma-ternal toxicity. Although such dose-effect analyses are common in other branches of toxicology, it is rare to find them in the teratologic literature.

Multigeneration reproductive studies have been advocated by regulatory officials[5] although an advisory panel has questioned their value beyond the second filial generation.[6] It is generally accepted that a complete evaluation of reproductive toxicity should include study of the reproductive performance in the F_1 animals which have been exposed continuously to the test substance from the time of conception and during the periods of embryogenesis, infancy, pu-berty, and reproductive maturity. This assessment requires observation of the growth and development of the F_2 generation through weaning.

Possible Reasons for Deficiences

DOSAGE

As previously discussed, meaningful interpretation of teratologic studies re-quires consideration of the relationship between the teratologic dose range and the maternal toxic dose range. Since abnormal fetal development is likely to result if the mothers are "sick," it is generally recommended that the highest dose level produce minimal, but measurable, maternal toxicity. Indirect "pseu-doteratogenicity" can occur if the treatment causes excessive depression of ma-ternal eating or drinking.[7,8]

PHARMACOKINETICS

The fraction of administered dose ultimately reaching sites of teratogenic ac-tion in the conceptus or placenta is governed by multiple kinetic factors including rates of absorption, biotransformation, placental passage, and maternal excre-tion. Inconsistent teratologic results between experiments, laboratories, species, and strains of animals can often be explained by variations in these factors. Keller and Blake[8] demonstrated a 400% difference in plasma levels of thalidomide in rabbits depending on the oral dosage formulation. The widely investigated strain-dependent susceptibility of mice to cortisone-induced anomalies correlates with slower material elimination of the drug in the more susceptible strain.[9] Although transport of chemicals across the placenta late in gestation has received a great deal of experimental attention, there is much less information on maternal-fetal exchange early in gestation when morphologic teratogenesis is induced. Moreover, there is a complete void in our knowledge of the amount of matenally-administered drug reaching the early human embryo at known levels of exposure. Thus, it is difficult to devise rational dosing regimens in animal experiments that would be relevant to the human situation.

Until recently, it was thought that the fetus lacked the enzyme activity re-sponsible for biotransformation of drugs and other xenobiotics. Through im-proved analytic methodology, it is now known that fetal liver, particularly in primates, possesses many of the metabolic capabilities of adult liver. Some of these metabolic transformations result in the formation of reactive metabolites that can bind to cellular macromolecules and thereby cause cancer, mutations, and cell death. Emerging evidence suggests that metabolites play a role in the mechanisms of embryopathy. Because the enzymatic activity responsible for these reactions is related to genotype and multiple environmental factors, it may also provide an explanation for species and other variations in teratologic results. The anticonvulsant phenytoin (Dilantin) is metabolized to a dihydrodiol metabolite via a reactive arene oxide intermediate. The arene oxide intermediate presumably binds covalently to fetal macromolecules and may be the cause of the well-documented teratogenic effect of the drug in mice.[10] Studies in our laboratory have shown a species correlation between susceptibility to phenytoin-induced teratogenesis and formation of the dihydrodiol metabolite in fetal liver.[11] There is also a strain-dependent embryopathic sensitivity to certain polycyclic aromatic hydrocarbons (PAH's) in mice which is related to the genotype determining inducibility of aryl hydrocarbon hydroxylase (AHH).[12] AHH converts PAH's to reactive toxic metabolites. We have found that fetal livers from four strains of mice activate benzo(a)pyrene to mutagenic metabolites at an efficiency that linearly correlates with their induced levels of AHH.[13] These findings provide a basis for the widely discussed genetic-environmental interactions that presumably explain multifactorial inheritance of susceptibility to birth defects.

A human genetic predisposition to phenytoin-induced birth defects has also been shown.[14] Lymphocytes from children exposed to phenytoin throughout gestation were challenged with phenytoin metabolites, looking for cell death. A positive challenge was highly correlated with major birth defects, suggesting that a genetic defect in arene oxide detoxification in the infant increased the risk of a major birth defect.

Predictability of Teratogenic Potential

The ultimate utility of any animal toxicologic testing procedure depends on the degree of extrapolatability to human beings. Thalidomide is the only chemical known to have a profound teratogenic effect in humans at non-toxic maternal dose levels and the failure to detect positive results with standard teratologic tests in mice and rats is well known. It was determined retrospectively that thalidomide was teratogenic in rabbits and monkeys but there is no assurance that these species would be better predictors for other human teratogens. Since there are only a few drugs with known human teratogenic potential,[1] it is difficult to evaluate predictability against known positives.

In contrast, there are numerous therapeutic drugs now known to have little or no human teratogenic risk.[1] This information is derived from a review of the data from the Perinatal Collaborative Project, a prospective and concurrent epidemiologic study of more than 50,000 pregnancies. The ascertainment of drug exposure in the first 4 months of pregnancy and uniformity of categorization of major structural anomalies is unparalleled by any other study to date. For many popular drugs, there were sufficient numbers of exposed cases to permit statistical confidence of the lack of teratogenic effect, at least under prevailing conditions of use. The results obtained for 16 drugs are listed in Table 1–1; values are given for the number of exposed cases (at least 100 for each drug selected) and the relative risk ratio after standardization for race and survival. A ratio of 1.0 indicates an identical frequency of congenital anomalies between exposed and non-exposed cases. The only drug on this list with a ratio significantly greater than unity is insulin. As maternal diabetes is known to be associated with an increased risk of congenital anomalies, this cannot be construed as cause and

Table 1–1. Predictability of Teratogenic Potential

Drug	Human[a]		Animal[b]	
	Number Exposed	Relative Risk	Species	Result
Analgesics:				
Aspirin	14,864	1.04	Rat	+
			Mouse	+
			Monkey	+
			Rabbit	−
Salicylamide	744	0.95	Hamster	+
Propoxyphene	686	0.99	Rat	−
			Mouse	−
			Rabbit	−
Antibacterials:				
Sulfisoxazole	796	1.04	Mouse	+
			Rat	+
Penicillins	3,546	1.07	Mouse	−
			Rat	−
Tetracycline	341	1.14	Mouse	+/−
			Rat	+/−
Anticonvulsants:				
Phenytoin	132	1.56	Mouse	+ +
			Rat	+/−
			Monkey	+/−
Phenobarbital	1,415	1.03	Mouse	+
			Rabbit	+
Antinauseants:				
Meclizine	1,014	1.21	Rat	+
			Ferret	+
Doxylamine	1,169	1.06	Rabbit	−
Prochlorperazine	877	1.18	Mouse	+
			Rat	+
Diphenhydramine	595	1.33	Rat	−
			Rabbit	−
			Mouse	+ (vitro)
Hormones				
Insulin	121	2.09 ($p < 0.01$)	Rat	+
			Mouse	+
			Rabbit	+
Norethynodrel	154	1.10	Rat	−
Stimulants:				
d-Amphetamine	367	1.11	Mouse	+
			Rabbit	+
Caffeine	5,378	0.98	Mouse	+/−
			Rat	+/−
			Rabbit	+/−

[a]From Heinonen et al[1]
[b]From Shepard[2]

effect. Also, shown in the table are the results of animal teratologic tests in various species taken from the reference text of Shepard.[2] A degree of subjective judgment was required to translate Shepard's comments into + or − categories and no consideration is given to the relevance of dose levels employed.

It can be seen that for 8 of 16 drugs (aspirin, salicylamide, sulfisoxazole, phenytoin, phenobarbital, meclizine, prochlorperazine and d-amphetamine), there was disagreement between animal tests and the human experience; the animal test results were positive (for at least one species) and the human experience negative. For 6 drugs, there was agreement; positive animal results correlating with a positive human result for 1 drug (insulin) and negative results with both animals and humans for 5 others (propoxyphene, penicillins, doxylamine, diphenhydramine, and norethynodrel). No decision could be reached for 2 drugs (tetracycline and caffeine) because of disagreement between studies with the same animal species. It should be realized that the reference source used for animal teratologic results is incomplete and other studies exist in the literature which would alter the comparability for a few of the drugs, particularly those with negative findings. In addition, the relative merits of individual animal studies could be argued extensively. These considerations aside, the obvious conclusion is that in vivo teratologic tests have poor predictability of human teratogenic potential. Generally stated, it would appear that most drugs can be found to be teratogenic in some animal models, while few drugs have a clinically significant teratogenic potential.

Isotretinoin

An example of a recently marketed drug whose teratogenic potential was predicted from subhuman primate testing is isotretinoin (Accutane). Isotretinoin is a significant human teratogen. This drug is marketed for treatment of cystic acne and thus has been taken inadvertently by teenagers who were not planning pregnancy.[15] When the drug was first marketed, it contained warnings that it had been shown to be teratogenic in subhuman primates and was contraindicated in pregnancy (FDA Category X). Of 154 exposed human pregnancies to date, there have been 21 reported cases of birth defects, 12 spontaneous abortions, 95 elective abortions, and 26 normal infants in women who were taking isotretinoin during early pregnancy.[16] The actual risk of anomalies was 14% in the prospective study of 36 exposed infants.

The 21 malformed infants had a characteristic pattern of craniofacial, cardiac, thymic, and central nervous system anomalies. They included microtia/anotia (absent ears) in 15 infants, micrognathia in 6, cleft palate in 3, heart defects in 8, thymic defects in 7, retinal or optic nerve anomalies in 4, and CNS malformations including hydrocephalus in 18.[4]

Isotretinoin is not stored in tissue, unlike vitamin A, so an exposure before pregnancy should not be a risk since the drug would not be detectable in serum 5 days after ingestion.

RECOMMENDATION

Hopefully through improvements in design and interpretation of animal tests and more appropriate selection of species based on comparability of metabolism, it may be possible in the future to improve on what currently must be regarded as unreliable toxicologic test procedure.

REFERENCES

1. Heinonen, O.P., Slone, D. and Shapiro, S.: Birth Defects and Drugs in Pregnancy, Littleton, Mass, Publishing Science Group, Inc, 1977.
2. Shepard, T.H.: Catalog of Teratogenic Agents. 2nd Ed, Baltimore, Johns Hopkins University Press, 1976.
3. Schumacher, H., Blake, D.A. Gurian, J.M., et al.: A comparison of the teratogenic activity of thalidomide in rabbits and rats. J Pharmacol Exp Ther, *160*:189, 1968.
4. Jusko, W.J.: Pharmacodynamic principles in chemical teratology: dose-effect relationships. J Pharmacol Exp Ther, *183*:469, 1972.
5. Kokoski, C.J.: Testimony at the Food and Drug Administration's public hearing on use of acrylonitrile for beverage packaging. Food Chem News, July 11, 8, 1977.
6. Anon: Food and Drug Administration Advisory Committee on Protocols for Safety Evaluation: Panel on reproduction report on reproduction studies in the safety evaluation of food additives and pesticide residues. Toxicol Appl Pharmacol, *16*:264, 1970.
7. Hemm, R.D., Arslanoglou, L. and Pollack, J.: Cleft palate following prenatal food restriction in mice: association with elevated maternal corticosteroids. Teratol, *15*:243, 1977.
8. Keller, G.R. and Blake, D.A.: Comparative studies on the absorption of thalidomide in rabbits and rats. Teratol, *4*:75, 1971.
9. Levine, A., Yaffe, S.J. and Back, N.: Maternal-fetal distribution of radioactive cortisol and its correlation with teratogenic effect. Proc Soc Exp Biol Med, *129*:86, 1968.
10. Martz, F., Failinger, C. and Blake, D.A.: Phenytoin teratogenesis: correlation between embryopathic effect and covalent binding of putative arene oxide metabolite in gestational tissues. J Pharmacol Exp Ther, *203*:231, 1977.
11. Blake, D.A., Martz, F., Failinger, C., et al.: Arene oxide mediated chemoteratogenesis. In Polynuclear Aromatic Hydrocarbons: Chemistry, Metabolism and Carcinogenesis, P.W. Jones and R.I. Freudenthal (eds), New York, Raven Press, 1978, pp. 401–411
12. Lambert, G.H. and Nebert, D.W.: Genetically mediated induction of drug-metabolizing enzymes associated with congenital defects in the mouse. Teratol, *16*:147, 1977.
13. Blake, D.A., Martz, F., Gery-Martz, A.M., et al.: Fetal tissues from various strains of induced mice metabolize benzo(a)pyrene to mutagenic metabolites. Teratol, *20*:377, 1979.
14. Strickler, S.M., Miller, M.A., Andermann, E., et al.: Genetic predisposition to phenytoin induced birth defects. Lancet, 2:746, 1985.
15. Rosa, F.: JAMA, *251*:3208, 1984.
16. Lammer, E.J., Chen, D.T., Hoar, R.M., et al.: Retinoic acid embryopathy. N Engl J Med, *313*: 837, 1985.

Chapter 2

Treatment of the Nausea and Vomiting of Pregnancy

Jennifer R. Niebyl and Keith D. Maxwell*

Nausea and vomiting are so common and predictable in pregnancy as to serve as one means of suspecting the presence of an early gestation. The spectrum of symptoms is wide, with some women experiencing only occasional mild nausea and others suffering severe nausea and vomiting throughout the first half of pregnancy. Because of different definitions of the syndrome of nausea and vomiting of pregnancy, the reported incidences vary widely, ranging from 25[1] to 88%.[2] To reconsider the status of drugs used for this condition, the Council on Pharmacy and Chemistry in 1956 found it necessary to attempt a precise definiton of the terminology:

> . . . although the term "nausea and vomiting of pregnancy" is applicable to both mild and severe forms, its use should be restricted to the condition, commonly observed during the first 14 to 16 weeks or pregnancy, that is characterized by some disturbance in appetite and reactions to food in a fairly large percentage of women. These reactions may vary from morning nausea to occasional emesis but are not accompanied by any signs of disturbed nutritional status. . . . The term hyperemesis gravidarum . . . should be applied to the condition occurring in the few patients who exhibit intractable vomiting and signs of disturbed nutritional status, such as alterations of electrolyte balance, 5% or more weight loss, ketosis, and acetonuria, with ultimate neurological disturbances, liver damage, retinal hemorrhage, and renal damage.[1]

Besides the problem of definition, the cause of nausea and vomiting of pregnancy has not been found, although many mechanical, endocrine, allergic, metabolic, toxic, and psychosomatic mechanisms have been proposed over the years (Table 2–1). Each theory of etiology has resulted in a new treatment (Tables 2–2 and 2–3), and success of a similar magnitude (70 to 100% cure or clinical improvement rate) has been claimed for each therapeutic regimen.[3] With so many sometimes contradictory treatments being touted as successful, it is clear that problems exist in the judging of the efficacy of therapy for this condition.

PROBLEMS ENCOUNTERED IN EVALUATION OF EFFICACY OF TREATMENTS

THE SYNDROME

Probably the greatest problem in judging the effect of a treatment is the protean nature of the syndrome itself. The onset is quite variable in its relationship to the time of conception. In one study, 23% of the patients had symptoms before they had missed a menstrual period, and others did not develop symptoms until the 14th week of pregnancy.[2] The condition is self-limiting, and an inves-

---

*Deceased

**Table 2–1.   Proposed Etiologies for the Nausea and
Vomiting of Pregnancy**[3,5]

Mechanical
  Congestion, Inflammation, Distention, Displacement, or Other Conditions
    of the Uterus and/or Cervix

Endocrinologic
  Sensitivity to Secretions of the Corpus Luteum of Pregnancy
    "Excessive" Estrogen or Progesterone
  Excessive Deportation of Chorionic Villi into Maternal Circulation
  Suppression of Ovarian Secretions
    Progesterone or Estrogen Deficiency
  Excessive HCG
  Relative Adrenocortical Insufficiency
  Secondary Hypopituitarism

Allergic
  Allergy to Secretions of Corpus Luteum or to Placental Proteins
  Allergy to Husband's Antigens
  Isoagglutinins
  Histamine Poisoning

Metabolic
  Intestinal Toxins
  Carbohydrate Deficiency
  Pyridoxine Deficiency

Psychosomatic
  Unconscious Repudiation or Aversion to Femininity, Pregnancy, Coitus, or
    the Husband
  Self-punishment
  Subconscious Desire for Abortion
  General Psychological Immaturity
  Hysteria
  Strong Mother-Dependence

tigator must be aware that a significant number of the subjects under study will become asymptomatic irrespective of any therapeutic measures undertaken. Symptoms may be intermittent, with the patient reporting a 1- or 2-day hiatus during which she has no symptoms, but after which her nausea and vomiting return unabated. Associated symptoms such as excessive salivation, constipation, and heartburn may be present.

Placebo Effect

Most, if not all, authorities on nausea and vomiting in pregnancy recognize a significant psychologic component[1,4] and numerous studies have shown that many sufferers (50% or more) will improve dramatically when given a placebo.[5-7] Because the placebo effect is significant, clinical investigations of drugs proposed for treatment must be double-blinded to yield meaningful results.[1]

The presence of the psychologic component in the nausea and vomiting of pregnancy should not be misconstrued as an indication of underlying mental illness. In a 3 1/2 year follow-up study of 48 women with hyperemesis gravidarum and 45 controls, the only chronic psychiatric illness that appeared significantly more frequently in the women with hyperemesis gravidarum was hysteria, 15% versus 2%.[8] In other words, even when the vomiting is sufficiently

Table 2–2. Treatments Proposed for Hyperemesis Gravidarum[3,7]

Hormonal
  Estrogens
  Progesterone
  Testosterone Propionate
  Adrenal Cortex
  ACTH, Cortisone
  Parathyroid Extract and Calcium
  Insulin
  Ovarian Extract
Vitamin
  B_1, B_6, B_{12}
  K
  C
  Liver Extract
Mineral
  Lugol's Iodine
  Calcium Gluconate
Other
  Glycerin and Boric Acid Tampons
  Autohemotherapy
  Injections of Husband's Blood
  Hibernotherapy
  Glucose
  Placental Extract
  Phosphorated Carbohydrated Solutions
  Multiple Intestinal Absorbents
  Intravenous Honey
  Oral Fructose, Glucose, and Orthophosphoric Acid
  Induction Current
  Intravenous Procaine
  Dextroamphetamine
  Blocking the Stellate Ganglion
  Hypnosis

Table 2–3. Drugs Used in Treatment of Nausea and Vomiting of Pregnancy[3,4]

Antihistamines
  Piperazines
    Meclizine (Antivert, Bonine)
    Cyclizine (Marezine)
    Buclizine (Bucladin)
  Ethanolamine
    Dimenhydrinate (Dramamine)
    Doxylamine and Pyridoxine (Bendectin)
    Trimethobenzamide (Tigan)

Phenothiazines
    Chlorpromazine (Thorazine)
    Prochlorperazine (Compazine, Combid)
    Promethazine (Phenergan)
    Promazine (Sparine)
    Triethylperazine (Torecan)

severe to be termed hyperemesis gravidarum, it is in the great majority of cases not a manifestation of clinical psychiatric disease.

Differential Diagnosis

Numerous conditions can be associated with nausea and vomiting during gestation,[4,5] including appendicitis, pyelonephritis, gastroenteritis, hepatitis, cholecystitic, pancreatitis, and many others. Thus, the clinician must remember that the diagnosis of nausea and vomiting of pregnancy is essentially one of exclusion.[4] Associated symptoms and signs must be considered before the nausea or vomiting is attributed to the pregnancy alone.

PROBLEMS ENCOUNTERED IN DETERMINING THE SAFETY OF A TREATMENT

Once one has designed a randomized, double-blind placebo-controlled study which might be sufficient to measure the efficacy of a new medication in treating the nausea and vomiting of pregnancy, one next must concern oneself with the safety of the proposed treatment. Deleterious effects of a drug can appear as an increased number of abortions, perinatal deaths, or congenital anomalies.[12] One confounding variable is that several investigators have reported a lower spontaneous abortion rate in women suffering from nausea and vomiting in the first trimester than in women with no symptoms.[9-14] One study indicated the relationship between nausea and vomiting and abortion to be an inverse one: the more severe the nausea and vomiting, the less the tendency to abort, and the patients who did abort had little or no nausea or vomiting.[10] Some investigators found not only a higher abortion rate, but also higher neonatal and perinatal mortality rates (due to a higher rate of smaller babies and shorter gestations) in pregnancies characterized by an absence of nausea in the first trimester.[13,14] Speert and Guttmacher found that the absence of nausea could be used to predict which patient with first trimester vaginal bleeding was destined to abort.[9]

Because of the inverse relationships between nausea and abortion, an adequate control group for the study of patients treated with a specific medication for the nausea and vomiting in pregnancy would have to consist of other patients suffering from nausea and vomiting; a control group consisting of asymptomatic pregnant patients would yield biased results, at least in terms of abortion rates.[12]

In a review of over 33,000 pregnancies complicated by nausea and vomiting, there was no evidence that vomiting or a diagnosis of hyperemesis gravidarum was associated with an increased (or decreased) incidence of malformations.[15] Thus, a drug with teratogenic effects could be identified with an adequately controlled, sufficiently large study.

TREATMENT OF NAUSEA AND VOMITING OF PREGNANCY

Since ancient times, the initial approach to the nausea and vomiting of pregnancy has consisted of numerous supportive measures: frequent, small feedings of bland, dry, mainly carbohydrate foods; liquids in small amounts; sufficient rest, especially after meals; avoidance of unpleasant odors and other irritating situations such as iron tablets; emotional support; and reassurance by the physician.[3-5] Protein-containing snacks at night and crackers by the bedside in the morning are helpful to some patients. For the majority of patients, these supportive measures suffice. For the remaining patients, symptoms will persist despite use of the non-pharmacologic measures. It is in these patients that the physician will consider the use of various antiemetics (Table 2–3).

In the small number of patients whose condition is severe enough to be hyperemesis gravidarum, the pressing need will be for hospitalization with intravenous hydration and correction of metabolic and electrolyte imbalances. Drug therapy will be of a secondary consideration. However, once the acute problems have been dealt with, the physician may choose to handle these patients on an outpatient basis with an antinauseant.

Antihistamines

Antihistamines constitute the most frequently used medications for nausea in pregnancy. Their usage has been controversial, with some authorities feeling that they were no more effective than placebos and attributing any effect to a sedative action rather than any specific inhibition of nausea and vomiting.

MECLIZINE

One of the most widely used and studied antihistamines is meclizine (Antivert, Bonine). After the United States Army, Navy, and Air Force Motion Sickness Team reported in 1956 that meclizine was the drug of choice in preventing motion sickness during long sea voyages,[16] that drug also gained wide acceptance for treatment of nausea and vomiting of pregnancy.

Uncontrolled studies reported complete or partial relief of symptoms in over 90% of patients, and mild side effects (drowsiness) in 4.3%.[17] The statistics contrasted favorably with the 29% failure rate and significant incidence of side effects reported with dimenhydrinate, another antihistamine.[6] In a small, randomized placebo-controlled study, meclizine gave significantly better results than a placebo.[2] The addition of pyridoxine failed to improve the results with meclizine alone. Thus, meclizine was accepted as an efficacious agent for treating the nausea and vomiting of pregnancy.

After the thalidomide tragedy in 1956, the use of drugs at the time of organogenesis came under close scrutiny.[4] Sporadic reports began to appear which reported congenital anomalies in infants born to mothers who had taken meclizine.[12,18,19] However, no adequate control group was available, the results were inconclusive and contradictory, and no definite pattern of anomalies as occurred with thalidomide could be detected.[12]

Despite these inadequacies of the available information, the Swedish National Board of Health withdrew meclizine from public sale in Sweden and warned doctors not to prescribe the drug for women in the early months of pregnancy,[20] and the Epidemic Observation Unit of the College of General Practitioners in England warned physicians of the "mounting evidence against the safety of meclizine."[18]

After studies in rats demonstrated a teratogenic effect of cyclizine (an antihistamine which approaches meclizine in its efficacy), congenital malformations were induced in the offspring of pregnant Sprague-Dawley rats by the administration of large doses of meclizine.[19] However, the meaning of these results for humans was questioned because the doses used were 25 to 50 times the recommended dose in humans, and the possibility of species-specificity of effect had not been ruled out.[12]

Because meclizine has been so widely used and because 2 to 3% of infants are born with major malformations, it is not surprising that some infants with anomalies are born to mothers who have taken meclizine at some point in their pregnancies.[20] However, prospective clinical studies have provided no evidence that meclizine is teratogenic in man.[12,20,21] In 1,014 patients in the Collaborative Perinatal Project[15] and an additional 613 patients from the Kaiser Health Plan,[21] no teratogenic risk was found.

BENDECTIN

Bendectin contained doxylamine succinate 10 mg and pyridoxine (vitamin B_6) 10 mg. In the placebo-controlled double blind study of 146 patients, treatment with the combination was significantly more effective than use of the placebo.[22] No teratogenic risk has been noted for either of these two components individually or in combination. Although some retrospective studies claimed teratogenicity, this was not confirmed in several large prospective controlled trials and the drug was approved by the FDA for use in the first trimester of pregnancy.

In 1,169 patients who took doxylamine succinate and 1,024 who took dicyclomine in the Collaborative Perinatal Project, no evidence for teratogencity was noted.[15] In addition, mean birth weight, perinatal mortality, and intelligence quotient scores of the children at age 4 were similar to the exposed and control groups.[23] In an additional 628 patients taking Bendectin in the Kaiser Health Plan,[21] again no evidence of teratogenicity was found. In England,[24] the incidence of major defects in 2,298 patients treated with Bendectin was compared to control patients and no evidence for teratogenicity was found. Thus, in a total of approximately 6,300 women studied whose infants were exposed to Bendectin in utero, no increaase in the incidence of birth defects has been found. As the incidence of congenital malformations is 2 to 3%[12] and approximately 10% of women had taken Bendectin in the first trimester of pregnancy, it is not surprising that sporadic cases were reported of infants with malformations who had been exposed to Bendectin in early pregnancy. Due to the cost of defending lawsuits alleging teratogenicity, the drug company manufacturing this combination decided in 1984 to stop the manufacture of Bendectin as it was simply not profitable to defend these legal cases (Fig.2–1)

However, the ingredients are available over the counter and vitamin B_6 has some efficacy alone. Doxylamine is available also over the counter as Unisom, 25 mg and so a combination similar to Bendectin can be made. One Unisom 25 mg and one vitamin B_6 25 mg is similar to two Bendectin which can be taken at bedtime, and half of each may be taken in the morning and afternoon in addition as necessary.

Other Antiemetics

Although there is no known teratogenicity of the other antiemetics, much less information is available about them.

TRIMETHOBENZAMIDE (TIGAN)

Trimethobenzamide is an antinauseant that is not classified as either an antihistamine or a phenothiazine and has been used for nausea and vomiting in pregnancy. In the Kaiser Health Plan study[21] of 193 patients exposed to trimethobenzamide, there was a suggestion of an excess of congenital anomalies (p <0.05). However, no concentration of specific anomalies or by anatomic sys-

Merrell Dow

MERRELL DOW PHARMACEUTICALS INC
Subsidiary of The Dow Chemical Company
Cincinnati, Ohio 45215. U S A

Telephone (513) 948-9111
Telex: 214320

July 20, 1984

Dear Doctor:

By the time you read this letter you may have already learned through the news media about the settlement of the massive litigation involving claims against Bendectin, formerly produced by Merrell Dow. Enclosed is our statement which was released to the press July 14, 1984. It may be helpful in clarifying questions you may have on this action.

As you can see from the press release, we remain confident in the safety of Bendectin. Unfortunately, we have been faced with escalating business costs which result from the complex legal system as it exists today in our country. This system affects all of us...industry, as well as you, the practicing physician. The settlement resolves this issue in the U.S.

In an effort to bring the Bendectin litigation to an end, we request that you no longer prescribe or dispense Bendectin from supplies that may still remain in your possession.

We appreciate your understanding of our action and invite any questions you may have.

Sincerely,

David B. Sharrock
President and General Manager
Merrell Dow Pharmaceuticals U.S.A.

DBS/jwr

Fig. 2–1. Letter sent to physicians reiterating the safety of Bendectin and noting that stopping manufacturing of the drug was a business decision.

tem was observed in these children and some of the mothers also took other drugs. In 340 patients in the Collaborative Perinatal Project,[15] no evidence for association between this drug and malformations was found.

DIPHENHYDRAMINE (BENADRYL)

Of 595 patients treated with diphenhydramine in the Collaborative Perinatal Project,[15] and 270 patients in one other study,[28] no increased teratogenic risk was observed.

DIMENHYDRINATE (DRAMAMINE)

No teratogenicity has been noted with dimenhydrinate, but a 29% failure rate and a significant incidence of side effects especially drowsiness have been reported.[6]

Phenothiazines

Because of the potential for severe side effects (liver damage, hematologic abnormalities) the phenothiazines have not been used routinely in the treatment of mild or moderate nausea and vomiting.[1] However, they have been used more extensively for the treatment of hyperemesis gravidarum. In one study, chlorpromazine (25 mg to 50 mg intramuscularly 2 or 3 times a day) resulted in excellent (13 patients) or good (4 patients) recovery in all patients.[25] The response usually occurred within 1 or 2 days. In 141 patients with vomiting less severe than hyperemesis gravidarum, 83% benefited from chlorpromazine. The most important side effect was drowsiness, a reaction which was therapeutically valuable in treating the patients with more severe symptoms.[25]

PROMETHAZINE (PHENERGAN)

Of 114 patients treated with promethazine in the Collaborative Perinatal Project, no teratogenicity was noted. Of 55 exposed mothers in France, no increased risk of anomalies was noted.[26]

Teratogenicity does not appear to be a problem with phenothiazines. In the Kaiser Health Plan study,[21] 976 patients were treated and in the Collaborative Perinatal Project,[15,27] 1,309 patients were treated with no evidence of association between these drugs and malformations. In one small study, however, which found no increased risk with prochlorperizine (Compazine) or promethazine (Phenergan),[26] of 133 infants exposed to chlorpromazine (Thorazine), 8 were malformed which was a significantly increased risk.

EMETROL

Emetrol is a phosphorated carbohydrate solution that acts locally on the wall of the gastrointestinal tract. It reduces smooth muscle contractions in direct proportion to the amount used. Recommended dosage in pregnancy is 1 to 2 tablespoons on arising, repeated every 3 hours or whenever nausea threatens.

RECOMMENDATIONS

Nausea and vomiting of pregnancy is a complex syndrome that presents in a spectrum of severity. Faced with a self-limited condition occurring at the time of organogenesis, the clinician is well advised to avoid the use of medications whenever possible and encourage supportive measures, such as frequent small feedings. When it is necessary to resort to pharmacologic measures, one should attempt to use relatively small amounts of those drugs which, in appropriate studies, have been found to be efficacious and unassociated with fetal malformations.

The drugs that have been evaluated in the largest numbers are the combination of doxylamine succinate and pyridoxine hydrochloride with no evidence of teratogenicity. As these drugs have also been shown to be effective compared to placebo, they are preferred when an antinauseant is indicated. Other antihistamines have been less well studied, but appear to have fair efficacy. If additional antiemetic therapy is needed, such as for hyperemesis gravidarum, no specific teratogenic effects have been noted with the use of the phenothiazines.

REFERENCES

1. Report of the Council on Pharmacy and Chemistry: Current status of therapy in nausea and vomiting of pregnancy. JAMA, *160*:208, 1956

2. Diggory, P.L.C. and Tomkinson, J.S.: Nausea and vomiting in pregnancy: A trial of meclozine dihydrochloride with and without pyridoxine. Lancet, *2*:370, 1962.
3. Fairweather, D.V.I.: Nausea and vomiting in pregnancy. Am J Obstet Gynecol, *102*:135, 1968.
4. Midwinter, A.: Vomiting in pregnancy. The Practitioner, *206*:743, 1971.
5. Dill, L.V.: Vomiting associated with pregnancy. Med Ann Dist Columbia, *18*:178, 1949.
6. Cartwright, E.W.: Dramamine in nausea and vomiting of pregnancy. Western J Surg Obstet Gynecol, *59*:216, 1951.
7. King, A.G.: The treatment of pregnancy nausea with a pill. Obstet Gynecol, *6*:332, 1955.
8. Guze, S.B., DeLong, W.B., Majerus, P.W., et al.: Association of clinical psychiatric disease with hyperemesis gravidarum: A three-and-a-half year follow-up study of 48 patients and 45 controls. N Engl J Med, *261*:1363, 1959.
9. Speert, H. and Guttmacher, A.F.: Frequency and significance of bleeding in early pregnancy. JAMA, *155*:712, 1954.
10. Medalie, J.H.: Relationship between nausea and/or vomiting in early pregnancy and abortion. Lancet, *2*:117, 1957.
11. Walford, P.A.: Antibiotics and congenital malformations. Lancet, *2*:298, 1963.
12. Yerushalmy, J. and Milkovich, L.: Evaluation of the teratogenic effect of meclizine in man. Am J Obstet Gynecol, *93*:553, 1965.
13. Brandes, J.: First-trimester nausea and vomiting as related to outcome of pregnancy. Obstet Gynecol, *30*:427, 1967.
14. Tierson, F.D., Olsen, C.L. and Hook, E.B.: Nausea and vomiting of pregnancy and association with pregnancy outcome. Am J Obstet Gynecol, *155*:1017, 1986.
15. Heinonen, O.P., Slone, D. and Shapiro, S.: Birth defects and drugs in pregnancy. Littleton, Mass, Publishing Sciences Group, Inc, 1977.
16. Evaluation of Drugs for Protection Against Motion Sickness Aboard Transport Ships: Report of study by Army, Navy, Air Force Motion Sickness Team. JAMA, *160*:755, 1956.
17. Lebherz, T.B. and Harris, J.H.: Bonamine: An effective new therapy in nausea and vomiting of pregnancy. Obstet Gynecol, *6*:606, 1955.
18. Watson, G.I.: Meclozine ("Ancoloxin") and foetal abnormalities. Br Med J, *2*:1446, 1962.
19. King, C.T.G: Teratogenic effects of meclizine hydrochloride on the rat. Science, *141*:353, 1963.
20. Smithells, R.W. and Chinn, E.R.: Meclozine and foetal malformations: a prospective study. Br Med J, *1*:217, 1964.
21. Milkovich, L. and Vandenberg, B.J.: An evaluation of the teratogenicity of certain antinauseant drugs. Am J Obstet Gynecol, *125*:244, 1976.
22. Geiger, C.J., Fahrenback, D.M. and Healey, F.J.: Bendectin in the treatment of nausea and vomiting in pregnancy. Obstet Gynecol, *14*:688, 1959.
23. Shapiro, S., Heinonen, O.P., Siskind, V., et al.: Antenatal exposure to doxylamine succinate and dicyclomine hydrochloride (Bendectin) in relation to congenital malformations, perinatal mortality rate, birth weight and intelligence quotient score. Am J Obstet Gynecol, *128*:480, 1977.
24. Smithells, R.W. and Sheppard, S.: Teratogenicity testing in humans: A method demonstrating safety of Bendectin. Teratol, *17*:31, 1978.
25. Benaron, H.B.W., Dorr, E.M., Roddick, W.J., et al.: The use of chlorpromazine in the obstetric patient: A preliminary report. Am J Obstet Gynecol, *69*:776, 1955.
26. Rumeau-Rouquette, C., Goujard, J. and Huel, G.: Possible teratogenic effect of phenothiazines in human beings. Teratol, *15*:57, 1977.
27. Slone, D., Siskind, V., Heinonen, O.P., et al.: Antenatal exposure to the phenothiazines in relation to congenital malformations, perinatal mortality rate, birth weight, and intelligence quotient score. Am J Obstet Gynecol, *128*:486, 1977.
28. Aselton, P., Jick, H., Milunsky, A., et al.: First-trimester drug use and congenital disorders. Obstet Gynecol, *65*:451, 1985.

Chapter 3

The Use of Mild Analgesics in Pregnancy

Jennifer R. Niebyl and Paul S. Lietman

Mild analgesics are widely used during pregnancy, both over the counter and by prescription. Of the 50,282 pregnancies studied in the Collaborative Perinatal Project between 1959 and 1965, 31% of mothers took analgesics and/or antipyretics during the first trimester of pregnancy, and 65% took these drugs sometime during pregnancy. Most of these patients took aspirin, and fewer women took propoxyphene (Darvon), but this study was done prior to its widespread availability. Codeine was taken by about 1%. Acetaminophen (Tylenol/Datril) was taken by only 0.5% at the time of this study, although it is probably the best mild analgesic if one is needed during pregnancy.

MECHANISM OF ACTION OF MILD ANALGESICS

The mild analgesics can be divided into two major categories. The first group are those that inhibit prostaglandin biosynthesis. These include aspirin, acetaminophen (Tylenol/Datril), and the other non-steroidal, anti-inflammatory agents such as ibuprofen, indomethacin, and naproxen. The other category includes those drugs which interact with opiate receptors, narcotics by definition. Propoxyphene (Darvon) and codeine are the two of these that are generally considered as mild analgesics.

Aspirin acts peripherally to block prostaglandin synthesis. Several of the prostaglandins, while they are not in themselves the cause of pain, make the patient hyperalgesic to a group of other chemicals. Aspirin also acts on the central nervous system, which mediates its antipyretic action. It inhibits prostaglandin synthesis in the part of the brain concerned with the thermostat, and stops the production of a pyrogenic prostaglandin.

The narcotic analgesics interact with opiate receptors in the central nervous system and change the perception of pain. The patient is still aware of having pain, but it is not as noxious as prior to the narcotic analgesic.

We shall focus on four drugs: aspirin and acetaminophen as examples of prostaglandin synthetase inhibitors; propoxyphene and codeine as examples of narcotics. These four drugs are similar in analgesic potency. If the dose of propoxyphene is at least 64 mg (not 32 mg), it is clearly better than a placebo and indistinguishable from codeine, acetaminophen, and aspirin with respect to pain relief. When carefully controlled studies of comparative doses were done, there was no evidence that there was any superiority of any of the mild analgesics.[2]

Only aspirin and acetaminophen are antipyretic, while propoxyphene and codeine have no antipyretic activity. Only aspirin possesses an anti-inflammatory effect, important in the treatment of rheumatic fever or rheumatoid arthritis (Table 3–1)

USE OF DRUG COMBINATIONS

Aspirin is normally eliminated by enzyme systems which are saturable, and at a certain blood level of aspirin the enzyme is overwhelmed. Although other mechanisms of elmination are nonsaturable, if one gives aspirin on a repetitive basis, the blood levels will rise rapidly after enzyme saturation occurs. Because of these pharmacokinetics, there is no rationale to using combinations of drugs for synergistic effect. With constant doses of the same drug, aspirin, a greater effect is achieved for a given dose of drug.

One of the arguments for using a combination of drugs is that the toxicity of each will be lessened. However, with acetaminophen the toxicity is nil at therapeutic doses, so it cannot be lessened. Thus, there is no good reason to either alternate acetaminophen and aspirin or give them together.

What about codeine plus aspirin? One might argue that a drug acting centrally and a drug acting peripherally might be synergistic since they act by different mechanisms. However, no one has ever shown that the combination of one drug of each type is any better than double the dose of the same type.

This chapter will address two aspects of mild analgesic use: 1. possible teratogenic effects, 2. perinatal effects when used later in pregnancy. Side effects of these drugs common to pregnant and non-pregnant women will also be discussed.

TERATOGENICITY

Is aspirin teratogenic in humans? By and large, animal data are not informative with regard to determining the teratogenicity of a drug in human beings. Any drug given at the right dose to the right species at the right time is teratogenic to some animals. Therefore, the fact that aspirin or any other drug can be shown to be teratogenic in animals does not answer the question of whether it is teratogenic in humans, as there are marked species differences.

There are two ways of studying teratogenicity in man. The retrospective way is to take a group of chldren who have malformations and to ask whether the ingestion of aspirin was greater in their mothers during the first trimester of pregnancy than in a control group who had no malformations. If more women whose children had malformations had taken aspirin, that would suggest that aspirin might be teratogenic. The prospective approach is to ascertain mothers who took aspirin during the first trimester of pregnancy and to ask whether the incidence of malformations in the children of mothers who took aspirin is dif-

Table 3–1.   Properties of Mild Analgesics

	Aspirin	Acetaminophen (Tylenol)	Propoxyphene (Darvon)	Codeine
Analgesic	+	+	+	+
Antipyretic (antiprostaglandin)	+	+	−	−
Anti-inflammatory	+	−	−	−

ferent from the incidence in mothers who took no aspirin. Both of these methods have been used with aspirin and the results are slightly conflicting.

There have been three retrospective epidemiologic trials. Richards,[3] and Nelson[4] selected a group of children with malformations of any type, and Saxen[5] selected a group with cleft lip ± cleft palate and asked if these mothers consumed aspirin with greater frequency than mothers of non-malformed children. In Richards' series, 22.3% of mothers who bore malformed children said they consumed aspirin in the first trimester of pregnancy, compared to ony 14.4% of the mothers of the control group. In Nelson's series, 3.5% of 458 mothers with malformed children said they consumed aspirin in the first trimester as opposed to 1.6% of the mothers of children who had no malformations. With regard to cleft lip with or without cleft palate, 14.9% of Saxen's group said they took aspirin if they had children with malformations compared with only 5.6% of the control group.

There are two major problems with these three studies which are inherent in retrospective studies. One is memory bias: the mother of a malformed child, having questioned over and over again what possibly could have caused this malformation, is much more likely to remember having taken aspirin during the first trimester than a mother of a perfectly normal child who has completely forgotten about the cold tablet containing aspirin that she took early in pregnancy. The second problem is the confounding variables, i.e., the indications for taking the drug. A viral illness or fever may have led to the aspirin ingestion, which might have a teratogenic risk in itself. With this kind of study it is impossible to separate confounding variables, and so it is difficult to know whether the aspirin is at fault or the reason the patient took the aspirin.

In a prospective study by Slone et al.,[6] aspirin users were identified and the incidence of malformations in the children of the users compared with the incidence of malformations in the children of non-users. Out of the 50,282 mother-child pairs studied, 35,418 women were not exposed to aspirin, 9,736 had intermediate exposure, and 5,128 women were heavily exposed during the first 4 lunar months of pregnancy. After controlling a wide range of potential confounding variables, the observed and expected numbers for a variety of malformations were similar in all three groups. Thus, the data suggest that aspirin is not teratogenic in humans. These numbers were so large that the statistical relative risk for aspirin users lies somewhere between 0.94 and 1.06, so that the worst aspirin could do is produce a risk only 1.06 times that for non-aspirin users.

None of these studies show that aspirin is absolutely not teratogenic. They can only fail to prove that aspirin is teratogenic. Therefore, it is still possible that one out of a thousand or one out of a million women for some genetic or environmental reason, when additionally exposed to aspirin, may have a malformed child. That may never be detected because of the enormity of the study required to detect things that happen one in a thousand times or one in a million times. Thus, one cannot say that the drug does not produce malformations. One can only say that if aspirin produces a teratogenic effect in humans, it must be rare.

Many patients will not describe their aspirin use as taking a drug and do not think of it as a drug. However, over 100 compounds contain aspirin of which patients may not be aware (Table 3–2) In one study,[7] salicylate levels above 1

Table 3–2.   Products Containing Aspirin

HEADACHE AND FEVER REMEDIES

ACA Capsules	Ascriptin	Cama Inlay	Measurin
ACA Capsules No. 2	Asphencaf	Capran	Manacet
Acetonyl Granular	Asperbu	Counterpain	Pabirin
Effervescent Salt	Asphyte	Dexensin	Pabirin Buffered
Acetophen	Aspireze	Dolcin	Persistin
Aidant	Aspirin (USP)	Dolor	Phenatin
Alka Seltzer	Aspirin Aluminum	Duragesic	Phencasal
Alubrin	Aspirin Suprettes	Ecotrin	Phensal
Aluprin	Aspodyne	Emagrin	Ponodyne
Anacin	Ban-O-Pain	Empirin	Pyrasal
Anadynos	Bayer	Emprazel	Sal-Aceto
Ansemco No. 1 & 2	Bayer Timed Release	Enpayne	Saleto
APC	Buff-A	Excedrin	Sal-Fayne
Aphodyne	Buffacet	Febrin	Salspirin
Arthra—Zene Capsules	Buffacetin	Fenadin	Sprin Buffered
ASA	Buffadyne	Fizrin	Stanback Tablets
ASA Compound	Buffadyne-25	Formasal Capsules	and Powders
Asalco No. 1	Buffaprin	and Tablets	St. Joseph Aspirin
Ascaphen	Bufferin	Haysma	Supac
Ascaphen Compound	Buffinol	Henasphen	Trigesic
As-ca-phen	Calurin	Hypan	Triocin
			Vanquish

COLD AND ALLERGY REMEDIES

Al-Ay	Coricidin Tablets	Hiscatab	Rhinex
Alka Saltzer Plus	Coricidin D Tablets	Histacamp Tablets	Rid-A-Col
Alumadrine	Co-ryd	Histadyl and ASA	Ryd
Aspir-B	Convangesie	Compound	Sine-Aid
Aspir-C	Dasikon	Histamead Forte	Sine-Off
Aspir-D Compound	Drinophen	His-Drist "MLT"	Soltice Cold Tablets
BiAct Cold Tablets	Dristamead	Novahistine w/APC	Super Afko-Hist
Cheracol Capsules	Dristan Tablets	P.A.A.M.	Super-Anahist
Cirin	Frogesic	Phencaset Improved	Toloxidyne
Cosamed	4-Way Cold Tablets	Pyroxate	Triaminicin
			Tussapap

CHILDREN'S PREPARATIONS

Aspirin Children's	Bayer Children's	Coricidin Medilets	St. Joseph Aspirin
Aspirjen Jr. Tablets	Cold	Febrinettes	for Children
Babylove	Congesprin	Liquiprin	St. Joseph Cold
Bayer Children's	Coricidin Demilets	Pedidyne	Tablets for Children

MENSTRUAL PROBLEM REMEDIES

Cope	Femcaps	Midol

MISCELLANEOUS

Aspergum	Excedrin P.M.	Phenodyne	Quiet World

ARTHRITIS REMEDIES

Anacin Arthritis	Bufferin Arthritis
Pain Formula	Strength

mg% were found in 9.5% of unselected consecutive cord sera, in which none of the patients had been treated by a physician with aspirin. Several patients denied aspirin use until specific trade names were mentioned. Thus the recording of aspirin ingestion requires careful history taking.

In summary, there is insufficient evidence to prove teratogenicity of aspirin in man. If aspirin is teratogenic, its risk must be small. Some rare individuals may be uniquely sensitive to aspirin, but we have no evidence for that. However, aspirin should be used, like all drugs in the first trimester, only when really indicated.

PERINATAL EFFECTS OF ASPIRIN

Aspirin has several effects on the mother and newborn around the time of delivery. As uterine contractions are mediated by prostaglandins, aspirin, a prostaglandin synthetase inhibitor, has an inhibitory effect on uterine contractility. In addition, aspirin causes an increase in maternal bleeding probably due to its inhibition of platelet agglutination, and also perhaps through an effect on uterine tone.

Aspirin has been shown to prolong the injection-abortion interval in nulliparous women undergoing elective mid-trimester abortion, when the dose of aspirin was 600 mg every 6 hours.[8] Also, chronic aspirin-takers have been shown to have a longer mean duration of gestation and a longer mean duration of labor than control patients.[9] In addition, patients have been reported to have a higher incidence of passing 42 weeks of gestation if they were constant aspirin takers compared to controls.[10] Thus, aspirin has an inhibitory effect on the triggering of labor and uterine contractility during labor, both in the mid-trimester and third trimester.

In one study, aspirin users had significantly more bleeding associated with delivery than non-users.[9] Another study showed that anemia of pregnancy, antepartum hemorrhage, postpartum hemorrhage, and the need for blood transfusion were greater in constant aspirin takers compared with intermittent takers or controls who took no aspirin.[10] Thus, maternal blood loss appears to be greater if aspirin is consumed late in pregnancy.

Furthermore, aspirin has a clear-cut effect on hemostasis of the newborn. In order for a clot to form, platelets must aggregate, and aspirin prevents platelet aggregation. In mothers and children who are exposed to aspirin in the last 2 months of pregnancy, there is a diminution or abolition of platelet aggregation in both the newborn and mother.[11] The newborn appears to be especially sensitive to this since aspirin taken prior to delivery continues to affect the newborn,[12] even if the mother has not taken any aspirin for the week immediately preceding delivery. The explanation for this long-acting effect is that aspirin affects one step in prostaglandin biosynthesis, the cyclooxygenase step, and irreversibly inactivates that enzyme.[14] As long as that enzyme is around in that platelet it can not function. All of the other nonsteroidal anti-inflammatory agents also act on that enzyme, but all act *reversibly* so that as soon as the blood levels are down and the drug is excreted, their effect is gone. Aspirin, however, permanently inactivates the enzyme for the rest of the life of that platelet. The only way that enzyme can reappear in the platelets of the mother or the newborn is for new platelets to be made in the bone marrow. This irreversible effect, then, carries over to the newborn even though small doses of the aspirin were given a week or more prior to the delivery. Thus, aspirin should seldom, if ever, be used in late pregnancy.

In addition to this effect on bleeding, other effects on the newborn occur as a result of transplacental passage of the aspirin. Aspirin is acetylsalicylic acid, and the newborn cannot convert that to salicylic acid readily. There is diminished protein-binding of aspirin by the newborn protein and therefore more is free in the newborn and available for entering cells and potentially causing pharmacologic effects. Aspirin transplacentally delivered can continue to persist in the newborn plasma and displace bilirubin causing hyperbilirubinemia. Also, aspirin is much more slowly eliminated in the newborn.

Prostaglandins also mediate the smooth muscle tone of the ductus arteriosus. Thus, the possibility exists that the administration of aspirin to pregnant women might result in in utero closure of the ductus arteriosus. In one patient who was treated with salicylates for 10 days prior to delivery at 37 weeks of gestation, the newborn had tricuspid insufficiency, severe heart failure and acidosis all of which disappeared the day after birth.[13] Hemodynamic studies at 4 hours of age demonstrated a cone-shaped ductus arteriosus arising from the pulmonary artery, but ending blindly at its aortic end, and the findings were considered to be consistent with closure of the ductus arteriosus before birth. This effect appears to be limited to infants at term, as the ductus is not as sensitive to oxygen or prostaglandin synthetase inhibitors in the premature age group. However, perinatal use of aspirin is not recommended for this reason as well.

ALTERNATIVE MILD ANALGESICS

Acetaminophen (Tylenol/Datril)

Acetaminophen, like aspirin, is contained in many combination products. Retrospective studies have also been done with acetaminophen looking for teratogenic risks. In one series of 458 malformed children, 0.8% were exposed to acetaminophen in the first trimester of pregnancy, whereas of 911 children having no malformations, 1% were exposed to it.[4] This retrospective controlled study provides no evidence for acetaminophen teratogenicity in humans.

In the Collaborative Perinatal Project[1] not enough patients took acetaminophen during the first trimester of pregnancy to resolve this issue. However, phenacetin is metabolized directly to acetaminophen and most of its analgesic and antipyretic properties are probably due to acetaminophen. Therefore, if acetaminophen is teratogenic, one would expect phenacetin also to be teratogenic and enough patients took phenacetin to evaluate the data. Of 50,282 pregnant women, 5,546 were exposed to phenacetin in the first trimester. Of these, 250 bore children with malformations; the relative risk for phenacetin was 0.97. The risk of malformations was no different whether the patient took phenacetin early in pregnancy or not. Because of the large number of patients studied, the 95% confidence limits were narrow, so one can be fairly confident that if phenacetin causes teratogenicity the risk must be small; presumably we can extrapolate to acetaminophen. Also, no teratogenicity of acetaminophen has been noted with 697 additional exposures.[16]

The discrepancy in toxicity between phenacetin and acetaminophen is due to differences in metabolism. Although most of the phenacetin is metabolized to acetaminophen, some is metabolized through another route. It is this metabolite by the other route which is responsible for methemoglobinemia in the newborn, which acetaminophen itself does not cause.

There are almost no known side effects of acetaminophen in anyone, including late in pregnancy. A few patients have had skin rashes associated with acetaminophen, but the causal relationship is nearly impossible to determine. Almost no other side effect has ever been reported at normal doses of acetaminophen. The inhibition of the cyclooxygenase step of prostaglandin biosynthesis by acetaminophen is reversible (rather than irreversible after aspirin[14]), and bleeding is not a problem even in the postoperative period associated with the use of this drug. The template bleeding time is significantly prolonged in pregnancy after consumption of 650 mg or 2 tablets of aspirin, but it is not prolonged after the same dose of acetaminophen.[15] Furthermore, acetaminophen can be given to the newborn and although he fails to eliminate it rapidly, it is non-toxic. Thus, acetaminophen is a far better choice for an analgesic and antipyretic in pregnancy than aspirin.

Acetaminophen pharmacokinetics are relatively unchanged in pregnancy,[17] The maximum plasma concentration occurred at 0.8 hours after an oral dose of 1000 mg at 36 weeks of gestation. The absorption, metabolism and renal clearance of acetaminophen were unchanged in late pregnancy.[17]

Propoxyphene (Darvon)

Much less is known about propoxyphene with respect to pregnancy. It is an acceptable alternative mild analgesic. With respect to teratogenesis, propoxyphene has been looked at in the prospective study.[1] Six hundred and eighty-six women were exposed to propoxyphene in the first trimester, and 31 or 4.5% of the infants had malformations. The relative risk of malformations for propoxyphene users was 0.90. However, because of the smaller numbers of patients taking propoxyphene, the assuredness of that 0.90 is less, and one can only say that one is 95% confident that the real relative risk is somewhere between 0.63 and 1.29. So it is possible that if the real risk were at the high end of the scale, that propoxyphene might have a risk, but there is no evidence for that risk.

However, propoxyphene should not be used for trivial indications, as the narcotic addiction potential of this drug has been estabished. Evidence of risk in late pregnancy comes from 2 case reports of infants of mothers who were addicted to propoxyphene, and had the typical narcotic withdrawal in the neonatal period.

Codeine

Little information is available about codeine with respect to pregnancy. Retrospective studies, in which malformed children are the starting point, suggest that there is little risk of teratogenicity. The first trimester exposure to codeine for malformed children was 2.2% of 458 mothers; in normal children the exposure was 1.7% of 911.[4] In the cleft lip/palate study, exposure occurred in 6.7% of those with clefts and 2.2% of normal children.[5] The prospective study, however, fails to show any significantly increased relative risk of malformations to codeine users. Five hundred and sixty-three mother-child pairs were exposed to codeine in the first trimester and 32 had malformations with a relative risk rate of 1.15. However, there is a broad range as far as confidence limits are concerned (0.84 to 1.57) and so codeine should be used only when necessary during pregnancy.

Since there is an alternative drug which is as effective as codeine and for which there is not even evidence suggestive of teratogenicity, that is propoxyphene, it makes sense to choose propoxyphene rather than codeine as a mild analgesic in the narcotic category if one is really indicated in the first trimester. Also, codeine can cause addiction and newborn withdrawal symptoms if used perinatally.

RECOMMENDATIONS

One of the first duties of the physician is to educate people not to take medicines needlessly, and nowhere is this more important than in obstetrics. Few pains during pregnancy justify the use of a mild analgesic. Pregnant patients should be encouraged to use nonpharmacologic remedies such as local heat and rest. Nevertheless, if a mild analgesic or antipyretic agent seems appropriate during pregnancy, acetaminophen is the drug of choice.

REFERENCES

1. Heinonen, O.P., Slone, D. and Shapiro, F.: Birth Defects and Drugs in Pregnancy. Littleton, Mass, Publishing Sciences Group, Inc, 1977, p. 261.
2. The Medical Letter, *18*:73, 1976.
3. Richards, I.D.G.: Congenital malformations and environmental influences in pregnancy. Br J Prev Soc Med, *23*:218, 1969.
4. Nelson, M.M. and Forfar, J.O.: Associations between drugs administered during pregnancy and congenital abnormalities of the fetus. Br Med J, *1*:523, 1971.
5. Saxen, I.: Associations between oral clefts and drugs taken during pregnancy. Int J Epidemiol, *4*:37, 1975.
6. Slone, D., Heinonen, O.P., Kaufman, D., et al.: Aspirin and congenital malformations. Lancet, *1*:1373, 1976.
7. Palmisano, P.A. and Cassady, G.: Salicylate exposure in the perinate. JAMA, *209*:556, 1969.
8. Niebyl, J.R., Blake, D.A., Burnett, L.S., et al.: The influence of aspirin on the course of induced midtrimester abortion. Am J Obstet Gynecol, *124*:607, 1976.
9. Lewis, R.B. and Shulman, J.D.: Influence of acetylsalicylic acid, an inhibitor of prostaglandin synthesis, on the duration of human gestation and labor. Lancet, *2*:1159, 1973.
10. Collins, E. and Turner, G.: Salicylates and pregnancy. Lancet, *2*:1494, 1973.
11. Bleyer, W.A. and Breckenridge, R.J: Adverse drug reactions in the newborn II. Prenatal aspirin and newborn hemostasis. JAMA, *213*:2049, 1970.
12. Corby, D.G. and Schulman, I.: The effects of antenatal drug administration on aggregation of platelets of newborn infants. J Pediatr, *79*:307, 1971.
13. Areilla, R.A., Thilenius, O.B. and Ranniger, K.: Congestive heart failure from suspected ductal closure in utero. J Pediatr, *75*:74, 1969.
14. Smith, W.L. and Lands, W.E.M.: Stimulation and blockade of prostaglandin biosynthesis. J Biol Chem, *246*:6700, 1971.
15. Waltman, T., Tricomi, V. and Tavakoli, F.M.: Effect of aspirin on bleeding time during elective abortion. Obstet Gynecol, *48*:108, 1976.
16. Aselton, P., Jick, H., Milunsky, A., et al.: First-trimester drug use and congenital disorders. Obstet Gynecol, *65*:451, 1985.
17. Rayburn, W., Shukla, U., Stetson, P., et al.: Acetaminophen pharmacokinetics: comparison between pregnant and nonpregnant women. Am J Obstet Gynecol, *155*:1353, 1986.

Chapter 4

Antibiotics in Pregnancy

Kamal A. Hamod and Victor A. Khouzami

Antibiotics are widely used in pregnancy, and most do not have teratogenic effects.

Antibiotic Kinetics in Pregnancy

The pharmacokinetics of antibiotic drugs during pregnancy are altered due to several factors (Table 4–1). The increase in maternal renal function, due to an increase in both renal blood flow and glomerular filtration rate,[1] results in a higher renal excretion of drugs excreted in the urine. The expansion of the maternal intravascular volume during the late stages of pregnancy[2] is another factor that affects the pharmacodynamics of antibiotic therapy. If the same dose of an antibiotic drug is given to both non-pregnant and pregnant women, lower serum levels are attained during pregnancy due to the distribution of the drug in a larger intravascular volume.[3]

The fetal-placental unit will also influence the maternal serum level of an antibiotic. The free circulating portion of most antibiotics crosses the placenta, resulting in lower maternal serum levels of the unbound portion of the drug.[4] The mechanism by which transplacental passage occurs is simple diffusion which in turn is affected by the molecular size, lipid solubility, degree of ionization and protein binding of the drug, as well as by the metabolic and functional changes of the placenta that occur during gestation. Antibiotics with low molecular weights, high lipid solubility, and low protein binding diffuse readily across the placenta. Also, the tissue layers interposed between maternal and fetal capillaries become progessively thinner with advancing gestation possibly expediting the transplacental transfer of drugs.[3,5]

Table 4–1. The Effect of Physiologic Alterations During Pregnancy on Antibiotic Kinetics

Physiologic Alteration	Effect on Antibiotic Kinetics
Increase in maternal renal function	Higher renal clearance
Expansion of maternal intravascular volume	Decreased maternal serum level
Transplacental transfer of drug	Decreased maternal serum level Perfusion of fetal tissues
Thinning out of feto-maternal barriers with advancing gestation	Increased transplacental diffusion (?)
Decreased fetal liver function and high blood/brain permeability	Increased fetal drug toxicity

The peak level of an antibiotic in the fetus is generally lower than that obtained in the mother. This is due to the fact that only the free portion of the maternal antibiotic diffuses through the placenta. The soft-tissue distribution of the drug is also different in the fetus. Blood flow to the fetal brain and kidneys is much greater than to the fetal lungs, resulting in higher tissue concentrations in the former mentioned sites. The fetal circulation pattern varies also throughout pregnancy. Early in pregnancy, the fetal brain receives a greater proportion of the cardiac output than near term. This could result in variation in the tissue concentrations of a given drug at different stages of gestation.

The antibiotic is ultimately excreted in the fetal urine and effective levels appear in the amniotic fluid. The delay in the appearance of different classes of antibiotics in the amniotic fluid depends primarily on the rate of transplacental diffusion, the amount of protein binding in fetal serum, and the adequacy of fetal enzymatic and renal functions. In general, several hours are needed for effective levels of an antibiotic to appear in the amniotic fluid. This delay could explain in part the relative failure of on-call prophylactic antibiotic administration in cesarean sections,[4] and the relative lack of efficacy of "fetal" therapy.

Adverse Fetal Effects

"Safety for use in pregnancy has not been established" is a well known label to all clinicians seeking information about the potential hazards of antibiotic usage in pregnancy. The fact that the fetus shares a sizable portion of the antibiotic prescribed to the pregnant woman constitutes a major ethical problem. During the preimplantation period which usually covers the first 14 days following conception, the embryo is relatively resistant to exogenous toxicity. If damage does occur during this time, it will usually result in the death and subsequent abortion of the embryo.

Teratogenicity, defined as the ability of an exogenous agent to produce congenital malformations grossly visible at birth, usually results from the administration of a drug during the embryonic period (day 15 to 55 after conception). The occurrence of congenital malformations secondary to antibiotic administration during pregnancy follows the interplay of four teratogenic principles listed by Eriksson et al. These are the nature of the antibiotic and its accessibility to the fetus, the time of its action, the level and duration of its dosage, and the fetal genetic makeup.[3]

Fetal growth and developmental anomalies are the main outcome of fetal drug toxicity during the second and third trimester of pregnancy.[6] A poor liver enzyme conjugating function coupled to a high blood brain permeability make the fetus an easy prey to the toxic effects of antibiotics during this period (Table 4–2). Although most organs are already formed prior to this period, it should be remembered that the central nervous system, the genitalia, and the teeth continue to mature and could, therefore, be particularly susceptible to the toxic effects of the drug.

Due to the intricate technical and ethical problems mentioned above, limited data are available on the kinetics of drugs in pregnancy. Most studies were carried out at the time of abortion and cesarean section and were limited to the investigation of the transplacental passage of a specific antibiotic. It should therefore be borne in mind when evaluating the results of such studies, that the data obtained may not be truly representative for all stages of pregnancy.[7]

Table 4–2. **Major Adverse Fetal Effects of Antibiotic Administration During Pregnancy**

Drug	Adverse Effects on Fetus and Newborn
Sulfonamides	Bony malformations (animal studies) Kernicterus
Penicillins	None reported
Tetracyclines	Retardation of skeletal growth Discoloration of teeth and hypoplasia of enamel
Aminoglycosides	Ototoxicity (streptomycin only)
Cephalosporins	None reported
Chloramphenicol	Gray-baby syndrome
Erythromycin and clindamycin	None reported

Antimicrobial Agents Commonly Used in Pregnancy

THE SULFONAMIDES

The sulfonamides are the first line of attack in the treatment of urinary tract infections early in pregnancy. They readily cross the placenta achieving fetal plasma levels 50 to 90% of those attained in the maternal plasma.[8] Ylikorkala et al. studied the pharmacokinetics of trimethoprim-sulfamethoxazole in 10 pregnant women at the time of abortion, and found the maternal serum levels of the drug to be comparable to non-pregnant individuals. The elimination half-life of this combination drug was shorter, however, in the pregnant women and trimethoprim was cleared faster from the maternal serum than sulfamethoxazole.[9]

Long acting sulfonamides and trimethoprim with sulfamethoxazole have been reported to cause congenital anomalies in experimental animals.[10,11] When high oral doses of these drugs were administered to pregnant rats, cleft palate and other skeletal abnormalities were noted in the offspring. However, among 1,455 human infants exposed to sulfonamides during the first trimester of pregnancy, no teratogenic effects were noted,[12] and controlled trials in humans of trimethoprim have failed to demonstrate any risk. The administration of sulfonamides should also be avoided in glucose-6-phosphate dehydrogenase deficient women. A dose-related toxic reaction may occur in these individuals resulting in red cell hemolysis.

While sulfonamides cause no known damage to the fetus in utero, they can have deleterious effects when present in the blood of the neonate. The sulfonamides complete with bilirubin for binding sites on albumin, thus raising the levels of free bilirubin in the serum and increasing the risk of kernicterus in the neonate.[13,14] For that reason, it is recommended that an alternate antibiotic be used in the third trimester, once fetal viability is attained.

THE PENICILLINS

The penicillins are probably the class of antibiotics most widely used in pregnancy. They have a wide margin of safety and lack of toxicity to both the pregnant woman and the fetus. Penicillin is also the antibiotic of choice in the treatment of numerous bacterial infections including gonorrhea and syphilis. Ampicillin, on the other hand, is one of the most frequently used drugs in the treatment of both lower and upper urinary tract infections in pregnancy.

In the Collaborative Perinatal Project, 3,546 mothers took penicillin derivatives in the first trimester of pregnancy, resulting in no teratogenic effects.[12]

Because of the safety of penicillin, the pharmacokinetics of the penicillin group of antibiotics have been relatively well studied. Several studies have revealed that the serum levels of these drugs are lower and their renal clearance is higher throughout pregnancy when compared ot the non-pregnant state.[7,15,17]

The transplacental passage of these drugs has also been extensively studied. The data obtained from several studies indicate that the maternal administration of penicillins with high protein binding, e.g. oxacillin, cloxacillin, dicloxacillin, and nafcillin result in lower fetal tissue and amniotic fluid levels than the administration of poorly bound penicillin, e.g. ampicillin and methicillin.[4,18,19]

THE TETRACYCLINES

Tetracyclines have a potential clinical usefulness in many types of infections, including gonorrhea, syphilis, and pyelonephritis. First trimester exposure to tetracycline was not found to have any teratogenic risk in 341 women in the Collaborative Perinatal Project,[12] or 174 women in another study.[53] However, tetracyclines are not recommended for use in pregnancy because of their adverse fetal and maternal effects.

Tetracyclines readily cross the placenta and are firmly bound by chelating to calcium to developing bone and tooth structures.[20] This produces fetal skeletal abnormalities, discoloration of the teeth, and possibly hypoplasia of the enamel. The yellowish-brownish staining of the teeth usually takes place in the second trimester of pregnancy after 24 weeks, while bone incorporation can occur as early as the first trimester. Depression of skeletal growth is particularly common among premature infants treated with tetracycline.[3]

THE AMINOGLYCOSIDES

This group of antibiotic drugs is commonly used, singly or in combination with penicillin and/or clindamycin in the treatment of postpartum endometritis, septic abortion, or amnionitis.

Animal studies failed to show any teratogenic effect associated with this group of drugs.[21] In 135 infants exposed to streptomycin in the first trimester, no teratogenic effects were observed.[12] Transplacental passage has been demonstrated and the fetal serum level is reported to be only 20 to 35% that of the maternal level.[22]

Maternal serum levels attained with these drugs have been shown to be consistently lower in pregnancy than in the non-pregnant state. The data were obtained from patients in labor or during cesarean sections and hysterectomies performed at different gestational ages.[23-25] Wide interpatient variation in gentamicin elimination rates have been observed in obstetric patients varying with the volume of distribution of the drug.[26] Serum levels should be monitored to assure therapeutic levels as well as avoid toxicity.[26]

Conway et al. demonstrated significant ototoxicity in children of mothers who received prolonged streptomycin treatment for tuberculosis during pregnancy.[16] Although the hearing loss appears to be dose-related and has not been reported with other aminoglycosides, these agents should be avoided if possible during pregnancy. In case these agents are required for serious infections due to organisms resistant to less toxic agents, their use should be restricted to as short a time as psosible and maternal serum levels should be carefully monitored.

THE CEPHALOSPORINS

The use of cephalosporins in obstetrics has been extensive. They have been used as prophylactic agents in cesarean section and in the treatment of septic abortion, pyelonephritis, and amnionitis. However, they are sufficiently new that no data about possible teratogenicity are available from the Collaborative Perinatal Project.

Maternal serum levels attained with these drugs during pregnancy are only a fraction of those in the non-pregnant state. This was shown to be true not only for well established cephalosporin drugs like cephalexin, cephalothin, and cephazolin,[27] but also for the newer cephalosporins, e.g. cephoxitin, cephradine, and cefuroxime.[28–30]

Transplacental transfer of these drugs is fairly rapid and adequate bactericidal concentrations are attained in both fetal soft tissues and the amniotic fluid.[28–30,31,32] Repeated high bolus doses of cephalosporins have been shown to result in higher levels in fetal serum and amniotic fluid than continuous intravenous infusions of the same amount of drug.[33]

Cephoxitin, a beta-lactamase resistant compound is highly effective in the treatment of both uncomplicated gonococcal cervicitis and penicillinase producing N. gonorrheae. Cephalothin has been shown to be as effective as ampicillin and chloramphenicol in the treatment of pyelonephritis in pregnancy.[34]

ERYTHROMYCIN

In 79 patients in the Collaborative Perinatal Project,[12] and 260 in one other study,[53] no teratogenic risk was noted.

This drug is the alternative of choice to penicillin in the treatment of gonorrhea or syphilis in pregnancy. Except for the estolate form, it is relatively non-toxic. Erythromycin estolate has been associated with subclinical, reversible hepatotoxicity during pregnancy.[35] Erythromycin is also a good substitute drug for the treatment of urinary tract infection in pregnancy provided the urine can be adequately alkalinized.[36]

Erythromycin base and its salts are not consistently absorbed from the gastrointestinal tract of pregnant women and their transplacental passage is unpredictable. Both maternal and fetal serum levels achieved after the administration of this drug during pregnancy are low and vary considerably from one individual to another.[37,38] Based on these observations, it is recommended that penicillin be administered to every newborn whose mother received erythromycin for the treatment of syphilis.[39]

CHLORAMPHENICOL

This drug is particularly useful in the treatment of anaerobic infections. Chloramphenicol has been associated, however, with drug-induced aplastic anemia. Its use, if ever, warrants therefore close hematologic supervision. Chloramphenicol has also been associated with the "gray baby syndrome" when used in the neonate. This toxicity is believed to be dose-related and a function of the relative immaturity of the enzymatic system of the neonate.[40]

Plomp et al. found serum levels of this drug in pregnant women to be comparable to non-pregnant individuals.[41] Furthermore, transplacental passage has been documented with fetal serum levels 30 to 80% that of maternal levels.[42,43]

In view of the toxicity in the neonate and especially the premature, once fetal viability is achieved, the presence of an acceptable alternate antibiotic is a relative contraindication to the use of chloramphenicol.

CLINDAMYCIN

Clindamycin is active against many aerobic gram-positive cocci and is highly effective in the treatment of infections caused by B. fragilis and other anaerobic bacteria. The greatest drawback to the use of this drug has been the frequently associated diarrhea in up to 20% of treated patients. In half of these patients, the diarrhea is secondary to a change in bowel flora, whereas pseudomembranous enterocolitis is the underlying disorder in the second half.[44] This colitis could be fatal and therefore, prompt diagnosis and immediate discontinuation of the drug when diarrhea develops are a must. Due to this potentially serious side effect, the use of clindamycin should be restricted to the treatment of obstetric infections near term where anaerobic bacteria are thought to be the causative organisms.

Serum levels of clindamycin in pregnant women were reported to be similar to those attained in non-pregnant individuals, although the serum half-life of the drug was shorter during pregnancy.[25,38] Transplacental passage occurs readily with clindamycin achieving adequate fetal tissue levels.[37] Animal studies have shown, however, that it is a poor substitute for penicillin in the treatment of syphilis during pregnancy.[45]

METRONIDAZOLE

Metronidazole has been used in obstetrics in the treatment of vaginal trichomoniasis and postpartum endometritis.[46] Controversy regarding its use in pregnancy started soon after the introduction of the drug to the U.S.A., when laboratory studies demonstrated that long-term administration of metronidazole in high doses resulted in an increased incidence of pulmonary adenomatosis in mice,[47] and mammary tumors and hepatocarcinomas in rats.[48] Metronidazole is mutagenic for bacteria by the Ames' test,[49] which correlates with carcinogenicity in animals.[50] Thus, if it is used during pregnancy, there may be potential for transplacental carcinogenicity.

However, several prospective and retrospective studies have failed to show any significant increase in the incidence of congenital defects among the newborns of mothers treated with metronidazole during early or late gestation.[51,52] Of 597 pregnant women exposed, 62 in the first trimester, 284 in the second trimester, and 251 in the third trimester, no adverse outcomes were noted. In one other study,[53] of 174 patients exposed in the first trimester, no teratogenic risk was noted. Further controlled studies involving larger numbers of patients are needed before all the doubts about the potential adverse effect of this drug are relieved. Until such final proof is obtained, it seems prudent to use metronidazole in pregnancy only when necessary.

Antibiotics are widely used during pregnancy. As pregnant patients are particularly susceptible to vaginal yeast infections, prophylaxis with antifungal agents may be advisable during the course of therapy.

REFERENCES

1. Sims, E.A.H. and Krantz, K.E: Serial studies of renal function during pregnancy and the puerperium in normal women. J Clin Invest, *37*:1764, 1958.
2. McLennan, C.E. and Thouin, L.G.: Blood volume in pregnancy, Am J Obstet Gynecol, *46*:63, 1943.
3. Eriksson, M., Catz, C.S. and Yaffe, S.J.: Drugs and pregnancy. Clin Obstet Gynecol, *16*:199, 1973.
4. Ledger, W.J.: Antibiotics in pregnancy. Clin Obstet Gynecol, *20*:411, 1977.
5. Ville, C.A.: Metabolism of the placenta. Am J Obstet Gynecol, *84*:1684, 1962.
6. Howard, F.M. and Hill, J.M.: Drugs in pregnancy. Ob Gyn Surv, *34*:643, 1979.
7. Philipson, A.: Pharmacokinetics of antibiotics in pregnancy and labour. Clin Pharmacokinetics, *4*:297, 1979.
8. Monif, G.F.G.: Infectious Diseases in Obstetrics and Gynecology. New York, Harper and Row, 1974, p. 26.
9. Ylikorkala, O., Sjostedt, E., Jarvinen, P.A., et al.: Trimethoprim-sulfonamide combination administered orally and intravaginally in the first trimester of pregnancy: its absorption into serum and transfer to amniotic fluid. Acta Obstet Gynecol Scand, *52*:229, 1973.
10. Goultschin, J. and Ulmansky, M.: Skull and dental changes produced by a sulfonamide in rats. Oral Surg, *31*:290, 1971.
11. Paget, G.E. and Thorpe, E.: A teratogenic effect of a sulfonamide in experimental animals. Br J Pharmacol, *23*:305, 1964.
12. Heinonen, O.P., Slone, D. and Shapiro, S.: Birth Defects and Drugs in Pregnancy. Littleton, Mass., Publishing Sciences Group, Inc, 1977.
13. Harris, R.C., Lucey, J.F. and MacLean, J.R.: Kernicterus in premature infants associated with low concentration of bilirubin in the plasma. Pediatr, *21*:878, 1950.
14. Nyhan, W.L.: Toxicity of drugs in the neonatal period. J. Pediatr, *59*:1, 1961.
15. Bastert, G., Muller, W.G., Wallhauser, K.H., et al.: Pharmacokinetische Untersuchungen zum Ubertritt von Antibiotika in das Fruchtwasser am Ende der Schwagerschaft. 3. Tiel: Oxacillin. Zietschrift fur Geburtshilfe und Perinatologie, *179*:346, 1975.
16. Conway, N. and Birt, B.D.: Streptomycin in pregnancy: effect on the foetal ear. Br Med J, *2*:260, 1965.
17. Philipson, A.: Pharmacokinetics of ampicillin during pregnancy. J Infect Dis, *136*:370, 1977.
18. Kunin, C.M.: Clinical pharmacology of the new penicillins. I. The importance of serum protein binding in determining antimicrobial activity and concentration in serum. Clin Pharmacol Ther, *7*:166, 1966.
19. Macaulay, M.A., Berg, S.A. and Charles, D.: Placental transfer of dicloxacillin at term. Am J Obstet Gynecol, *102*:1162, 1968.
20. Kline, A.H., Blattner, R.J. and Lunin, M.: Transplacental effects of tetracycline on teeth. JAMA, *118*:178, 1964.
21. Welles, J.S., Emerson, J.L, Gibson, W.R., et al.: Preclinical toxicology studies with tobramycin. Toxicol Appl Pharmacol, *25*:398, 1973.
22. Yoshioka, H., Monma, T. and Matsuda, S.: Placental transfer of gentamicin. J Pediatr, *80*:121, 1972.
23. Bernard, B., Abate, M., Thielen, P.F., et al.: Maternal-fetal pharmacological activity of amikacin. J Infect Dis, *135*:925, 1977.
24. Good, R.G. and Johnson, G.: The placental transfer of kanamycin during later pregnancy. Obstet Gynecol, *38*:60, 1971.
25. Weinstein, A.J., Gibbs, R.S. and Gallagher, M.: Placental transfer of clindamycin and gentamicin in term pregnancy. Am J Obstet Gynecol, *24*:688, 1976.
26. Zaske, D.E., Cipolle, R.J., Strate, R.G., et al.: Rapid gentamicin elimination in obstetric patients. Obstet Gynecol, *56*:559, 1980.
27. Morrow, S., Palmisano, P. and Cassady, G.: The placental transfer of cephalothin. J Pediatr, *73*:262, 1968.
28. Dubois, M., Delapierre, D., Dresse, A., et al.: Transplacental transfer of cefuroxine, 11th International Congress of Chemotherapy and 19th Interscience Conference on Antimicrobial Agents and Chemotherapy. Boston, Mass., 1979.
29. Dubois, M., Delapierre, D., Demonty, J., et al.: Transplacental and mammary transfer of cephoxitin. 11th International Congress of Chemotherapy and 19th Interscience Conference on Antimicrobial Agents and Chemotherapy. Boston, Mass., 1979.
30. Philipson, A. and Stiernsted, T.G.: Pharmacokinetics of cephradine in pregnancy. 11th International Congress of Chemotherapy and 19th Interscience Conference on Antimicrobial Agents and Chemotherapy. Boston, Mass., 1979.

31. Craft, I., Mullinger, B.M. and Kennedy, M.R.K.: Placental transfer of cefuroxine, 11th International Congress of Chemotherapy and 19th Interscience Conference on Antimicrobial Agents and Chemotherapy. Boston, Mass., 1979.
32. Macaulay, M.A. and Charles, D.: Placental transfer of cephalothin. Am J Obstet Gynecol, *100*:940, 1968.
33. Hirsch, H.A., Herbst, S., Lang, R., et al.: Transfer of a new cephalosporin antibiotic to the foetus and the amniotic fluid during a continuous infusion (steady state) and single repeated intravenous injections to the mother. Arch fur Gynakologie, *216*:1, 1974.
34. Cunningham, F.G., et al.: Acute pyelonephritis of pregnancy: A clinical review. Obstet Gynecol, *42*:112, 1973.
35. McCormack, W.M., George, H., Donner., A., et al.: Hepatotoxicity of erythromycin estolate during pregnancy. Antimicrob Agents Chemother, *12*:630, 1977.
36. Sabath, L.D., Gerstein, D.A., Loder, P.B., et al.: Excretion of erythromycin and its enhanced activity in urine against gram negative bacilli with alkalinization. J Lab Clin Med, *72*:916, 1968.
37. Philipson, A., Sabath, L.D., and Charles, D.: Erythromycin and clindamycin absorption and elimination in pregnant women. Clin Pharmacol Ther, *19*:68, 1976.
38. Philipson, A., Sabath, L.D. and Charles, D.: Transplacental passage of erythromycin and clindamycin. N Engl J Med, *288*:1219, 1973.
39. South, M.A., Short, D.H. and Knox, J.M.: Failure of erythromycin estolate therapy in in utero syphilis. JAMA, *190*:70, 1964.
40. Lietman, P.S.: Chloramphenicol and the neonate—1979 view. Clin Pharmacol, *6*:March, 1979.
41. Plomp, T.A., Maes, R.A.A.A., Thiery, M., et al.: Placental transfer of thiamphenicol. Zeitschrift fur Geburtshilfe und Perinatologie, *180*:149, 1979.
42. Ross, S., Burke, R.G, Sites, J., et al.: Placental transmission of chloramphenicol (Chloramycetin). JAMA, *142*:1361, 1950.
43. Scott, W.C. and Warner, R.F: Placental transfer of chloramphenicol (Chloramycetin). JAMA, *142*:1331, 1950.
44. Tedesco, F.J., Stanley, R.J. and Alpers, D.H.: Diagnostic features of clindamycin associated pseudomembranous colitis. N Engl J Med, *290*:841, 1974.
45. Brause, B.D., Borger, J.S. and Roberts, R.B.: Relative efficacy of clindamycin, erythromycin and penicillin in treatment of treponema pallidum in skin syphilomas of rabbits. J Infect Dis, *134*:93, 1976.
46. Brogden, R.N., Heel, R.C., Speight, T.M., et al.: Metronidazole in anaerobic infections: a review of its activity, pharmacokinetics and therapeutic use. Drugs, *16*:387, 1978.
47. Rustia, M. and Shubik, P.: Reduction of lung tumors and malignant lymphomas in mice by metronidazole. J Nat Cancer Inst, *48*:221, 1972.
48. Rustia, M. and Shubik, P.: Experimental reduction of hepatomas, mammary tumors and other tumors with metronidazole in non-inbred Sas: MRC(WI)BR rats. J Nat Cancer Inst, *63*:863, 1979.
49. Rosenkrantz, H.S. and Speck, W.T.: Mutagenicity of metronidazole: activation by mammalian liver microsomes. Biochem Biophys Res Commun, *66*:520, 1975.
50. McCann, J. and Ames, B.N.: Detection of carcinogens as mutagens in the Salmonella/microsome test: assay of 300 chemicals. Proc Natl Acad Sci USA, *73*:950, 1976.
51. Peterson, W.F., Stauch, J.E. and Ryan, E.D.: Metronidazole in pregnancy. Am J Obstet Gynecol, *94*:343, 1966.
52. Morgan, I.F.K.: Metronidazole treatment in pregnancy. Phillips, I and Collier, J (eds) Metronidazole. London, Academic Press, 1979, p. 215.
53. Aselton, P., Jick, H., Milunsky, A., et al.: First-trimester drug use and congenital disorders. Obstet Gynecol, *65*:451, 1985.

Chapter 5

Treatment of Tuberculosis in Pregnancy

Frank R. Witter

The concurrence of tuberculosis and pregnancy which was once dreaded can now be adequately treated with the same success as in the non-pregnant patient.[1,2] The incidence of relapse in adequately treated patients, even those with inactive persisting pulmonary cavities, is not increased by pregnancy.[3] Further, lactation does not affect the course of adequately treated tuberculosis,[2,4] and may be permitted with the reservations listed below.

The evaluation of patients suspected of having tuberculosis during pregnancy does not vary from that in the non-pregnant patient. It consists of history, physical examination, PPD placement, sputum cultures and stains for acid fast bacilli, and chest x ray after 20 weeks' gestation. It has been shown that tuberculin skin testing (PPD placement) is valid throughout the course of pregnancy.[5] Skin testing is recommended for all pregnant women unless they have been vaccinated with Bacille Calmette-Guérin (BCG) vaccine or are known to be PPD reactive. Patients who are PPD positive with known prior negative reaction, are PPD positive with a time of conversion unknown, or have a suspicious history or physical examimation irrespective of PPD status, should have at least three sputum specimens sent for cultures and stains for acid fast bacilli, and have a chest x ray after 20 weeks' gestation. Patients who have positive sputum specimens should have sensitivity testing done on the bacilli isolated, and should have a chest x ray done irrespective of the weeks of gestation. The radiation dose to the fetus and gonads with modern x-ray equipment is from 2.5 to 5 mrads which is far below 1 to 5 rads needed for a radiation effect.[5]

The rate of activation of tuberculosis in PPD converters is not altered by pregnancy.[2] History and physical examination findings suspicious for tuberculosis in pregnancy include: history of an exposure to a case of active tuberculosis, recent immigration from Korea or Southeast Asia, chronic cough, weight loss, fever, malaise, fatigue, and hemoptysis. Only 19% of active pulmonary tuberculosis presenting in pregnancy will be asymptomatic.[6] Attention should be paid to physical findings and symptoms arising from lymph nodes, bones, and kidneys as these are the most common extrapulmonary sites of involvement with tuberculosis in pregnancy.[6] Routine lumbar puncture is not necessary in evaluating the pregnant patient with tuberculosis, as tuberculosis meningitis is extremely rare in pregnancy. If neurologic signs or symptoms are present, evaluation for tuberculosis meningitis is indicated. Pregnant patients with drug resistant disease present with the same symptoms and signs as non-drug resistant patients; however, the incidence of extensive pulmonary disease is higher with drug resistant tuberculosis.[6]

Drugs Available for the Treatment of Tuberculosis

All of the drugs available for the treatment of tuberculosis in pregnancy cross to the fetus.[7]

ISONIAZID (INH)

Isoniazid (INH) remains the drug of choice for the treatment of tuberculosis, not only as a single agent for recent PPD converters, but also in multidrug combinations for active disease. It has not been shown to be teratogenic in humans,[6,8–10] and is not associated with any increase in perinatal mortality.[11,12] Although there is one case report of breast hypertrophy,[13] and one case report of a pellegra-like syndrome,[14] most series show no adverse fetal or maternal effects.[1,7] However, as with any patient receiving INH, there is a risk in the pregnant patient of gastrointestinal disturbance, peripheral neuropathy, and hepatitis.[6] Infants exposed to INH in utero are not at increased risk of childhood cancer.[15] There is one reported case of arthrogryposis multiplex congenita in association with a massive INH overdose taken as a suicide attempt.[16] This patient ingested greater than 50 INH tablets at 12 weeks' gestation. As arthrogryposis multiplex congenita can be produced by even brief immobilization in utero, it is possible that the potential neurotoxicity from this extremely high dose of INH was responsible for the congenital anomaly. This case underscores the need to give pyridoxine to prevent fetal and maternal neurotoxicity from INH.[2,17]

The elimination half-life for INH is 3.0 hours in the pregnant woman, while in the neonate it may vary between 7.8 hours and 19.8 hours.[18] At birth under chronic dosing conditions, the maternal and fetal serum INH concentrations are nearly identical. On the basis of the elimination half-life, the neonate would be classified as a slow acetylator of INH.[18] The milk-plasma ratio for INH in human milk is 1.0.[19] The risk to infants of nursing mothers is low, as only 20% of the usual therapeutic dose for infants will get into the breast milk and be received by the infant.[2] The infant should, however, receive supplemental pyridoxine.

ETHAMBUTOL

Ethambutol is another highly effective, first line drug for tuberculosis. No teratogenic effect has been shown for ethambutol.[9,11,12,20,21] Ethambutol is probably the safest drug next to INH for the treatment of tuberculosis from the standpoint of fetal anomalies as the rate of anomalies is low and does not differ from the general population.[7] Although it may produce optic neuritis, hepatitis, and peripheral neuritis in the adult, no adverse fetal effects have been seen.[1,22,23] Optic neuritis has not been seen in the neonate.[12]

The concentrations of ethambutol achieved with the recommended dosage (15 mg/kg/day at 30 hours after dosing) are 5.5 μg/L in the maternal blood, 5.0 μg/L in the placental blood, 4.1 μg/L in cord blood and 9.5 μg/L in amniotic fluid.[24] As 1 to 5 μg/L will inhibit the tuberculosis bacillus, present doses should adequately treat the fetus in utero. Data are not available on the safety of ethambutol during breastfeeding.

RIFAMPIN

Rifampin is an excellent anti-tuberculous drug for which no adverse fetal affects have been seen in humans to date,[1,9,21] although it is teratogenic in mice.[11,12] The incidence of anomalies among infants exposed in utero is 4.4% which is similar to the general population.[10] There may be a nonsignificant increase in limb abnormalities.[7] In any event the anomaly rate may be higher than with INH and ethambutol[10] and therefore should only be used in patients with extensive disease requiring triple drug therapy.

Rifampin enters breast milk with a milk plasma ratio of 0.2 to 0.6,[19] achieving levels of 1 to 3 mg/ml.[10] These levels do not pose a threat to the nursing infant and breast feeding may be permitted with rifampin therapy.[2]

When treating women with rifampin it should be born in mind that rifampin lowers the contraceptive effectiveness of concurrently administered oral contraceptives,[2] and so unexpected pregnancies may occur. Alternative contraception is recommended during therapy.

STREPTOMYCIN

Streptomycin is one of the oldest effective antituberculous agents. It has not been associated with increased fetal anomalies.[1,8] However, it crosses the placenta and reaches levels in the fetus of up to 50% of the maternal blood levels.[9,25] Streptomycin is associated with mild auditory and vestibular defects in the newborn exposed as a fetus.[9,21] Although cases of deafness have been reported,[7,25] most damage is only detectable on laboratory testing and hearing loss is in the high frequency, non-speech area of the auditory spectrum.[12,25] The risk of ototoxicity extends throughout pregnancy.[7] However, the incidence of auditory damage is low.[10,17] Because of the risk of eighth nerve damage, Streptomycin should be reserved in pregnancy for those cases of extensive disease where resistance ot rifampin is documented.

Streptomycin crosses into breast milk with a milk-plasma ratio of 0.5 to 1.0.[10] However, due to its poor oral absorption, it poses no threat to the breastfeeding infant and is not contraindicated during breastfeeding.

Kanamycin is another aminoglycoside used to treat tuberculosis. It also produces fetal hearing loss[26] and crosses into breast milk with a milk-plasma ratio of 0.05 to 0.40.[19] The same considerations which apply to Streptomycin apply to kanamycin. Streptomycin is to be preferred over kanamycin in the treatment of tuberculosis in pregnancy.

PARA-AMINOSALICYLIC ACID (PAS)

Para-aminosalicylic acid (PAS) is no longer a first line drug for the treatment of tuberculosis due to its low efficacy and gastrointestinal side effects. The gastrointestinal side effects make it even less desirable during pregnancy.[2] PAS has not been associated with adverse fetal effects.[1,8] and is considered nonteratogenic.[21] It does not enter breast milk and is therefore safe for the nursing infant.[27] PAS has, however, been replaced by more efficacious medications.

CYTOSERINE

Cytoserine is not a first line drug for the treatment of tuberculosis. The teratogenic potential of cytoserine is unknown.[6] Because of the psychoses induced by cytoserine, its use in pregnanacy is undesirable.[2,5] Cytoserine crosses into breast milk with a milk-plasma ratio of 0.67 to 0.75[2] It is also best avoided during lactation.

ETHIONAMIDE

Ethionamide is not a first line drug for the treatment of tuberculosis. Ethionamide has been reported to be teratogenic.[2,5] It should be considered contraindicated in pregnancy. No information is available on breastfeeding.

PYRAZINAMIDE

Pyrazinamide is not a first line drug for the treatment of tuberculosis. The effects of pyrazinamide on the fetus and nursing infant are unknown.[5,6] The possibility of maternal hepatotoxicity makes it an unattractive drug for use in pregnancy.

CAPREOMYCIN

Capreomycin is not a first line drug for the treatment of tuberculosis. Capreomycin is teratogenic in animals and has been reported to cause fetal ototoxicity.[6] Its effects on the breastfed infant are unknown. It is best avoided in pregnancy and lactation.

Table 5–1 lists the major maternal side effects from the drugs used for tuberculosis in pregnancy.

Table 5–1.   Adverse Maternal Effects

Isoniazid	Gastrointestinal disturbance Peripheral neuropathy Hepatitis
Ethambutol	Optic neuritis
Rifampin	Gastrointestinal disturbance Headache Hepatitis (rarely)
Streptomycin	Ototoxicity (vestibular and cochlear) Headache Pain at site of injection Nephrotoxicity (rarely)
Kanamycin	Ototoxicity (auditory) Nephrotoxicity
Para-aminosalicylic acid	Nausea and vomiting Diarrhea Myxedema (rarely)
Cytoserine	Central nervous system (psychoses) Drowsiness Headache Convulsions
Ethionamide	Gastrointestinal disturbances Hepatitis Optic and peripheral neuritis
Pyrazinamide	Hepatic toxicity Hyperuricemia
Capreomycin	Nephrotoxicity Ototoxicity

RECOMMENDATIONS

Recommendations for Therapy of the Mother

Three groups of patients may require antituberculosis therapy during pregnancy. The first of these is the recent PPD converter. This group consists of those patients who are PPD positive with a known prior negative reaction, or with the time of conversion unknown and who have three negative sputums for culture and stain for acid-fast bacilli, and negative chest x rays. These patients should be treated with 6 months to 1 year of 300 mg per day of oral INH plus 50 mg per day of oral pyridoxine to prevent maternal and fetal neurotoxicity.[7] Therapy may be safely deferred until after delivery. If, however, follow-up is uncertain in the time period after delivery, therapy should be started antepartum.

The second group of patients are those with non-extensive disease. Non-extensive disease is defined as non-cavitary tuberculosis confined to one lung field. These patients should be treated with 300 mg per day of oral INH for 18 months, plus 25 mg/kg per day of oral ethambutol for the first month followed by 15 mg/kg per day of oral ethambutol for a total of 18 months.[7] The initial higher dose of ethambutol is to avoid emergence of drug resistant bacilli. Pyridoxine at a dose of 50 mg per day orally should be given during the entire 18 months of therapy to prevent maternal and fetal INH-induced neurotoxicity.

The third group of patients consists of those with extensive disease and consists of all patients with tuberculosis not in the first two groups. Patients with extensive disease should be treated with 300 mg per day of oral INH plus 15 mg/kg per day of oral ethambutol, plus 600 mg per day of oral rifampin.[7] The duration of the therapy should be 9 months or for 6 months after sputum conversion, whichever is longer. The rifampin dose should be adjusted down to 450 mg per day for those patients weighing less than 50 kg. Pyridoxine in a dose of 50 mg per day orally is once again used to avoid INH-induced maternal and fetal neurotoxicity.

Therapy should be adjusted based on drug sensitivity determined from cultures. Patients with more extensive disease especially with more than one cavity involving more than one lobe of the lungs are at increased risk of having drug-resistant bacilli.[6] In those cases where drug resistance to rifampin occurs, or where rifampin is contraindicated due to maternal sensitivity, streptomycin is the next drug of choice.[7] The non-first line drugs for tuberculosis therapy have been used insufficiently in pregnancy and lactation for their safety for the fetus and nursing infant to be assessed. However, if drug-resistant disease is present, these drugs may be used when indicated because the benefit to the mother outweighs the unknown risk to the fetus. The usual adult dosages of the antituberculosis drugs are listed in Table 5-2.[6]

Recommendations for the Therapy of the Neonate of a Mother with Tuberculosis

Since the introduction of INH in 1952, congenital tuberculosis has become very rare with only 27 reported cases in the English literature.[28] However, as the infants of mothers with tuberculosis carry a 50% risk of acquiring tuberculosis within the first year of life without prophylaxis,[5] some form of prophylaxis should be given.

Table 5–2.   Usual Adult Dosages

		Route of Administration
Isoniazid	300 mg/day	Orally
Ethambutol	25 mg/kg/day for 1 month, then 10–15 mg/kg/day	Orally
Rifampin	600 mg/day	Orally
Streptomycin	0.75–1 g/day for 14 to 21 days, then 1 g 3 times/ week	IM
Kanamycin	15 mg/kg 3–5 times/week	IM
Para-amino-salicylic acid	10–12 g/day	Orally
Cytoserine	250 mg bid not to exceed 1 g/day	Orally
Ethionamide	0.5–1 g/day in divided doses	Orally
Pyrazinamide	20–35 mg/kg/day	Orally
Capreomycin	0.75–1 g/day for 60–120 days, then 1 g 3 times/wk	IM

The first step in prevention of neonatal transmission is isolation from the potential source. If maternal disease is inactive or if active and under treatment for 3 weeks, contact with the neonate may be permitted.[4] In any event, the infant should be isolated from the mother until she is no longer infectious.[28] A longer period of isolation may be necessary for mothers with drug resistant disease.[6]

Several methods of neonatal prophylaxis have been suggested. The first is INH prophylaxis with 10 mg/kg for 3 to 6 months with monitoring of the PPD reaction at 3 and 6 months.[29] If the PPD turns positive, then INH should be given for a full year. A problem with this form of prophylaxis is compliance.[28]

A second method of prophylaxis is Bacille Calmette-Guérin (BCG) vaccination. This method is advocated by some experts as the method of choice,[11] and is indicated if compliance appears unlikely.[29] Unfortunately, it takes 6 weeks to confirm vaccination with a positive PPD and the mother must be isolated from the infant during this time.[28]

A third method of neonatal prophylaxis in selected cases is continued surveillance with repeated PPD placement.[28] PPD's should be placed at 3 and 12 months and only reliable mothers with inactive disease should be considered for this method.

CONCLUSIONS

The therapy of tuberculosis in pregnancy should be adjusted based on the extent of disease and the sensitivity of the organisms. Preferred drugs are INH, ethambutol, rifampin, followed by Streptomycin. Infants of mothers with tuberculosis should receive antituberculosis prophylaxis either with INH or BCG vaccine.

REFERENCES

1. Wilson, E.A., Thelin, T.J. and Dilts, P.J.: Tuberculosis complicated by pregnancy. Am J Obstet Gynecol, *115*:526, 1973.

2. Snider, D.: Pregnancy and tuberculosis. Chest, *86*(3 suppl):10S, 1984.
3. deMarch, P.: Tuberculosis and pregnancy, five-to-ten-year review of 215 patients in their fertile age. Chest, *68*:800, 1975.
4. Fishburne, J.I.: Physiology and disease of the respiratory system in pregnancy. J Reprod Med, *22*:177, 1979.
5. Weinberger, S.E., et al.: Pregnancy and the lung. Ann Rev Respir Dis, *121*:559, 1980.
6. Good, J.T., et al.: Tuberculosis in association with pregnancy. Am J Obstet Gynecol, *140*:492, 1981.
7. Snider, D.E., Layde, P.M., Johnson, M.W. and Lyle, M.A.: Treatment of tuberculosis during pregnancy. Am Rev Respir Dis, *122*:65, 1980.
8. Marcus, J.C.: Non-teratogenicity of antituberculous drugs. S Afr Med J, *41*:758, 1967.
9. Scheinhorn, D.J. and Angelillo, J.A.: Antituberculous therapy in pregnancy. West J Med, *127*:195, 1977.
10. Briggs, G.G., Bodendorter, T.W., Freeman, R.K., and Yaffe, S.J.: Drugs in Pregnancy and Lactation. Baltimore, Williams & Wilkins, 1983.
11. DeSwiet, M.: Diseases of the respiratory system, Clin Obstet Gynaecol, *4*:287, 1977.
12. DeSwiet, M.: Respiratory disease in pregnancy. Postgrad Med J, *55*:325, 1979.
13. Van der Meulen, A.J.: An unusual case of massive hypertrophy of the breasts. S Afr Med J, *48*:1465, 1974.
14. DiLorenzo, P.A.: Pellagra-like syndrome associated with isoniazid therapy. Acta Derm Venereol (StachH), *47*:318, 1967.
15. Sanders, B.M. and Draper, G.J.: Childhood cancer and drugs in pregnancy. Br Med J, *1*:717, 1979.
16. Lenke, R.R., Turkel S.B. and Monsen, R.: Severe fetal deformities associated with ingestion of excessive isoniazid in early pregnancy. Acta Obstet Gynecol Scand, *64*:281, 1985.
17. Warkany, J.: Antituberculous drugs. Teratology, *20*:133, 1979.
18. Miceli, J.N., Olson, W.A. and Cohen, S.N.: Elimination kinetics of isoniazid in the newborn infant. Dev Pharmacol Ther, *2*:235, 1981.
19. Wilson, J.T., et al.: Drug excretion in human breast milk. Clin Pharmacokinetics, *5*:1, 1980.
20. Lewit, T., Nebel, L., Terracina, S. and Korman, S.: Ethambutol in pregnancy: observations on embryogenesis. Chest, *66*:25, 1974.
21. Shepart, T.H.: Cataloge of Teratogenic Agents. 3rd Ed. Baltimore, Johns Hopkins University Press, 1980.
22. Bobrowitz, I.D.: Ethambutol in pregnancy. Chest, *66*:20, 1974.
23. Council on Drugs: Evaluation of a new antituberculous agent ethambutol hydrochloride (Myambutol). JAMA, *208*:2463, 1969.
24. Shneerson, J.M., and Francis, R.S.: Ethambutol in pregnancy—foetal exposure. Tubercle, *60*:167, 1979.
25. Donald, P.R. and Sellars, S.L.: Streptomycin ototoxity in the unborn child. S Afr Med J, *60*:316, 1981.
26. Gladtke, E.: Effect on the child of drugs taken in late pregnancy. Germ Med, *3*:135, 1973.
27. Lawrence, R.A.: Breastfeeding. St. Louis, C.V. Mosby Co., 1980.
28. Lorin, M.I., Hsu, K.H.K. and Jacob, S.C.: Treatment of tuberculosis in children. Pediatr Clin North Am, *30*:333, 1983.
29. Bailey, W.C., et al.: Treatment of tuberculosis and other mycobacterial diseases. Am Rev Respir Dis, *127*:790, 1983.

Chapter 6

Anticonvulsants in Pregnancy

Anthony R. Scialli

EPILEPSY AND PREGNANCY

One in every 200 individuals is affected with a seizure disorder and close to the same incidence of epilepsy is seen among pregnant women. Epilepsy refers to a group of disorders of different causes characterized by paroxysmal depolarization of neurons in the central nervous system. The location and number of neurons involved give rise to the different manifestations of seizure disorders.

Types of Seizure Disorders

The most easily recognized seizures are the tonic-clonic convulsions of grand mal epilepsy. These are examples of generalized epilepsy, characterized by bilateral and symmetrical involvement. Another generalized seizure is the absence or petit mal seizure which consists of staring or blinking with little or no other motor activity. In both grand and petit mal epilepsy there is loss of awareness. Grand mal seizures are also followed by prolonged depression of cerebral function during the postictal period. Other generalized convulsions include atonic seizures, with loss of postural muscle tone and myoclonic epilepsy, in which there are isolated clonic jerks. Young children may demonstrate clonic seizures with loss of consciousness and autonomic features, tonic seizures with opisthotonus, and infantile spasms with progressive mental deterioration.

Although generalized seizures are clinically the most dramatic forms of epilepsy, of equal importance are the partial seizures. These are characterized by focal involvement of the central nervous system and may be confused with other illnesses such as transient ischemic attacks. Partial seizures are classified as simple and complex. The simple seizure disorders are also called Jacksonian epilepsies and produce elementary symptoms, often involving sensation or the motor function of a single limb. Simple partial seizures may include autonomic or psychic symptoms but do not involve loss of consciousness. Complex partial seizures, called psychomotor epilepsy, may start out with simple manifestations and progress to generalized involvement with loss of awareness and bizarre behavior.

Effects of Pregnancy on Epilepsy

There does not appear to be a uniform effect of the gravid state on the tendency to have seizures. Pregnant experimental animals have been found both more[1] and less[2] susceptible to the induction of convulsions and it has been proposed that progesterone may increase the seizure threshold.[2] In humans, pregnancy has no effect on the frequency of convulsions in 50% of all epileptic women, with an increase in seizure frequency in 40 to 45% and a decrease in seizure frequency in 5 to 10%.[3,4] The increase in seizure incidence during pregnancy may be due to a decrease in blood levels of anticonvulsant medication. Such a decrease may result from the hemodilution normally seen during gestation. In addition, some drugs (e.g., phenytoin, phenobarbital, carbamazepine) are cleared more rapidly during pregnancy. Pregnant women may omit doses or discontinue drug therapy due to pregnancy-related nausea or because they are worried that the therapy will cause damage to the conceptus. The measurement of blood levels of anticonvulsant medication is, therefore, important to avoid loss of seizure control during therapy.

Effects of Epilepsy on Pregnancy

Although it has been reported that epileptic gravidas have an increased incidence of vaginal bleeding,[5] an increase in spontaneous abortion has not been found to be associated with maternal epilepsy.[3] Pregnancy outcome among epileptics has, however, been of concern with regard to congenital anomalies. A number of studies have found that the offspring of epileptic women have a reproducibly higher incidence of birth defects than do those of nonepileptic controls. Information from the national registry of births in Norway, for example, showed a diagnosis of epilepsy in the mother to be associated with a doubling of the incidence of birth defects in the offspring.[5] A case control study from Finland and data from the Collaborative Perinatal Project in the United States gave similar results.[6] Epilepsy in a child's father was not associated with a statistically significant increase in the congenital anomaly rate[6,7] suggesting that a purely genetic effect of parental epilepsy is not involved. Attempts have been made to determine whether the effects of maternal epilepsy on the offspring are attributable to anticonvulsant medications. Certainly, case reports of women using anticonvulsants during the first trimester have yielded high rates of congenital anomalies.[8] Controlled studies examining epileptic women on drugs compared to those not receiving therapy show an increase in birth defects in the offspring in the drug-using group.[7,9] In some studies, no increase in incidence of birth defects was found in the offspring of epileptic women not on drug therapy when compared to the offspring of normal women.[7,9] In the CPP data, the disease itself without any drug increased the risk of anomalies.[14] Most of the medication-associated malformations identified in these studies are facial clefts, neural tube defects, and congenital heart disease. The presence or absence of seizures during the pregnancy does not influence the incidence of anomalies in the offspring.

In spite of the evidence that maternal drug therapy for epilepsy appears to be a factor determining an increase in birth defects in the offspring, the data cannot be regarded as conclusive. Women with epilepsy who are not treated with medication are almost certainly more mildly affected than women who require drug therapy. It has not been possible to show that in women with equally severe disease, a difference in pregnancy outcome is related to drug therapy alone. It is believed that epilepsy itself may predispose to congenital anomalies with a disease-associated increase in birth defects to about twice the baseline rate in the population.[4] An effect of epilepsy on birth defects is likely to be in part genetically mediated. In fact, it is possible that epilepsy is in some cases a manifestation of a congenital anomaly of the central nervous system in the mother. The offspring of a woman with birth defects will be more likely to have an anomaly than the offspring of a normal women. If this is the case, however, an increase in birth defects in the offspring of epileptic fathers would be expected. In fact, there is one report suggesting a similar increase in the incidence of birth defects in children whether epilepsy affects the father or the mother.[10] Those studies[6,7] which do not show a statistically significant increase in birth defects associated with paternal epilepsy nonetheless show a higher rate which might be statistically significant with a larger number of subjects.

The genetic argument notwithstanding, it is clear that the greater part of the increase in the congenital anomaly rate seen in the offspring of epileptic women is associated with drug therapy. At the same time, the use of drugs to control seizures during pregnancy is desirable since convulsions may be associated with maternal injury, aspiration, and/or hypoxia.

USE OF ANTICONVULSANT THERAPY

The prescribing of anticonvulsant medication during pregnancy should adhere to guidelines similar to those for nonpregnant individuals. The choice of drug is based on the type of seizure disorder to be controlled. If a woman has not had seizures for many years, it may be possible to discontinue her anticonvulsant therapy prior to pregnancy; however, many epileptics will become pregnant when they are already under therapy. Much has been written on the matter of which anticonvulsants should be avoided during pregnancy. There is general agreement that the oxazolidinediones (trimethadione and paramethadione) should not be given. These agents are used in absence seizures where therapy with ethosuximide is more effective and poses less risk of toxicity to the fetus. The potential for reproductive toxicity of these and other agents will be discussed below; however, except for the oxazolidinediones, there is no consensus on which other of these drugs should be avoided. For example, although phenytoin has been associated with a syndrome of anomalies by many reports, not all authorities agree that important fetal toxicity is due to this drug and many do not recommend switching pregnant epileptics from this agent.[4] The plan of anticonvulsant management should include consideration of the estimated rate and severity of fetal toxicity associated with a drug (discussed below), the alternative medications available and the wishes of the pregnant epileptic and her partner. As a rule, therapy with one agent is preferred to therapy with multiple agents, not only to enhance compliance but to reduce toxicity which may be synergistic among these agents.

When a course of therapy is elected, it should be anticipated that drug levels in the blood may decrease during gestation. Monitoring of these levels should be considered every 2 to 4 weeks. Postpartum increases in drug levels may also occur and checking blood levels during this period will help to prevent drug toxicity. The patient's cooperation with the treatment plan should be reinforced at frequent intervals. In addition, factors known to increase seizure frequency, such as fatigue and sleep deprivation, should be minimized. Many anticonvulsants are associated with the induction of enzymes that metabolize folic acid; therefore, folate supplementation at a dose of 1 mg/day during pregnancy should be recommended. In addition, prolonged therapy with phenytoin may result in vitamin D deficiency which may be corrected by oral supplementation. The use of the hydantoins and barbiturates during pregnancy is associated with a bleeding disorder in the neonate. This may be corrected by administration of vitamin K to the newborn. The use by the pregnant epileptic of oral vitamin K at a dose of 10 mg/day during the last month of pregnancy has also been recommended.[11]

Barbiturates

All barbiturates appear to have anticonvulsant activity; however, the clinical usefulness of an agent depends on whether an anticonvulsant effect occurs at doses that are not excessively hypnotic. Of the barbiturates, phenobarbital, mephobarbital, and methabarbital have been used for seizure disorders. A barbiturate derivative, primidone, is also considered with this group of drugs.

Phenobarbital is one of the oldest anticonvulsants in use and is by far the most common of the barbiturate antiseizure medications. This drug is used in grand mal epilepsy and in focal cortical seizures. During pregnancy, the clearance of phenobarbital from the blood is increased in most patients; however, the clearance may also decrease or remain unchanged.[12] Therapeutic plasma phenobarbital levels are 10 to 25 μg/mL although levels as high as 35 μg/mL have been recommended.[4] These levels are obtainable with doses of 1 to 5 mg/kg/day. It takes several hours for orally administered phenobarbital to result in peak plasma levels.

The barbiturates are capable of causing birth defects in animals, although these drugs are not potent teratogens and the defects caused are usually minor.[13] Studies on the use of phenobarbital in human pregnancy have often been confounded by the common use of combination therapy with phenytoin. Cases have been reported in which hydantoin-like effects in the offspring were associated with maternal phenobarbital alone; however, controlled studies establishing phenobarbital as a cause of these effects are unavailable. Although the Collaborative Perinatal Project found an association between phenobarbital use during pregnancy and congenital heart disease in the offspring,[14] phenobarbital is considered one of the safest of the anticonvulsants for use during pregnancy. As discussed above, a vitamin K-responsive bleeding abnormality may be seen in the neonate after maternal phenobarbital therapy. Newborns may also exhibit a phenobarbital withdrawal syndrome characterized by hyperactivity and tremors.

An interesting area of research is the production of behavioral abnormalities in the offspring of animals treated with barbiturates during pregnancy. Phenobarbital has been investigated as a possible behavioral teratogen; however, studies have given opposite results on the possible effects of this agent, even when used in the same species.[15,16]

Primidone is metabolized to phenobarbital and phenylethylmalonamide. The parent compound and both metabolites have anticonvulsant activity and primidone may control seizures that are refractory to phenobarbital. The therapeutic blood levels of 5 to 10 μg/mL are achieved with doses of 500 to 2000 mg/day. Pregnancy does not impose a consistent change in primidone pharmacokinetics although there may be a decreased rate of metabolism of the drug to phenobarbital.[12,17] It is not known whether this decreased conversion of the parent compound is associated with a clinically important change in drug activity.

It is unclear whether primidone alone may be responsible for congenital anomalies. There have been a number of case reports of children born with features of the fetal hydantoin syndrome where the mother was exposed only to primidone.[13,18] There are no data which permit a prediction of the frequency with which primidone therapy of the mother might lead to an abnormal child. As with phenobarbital therapy, administration of primidone to the mother may result in a bleeding abnormality and/or a withdrawal syndrome in the newborn.

Hydantoins

This group of agents is represented almost exclusively by phenytoin, an anticonvulsant widely used for all types of seizures except petit mal epilepsy. Therapeutic levels of 10 to 20 μg/mL are obtained with doses of 300 to 600 mg/day. Phenytoin toxic effects include nystagmus, ataxia, and lethargy; these effects are generally seen above blood concentrations of 20 μg/mL. Oral availability of phenytoin remains excellent during pregnancy;[19] however, the volume of distribution of the drug increases by about 20% in proportion to body weight.[20] This may require much larger doses of medication to achieve the same blood level and up to 1200 or 1300 mg/day of phenytoin therapy during pregnancy has been described.[4,20] Clearance of the drug is increased in most pregnant women but is decreased in some.[12,19] Phenytoin in the circulation is largely bound to proteins. A decrease in drug binding in pregnancy may be seen and could theoretically lead to an increase in drug effect. In mice, however, an increase in brain concentration of phenytoin, attributed to the increased serum concentration of free drug, does not result in an increase in anticonvulsant activity.[2] A similar increase in free phenytoin levels accompanying pregnancy in rats is also not associated with an increase in protection from seizures.[1]

Phenytoin is teratogenic in mice, rats, and rabbits. Although multiple defects have been reported from animal teratogenicity studies, abnormalities particularly associated with phenytoin include cleft palate, micromelia, kidney defects, and hydrocephalus.[13] Mephenytoin, a similar agent, is teratogenic in mice.[21] Human infants exposed to phenytoin and other hydantoins in utero have been reported to show a number of different abnormalities, especially heart defects and facial clefts. Up to 10% of exposed pregnancies may give rise to an infant with major birth defects.[22]

A constellation of lesser abnormalties, called the fetal hydantoin syndrome, is seen in some exposed infants. The syndrome includes dysmorphic facies (short nose, low bridge, epicanthic folds, hypertelorism, abnormal ears, wide mouth), hypoplasia of distal phalanges (especially involving the nails), fingerlike thumbs, short or webbed neck, low hairline, and abnormalities of growth and of mental and/or motor development. A number of additional anomalies have appeared in case reports of children with the fetal hydantoin syndrome.[23] It should be recognized that not all studies have been able to confirm an increase in human birth defects associated with maternal phenytoin use.[4,6] It has been proposed, for example, that an increase in adverse fetal outcome in phenytoin-exposed pregnancies may be due to maternal toxicity of the drug (as in decreasing appetite) rather than to a direct effect of phenytoin on fetal development.[24]

It was at one time felt that the mechanism of action of phenytoin-induced birth defects involved the reduction in folic acid associated with hydantoins. Folic acid antagonists such as aminopterin and methotrexate are teratogenic and it would be consistent for anticonvsulant-mediated folic acid deficiency to result in similar fetal toxicity. Although phenytoin has been shown to decrease maternal plasma folate levels in mice, total embryo folate is not decreased in this species.[25] In addition, animal work involving supplemental folate has not shown a role for this agent in preventing hydantoin-induced fetal abnormalities.[13]

It appears more likely that the fetal toxicity of phenytoin and similar agents is due to the generation of reactive intermediates. Arene oxides of phenytoin are unstable metabolites produced by cytochrome p450-associated monooxygenases. These arene oxides may covalently bind cell macromolecules theoretically leading to derangements of cell function and perhaps to cell death or mutation. Arene oxides are metabolized by epoxide hydrolase, an enzyme normally present in low amounts in the fetus. It would be expected that genetic variability in the amount of available epoxide hydrolase would influence the susceptibility of the fetus to phenytoin toxic effects. This has, in fact, been shown in an investigation of the sensitivity of lymphocytes to phenytoin toxicity: the presence of major phenytoin-associated birth defects in a child correlates with an inability of that child's lymphocytes to detoxify phenytoin metabolites.[22] The importance of genetic susceptibility to phenytoin fetal toxicity is also suggested by a report of heteropaternal twins born to a phenytoin-using woman. The twins were discordant for manifestations of the fetal hydantoin syndrome.[26]

The use of phenytoin during pregnancy may increase the risk of childhood neuroectodermal tumors in the offspring. There have been 9 reported cases of tumors in children with intrauterine exposure to phenytoin (often with barbiturate cotherapy).[27] The reported malignancies include ependymoma, mesenchymoma, neuroblastoma, ganglioneuroblastoma, melanotic ectodermal tumor, and Wilms' tumor. Although controlled studies are not available to establish the magnitude, if any, of transplacental carcinogenicity risk associated with anticonvulsants, the association between these unusual childhood neoplasms and maternal therapy appears greater than expected by chance.[28]

In view of the number of reports on possible adverse effects attributed to phenytoin, it is difficult for many clinicians to feel comfortable prescribing this agent during pregnancy. It should be borne, in mind, however, that an increase in serious fetal toxicity imposed by phenytoin is disputed, that such an increase (if present) is of low order, and that seizure control may not be possible without this agent. Several investigators have concluded that there is no justification in withholding phenytoin from pregnant epileptics who require the drug to remain seizure free.[4,13]

Succimides

This class of agents is used in absence seizures and includes phensuximide, methsuximide, and ethosuximide. Ethosuximide, the most widely used of these drugs, is given in doses of 500 to 2000 mg/day to yield therapeutic plasma levels of 40 to 100 μg/mL. The effects of pregnancy on maternal serum drug levels are variable[29] and dosage regimens must be tailored to individual requirements.

The succimide anticonvulsants are teratogenic in mice and ethosuximide is also teratogenic in rats, hamsters, and rabbits.[13] These agents do not appear to be teratogenic in humans, however, and are considered drugs of choice for therapy of petit mal epilepsy during pregnancy.[29,30] Ethosuximide appears in breast milk at levels nearly equal to those in plasma. The possibility of sedation related to succimide ingestion should be considered in nursing infants exposed to this group of drugs.

Oxazolidinediones

Trimethadione and paramethadione are similar agents which have been used in the treatment of petit mal epilepsy. These drugs are best avoided during pregnancy because of their association with a syndrome of abnormalities in the offspring. This "fetal trimethadione syndrome" consists of developmental delay, mental retardation, low-set ears, palate defects, irregular teeth, V-shaped eyebrows, and speech disturbances.[31] An analysis of reports concerning 36 trimethadione-exposed pregnancies in 9 families revealed a congenital anomaly rate of 69%.[23] Three of these families produced 5 normal pregnancies after discontinuation of the anticonvulsant.

Benzodiazepines

Most drugs in this group have some anticonvulsant activity; however, only clonazepam is used to any extent in the long-term therapy of epilepsy. Diazepam may be used to control acute episodes of convulsions, especially during labor, and for status epilepticus (discussed below).

Clonazepam may be used for petit mal and myoclonic epilepsy. Dosage ranges from 1.5 to 20 mg/day to give therapeutic plasma levels of 0.01 to 0.07 μg/mL. Clonazepam is teratogenic in mice but not in rats or rabbits.[13] There are no available human studies on possible teratogenicity of this agent. Toxicity of this drug for the neonate is suggested by a report of an infant with apnea, hypotonia, and cyanosis at 6 hours of age.[32] The serum concentration of clonazepam in the mother at birth was 0.032 μg/mL (within the therapeutic range) with a corresponding cord blood clonazepam level of 0.019 μg/mL. The milk:plasma ratio was 1:3. This one case does not establish a hazard of maternal clonazepam therapy for the neonate but makes advisable the close observation of exposed infants.

Diazepam administered intravenously at a dose of 2 mg/min to a maximum of 10 to 20 mg will arrest many tonic-clonic seizures, including those of eclampsia. Diazepam was used in the past with other anticonvulsants as an adjunct in the long-term treatment of epilepsy. The chronic use of diazepam during pregnancy has been discouraged because of associations between minor tranquilizer use by pregnant women and birth defects in the offspring. Retrospective studies from the 1970s showed an increased incidence of cleft palate and/or cleft lip in the offspring of women using diazepam or similar drugs.[33,34] A decade later, controlled epidemiologic studies involving large numbers of diazepam-exposed pregnancies were unable to show an association between use of this drug and oral clefts or any other abnormality in the offspring.[35,36]

Maternal treatment with diazepam chronically during the third trimester or with high doses (>30 mg) shortly before delivery may be associated with a "floppy infant syndrome" in the neonate. Affected babies are hypotonic with apnea and impaired response to cold stress. Diazepam is metabolized to oxazepam and desmethyldiazepam both of which are pharmacologically active. In reported cases of the floppy infant syndrome, diazepam and desmethyldiazepam have been detectable in significant amounts in the neonate for 8 to 14 days after birth.[37,38]

Carbamazepine

Carbamazepine is an iminostilbene with activity in all seizure disorders other than petit mal epilepsy. This drug is used particularly in patients with psychomotor (temporal lobe) and grand mal epilepsy. Doses of 200 to 1200 mg/day give rise to therapeutic plasma levels of 4 to 8 μg/ml. Clearance of this agent has been reported to increase during pregnancy.[12]

Reports concerning the use of carbamazepine in 531 human pregnancies have been reviewed.[23] Use of this drug alone during pregnancy has not been shown to cause an increase in the incidence of birth defects in the offspring; however, interpretation of the data is limited by the frequency with which combination therapy is used. It has been proposed that the inclusion of the carbamazepine in combination therapy may increase the risk of anticonvulsant teratogenesis due to an accumulation of carbamazepine epoxide.[39] Whether the presence of this epoxide in carbamazepine monotherapy is associated with an increase in adverse fetal effects has not been established.

Valproic acid

Valproic acid is used in simple and complex absence seizures. A dose of 15 to 60 mg/kg/day is used to achieve therapeutic plasma levels of 50 to 100 μg/mL. Clearance of the drug is increased during pregnancy.[12] Valproic acid levels in cord serum are 1.1 to 4.6 times the levels in maternal serum at term.[40] This is attributed to displacement of the drug from binding sites on maternal protein by free fatty acids and more avid binding in the fetal compartment.[40,41] Since hepatotoxicity with valproic acid occurs in a dose-related fashion, a risk of liver damage in fetuses concentrating this drug has been suggested.[23] The magnitude of such a risk is unknown.

Sodium valproate, an equivalent form of valproic acid, is teratogenic in mice, rats, and rabbits, but not in monkeys.[13] A human "fetal valproate syndrome" has been described:[42] many of the features are similar to those seen in the fetal hydantoin syndrome. Of particular concern, however, are data from questionnaire studies and registries associating valproic acid with neural tube defects.[43,44] A review of these data and other reports suggests that there is a 1% incidence of neural tube defects in the offspring of women who take valproic acid during pregnancy.[45]

STATUS EPILEPTICUS

Status epilepticus, in which major convulsions are continuous or interrupted only by brief periods of incomplete recovery, is a medical emergency. Untreated status epilepticus may lead to permanent neurologic injury or death. Treatment during pregnancy is similar to that for nonpregnant individuals: it is not appropriate to withhold necessary drugs because of concern about teratogenic risks to the fetus. An intravenous line is started and 50 mL of 50% dextrose is administered. This is followed by diazepam at 2 mg/min until seizures stop or until 20 mg has been given. Phenytoin is then given at a rate not to exceed 50 mg/min to a dose of 18 mg/kg (750 to 1000 mg for most women).

If seizures are not arrested by this therapy, a diazepam or phenobarbital infusion may be started. Diazepam is administered at a rate of 4 to 8 mg/hr and phenobarbital at a rate not faster than 100 mg/min until seizures stop or until a total dose of 20 mg/kg has been given.

If seizures continue after a diazepam or phenobarbital infusion has been given, general anesthesia is induced with halothane or a similar agent plus neuro-muscular blockade.

During the therapy of status epilepticus, attention must be directed to maintaining adequate ventilation, to support of the blood pressure if necessary, and to correction of fluid and electolyte abnormalities. Continuous electrocardiographic monitoring is often helpful, especially when phenytoin is given. After resolution of status epilepticus, a cause for this condition should be sought. Status epilepticus may, for example, be precipitated by the abrupt discontinuation of prescribed anticonvulsant medication. Education of the pregnant epileptic on the importance of maintaining therapy should help to avoid this complication.

Seizures occurring during pregnancy or shortly after delivery may, of course, be signs of eclampsia. Specific treatment of the hypertensive disorders of pregnancy is considered elsewhere in this book (Chapter 7). The initial management of the seizing gravida, however, may follow that outlined above for status epilepticus since control of the convulsions, adequate oxygenation, and correction of glucose and electrolyte abnormalities are as important in eclampsia as they are in epilepsy.

REFERENCES

1. Chou, R.C. and Levy, G.: Kinetics of drug action in disease states, III: Effect of pregnancy on the relationship between phenytoin concentration and antiseizure activity in rats. J Pharm Sci, *73*:1348, 1984.
2. Nau, H., Kuhnz, W. and Löscher, W.: Effect of pregnancy on seizure threshold and the disposition and efficacy of antiepileptic drugs in the mouse. Life Sci, *36*:663, 1985.
3. Knight, A.H. and Rhind, E.G.: Epilepsy and pregnancy: a study of 153 pregnancies in 59 patients. Epilepsia, *16*:99, 1975.
4. Dalessio, D.J.: Current concepts: Seizure disorders and pregnancy. N Engl J Med, *312*:559, 1985.
5. Bjerkedal, T. and Bahna, S.L: The course and outcome of pregnancy in women with epilepsy. Acta Obstet Gynecol Scand, *52*:245, 1973.
6. Idänpään-Heikkilä, J., Härö, S. and Saxén, L.: Anticonvulsants and parental epilepsy in the development of birth defects. Lancet, *1*:272, 1976.
7. Annegers, J.F., et al.: Congenital malformations and seizure disorders in the offspring of parents with epilepsy. Int J Epidemiol, *7*:241, 1978.
8. Biale, Y., Lowenthal, H., and Ben Aderet, N.: Congenital malformations due to anticonvulsant drugs. Obstet Gynecol, *45*:439, 1975.
9. Lowe, C.R.: Congenital malformations among infants born to epileptic women. Lancet, *1*:9, 1973.
10. Shapiro, S., et al.: Anticonvulsants and parental epilepsy in the development of birth defects. Lancet, *1*:272, 1976.
11. Hadi, H.A. and Mashini, I.S.: Management of epilepsy during pregnancy. Female Patient, *11*:131, 1986.
12. Levy, R.H. and Yerby, M.S.: Effects of pregnancy on antiepileptic drug utilization. Epilepsia, *26*[Suppl. 1]:S52, 1985.
13. Schardein, J.I..: Chemically Induced Birth Defects, New York, Marcel Dekker, Inc., 1985.
14. Heinonen, O.P., Slone, D. and Shapiro, S.: Birth Defects and Drugs in Pregnancy, Littleton, Mass., Publishing Sciences Group, Inc., 1977.
15. McBride, M.C. and Rosman, N.P.: Absence of behavioral effects of intrauterine phenobarbital exposure in rats. Exper Neurol, *86*:53, 1984.
16. Martin, J.C., et al.: Maternal barbiturate administration and offspring response to shock, Psychopharmacol, *85*:214, 1985.
17. Battino, D., et al.: Changes in primidone/phenobarbitone ratio during pregnancy and the puerperium. Clin Pharmacokinet, *9*:252, 1984.
18. Krauss, C.M., Holmes, L.B., VanLang, Q.N. and Keith, D.A.: Four siblings with similar malformations after exposure to phenytoin and primidone. J Pediatr, *105*:750, 1984.
19. Lander, C.M., et al.: Bioavailability and pharmacokinetics of phenytoin during pregnancy. Eur J Clin Pharmacol, *27*:105, 1984.

20. Freed, C.R., Gal, J. and Manchester, D.K.: Dosage of phenytoin during pregnancy, Lancet, *1*:2833, 1985.

21. Kao, J., Brown, N.A., Shull, G. and Fabro, S.: Chemical structure and teratogenicity of anti-convulsants. Fed Proc, *38*:438, 1979.

22. Strickler, S.M., et al.: Genetic predisposition to phenytoin-induced birth defects. Lancet, *2*:746, 1985.

23. Briggs, G.G., Freeman, R.K. and Yaffe, S.J.: Drugs in Pregnancy and Lactation, 2nd Ed., Baltimore, Williams & Wilkins, 1986.

24. Khera, K.S.: Phenytoin and trimethadione: pharmacokinetics, embryotoxicity, and maternal toxicity. Prog Clin Biol Res, *163C*:317, 1985.

25. Hansen, D.K. and Billings, R.E.: Phenytoin teratogenicity and effects on embryonic and maternal folate metabolism. Teratology, *31*:363, 1985.

26. Phelan, M.C., Pellock, M.M. and Nance, W.E.: Discordant expression of fetal hydantoin syndrome in heteropaternal dizygotic twins. N Engl J Med, *307*:99, 1982.

27. Lipson, A. and Bale, P.: Ependymoblastoma associated with prenatal exposure to diphenylhydantoin and methylphenobarbitone. Cancer, *55*:1859, 1985.

28. Fabro, S. and Brown, N.A.: Anticonvulsant-induced transplacental carcinogenesis. Repro Toxicol Med Lett, *1*:1, 1982.

29. Kuhnz, W., et al.: Ethosuximide in epileptic women during pregnancy and lactation period. Placental transfer, serum concentrations in nursed infants and clinical status. Br J Clin Pharmacol, *18*:671, 1984.

30. Fabro, S. and Brown, N.A.: Teratogenic potential of anticonvulsants. N Engl J Med *300*:1280, 1979.

31. Zackai, E.H., Mellman, W.J., Neiderer, B. and Hanson, J.W.: The fetal trimethadione syndrome. J Pediatr, *87*:280, 1975.

32. Fisher, J.B., Edgren, B.E., Mammel, M.C. and Coleman, J.M.: Neonatal apnea associated with maternal clonazepam therapy: a case report. Obstet Gynecol, *66*:34S, 1985.

33. Saxén, I. and Saxén, L.: Association between maternal intake of diazepam and oral clefts. Lancet, *2*:498, 1975.

34. Safra, M.J. and Oakley, G.P.: Association between cleft lip with or without cleft palate and prenatal exposure to diazepam. Lancet, *2*:478, 1975.

35. Rosenberg, L., et al.: Lack of relation of oral clefts to diazepam use during pregnancy. N Engl J Med, *309*:1282, 1983.

36. Shiono, P.H. and Mills, J.L.: Oral clefts and diazepam used during pregnancy. N Engl J Med, *311*:919, 1984.

37. Cree, J.E., Meyer, J. and Hailey, D.M.: Diazepam in labour: its metabolism and effect on the clinical condition and thermogenesis of the newborn. Br Med J, *4*:251, 1973.

38. Gillberg, C.: "Floppy infant syndrome" and maternal diazepam. Lancet, *2*:244, 1977.

39. Lindhout, D., Höppener, R.J.E.A. and Meinardi, H.: Teratogenicity of antiepileptic drug combinations with special emphasis on epoxidation (of carbamazepine). Epilepsia, *25*:77, 1984.

40. Froescher, W., Gugler, R., Niesen, M. and Hoffman, F.: Protein binding of valproic acid in maternal and umbilical cord serum, Epilepsia, *25*:244, 1984.

41. Albani, F., et al.: Differential transplacental binding of valproic acid: influence of free fatty acids. Br J Clin Pharmacol, *17*:759, 1984.

42. DiLiberti, J.J., Farndon, P.A., Dennis, N.R. and Curry, C.J.R.: The fetal valproate syndrome. Am J Med Genet, *19*:473, 1984.

43. Robert, E., Löfkvist, E. and Mauguiere, F.: Valproate and spina bifida. Lancet, *2*:1392, 1984.

44. Lindhout, D. and Meinardi, H.: Spina bifida and in-utero exposure to valproate. Lancet, *2*:396, 1984.

45. Gram, L. and Drachmann Bentsen, K.: Valproate: an updated review. Acta Neurol Scand, *72*:129, 1985.

Chapter 7

Pharmacologic Management of Hypertension in Pregnancy

John T. Repke

The management of pregnancy-induced hypertension has undergone many changes over the past 20 years, as the physician's choice of drugs has expanded and as the prognosis for the premature infant has improved. As obstetricians and perinatologists have become increasingly comfortable with the idea of managing the pregnancies of women with underlying hypertensive disease, the issue of which drugs to use during pregnancy has achieved a new importance. While the woman with chronic hypertension is still at high risk for adverse perinatal outcome, the prognosis for her and her child is improving as we understand more about the pathophysiology of hypertension, how it complicates pregnancies, and what impact pharmacotherapy will have on the maternal and uteroplacental circulation.

ETIOLOGY

Multiple causes have been proposed for the development of pregnancy-induced hypertension. For many years, the prevailing viewpoint was that uteroplacental ischemia led to the development of hypertension in pregnancy. Hodgkinson and Hodari,[1] and Berger and Cavanaugh[2] experimentally demonstrated that iatrogenically produced uteroplacental ischemia would result in the development of hypertension in laboratory animals. In some instances, this was reversible when the ischemia was corrected. A suggestion that this uteroplacental ischemia would accelerate the degradation of monoamine oxidase, thus potentiating the effect of circulating catecholamines seemed reasonable. Indeed, we know that maternal catecholamine levels may, in fact, play a role in the regulation of normal blood pressure in the pregnant state.[3,4] The association of nutritional characteristics in the development of preeclampsia has been studied extensively.[5] It is a particularly serious complication when the chronically hypertensive patient develops superimposed pregnancy-induced hypertension. The physician must carefully select pharmacologic agents that will maximally benefit mother and fetus as well as make certain that a diagnosis of superimposed preeclampsia is not overlooked so that definitive therapy (delivery) is not inappropriately delayed.

EPIDEMIOLOGY

Pregnancy-induced hypertension occurs with increased frequency among black women, even after correction for age and parity. Patients at risk for pregnancy-induced hypertension tend to come from lower socioecomic groups, tend to be young, primigravid, and usually of relatively poor nutritional status. Although various hypotheses have, at varying times, seemed to be attractive, there is no definitive way, at present, to predict those patients who will become preeclamptic on the basis of epidemiologic variables.

PATHOPHYSIOLOGY

The pathophysiology of essential hypertension and pregnancy-induced hypertension is not completely understood. Extensive investigations, however, have led to the general acceptance of the hypothesis that pregnancy-induced hypertension is most likely the result of altered vascular reactivity. Gant and co-workers,[6–8] using a series of hypothetical models, have demonstrated that it is the change in vascular reactivity that accounts for the alteration in blood pressure in those patients with pregnancy-induced hypertension. This has been demonstrated by studying the sensitivity to angiotensin II as a possible predictor of which patients will go on to develop preeclampsia. These elegant investigations also held for those patients with chronic hypertension, with those individuals going on to develop superimposed preeclampsia being identified by their increasing sensitivity to angiotensin II as their pregnancy progressed. An intricate relationship exists between circulating angiotensin II concentration and the concentration of prostacyclin and prostaglandin E-II. The opposite effects of these substances contribute to the maintenance of normal blood pressure in a hyper-reninemic state with the maintenance of adequate uteroplacental perfusion. Locally produced prostaglandins and cyclic nucleotides contribute to the maintenance of this exquisite homeostasis. The final common path in the regulation of blood pressure seems to involve a calcium-mediated mechanism. Alteration of the concentration of intracellular free calcium has been demonstrated to have an effect on systemic arterial pressure.[9] In fact, whatever the mechanism of pregnancy-induced hypertension, it is probably finally mediated through this mechanism, that is altering intracellular free calcium. Some investigators have suggested that this may be, in part, mediated through the effects of parathyroid hormone.[10] In any case, the exact mechanism involved in the development of pregnancy-induced hypertension is incompletely understood. What is important is to recognize which patients should be offered pharmacotherapy, which patients should be expeditiously delivered, and, when pharmacotherapy is chosen, what agents will provide the best outcome for mother and fetus with a minimum of adverse side effects.

TREATMENT

The first step in the treatment of hypertension during pregnancy is to determine whether, in fact, one is treating underlying chronic hypertensive disease or developing preeclampsia. In the latter case, the only definitive treatment is delivery of the infant. In the case of chronic hypertension there are several avenues of treatment available to the obstetrician. Drug therapy will be categorized into those for treatment of chronic hypertension, preeclampsia, and for hypertensive emergencies.

Nonpharmacologic Therapy of Chronic Hypertension

Whenever possible, treatment of the pregnant hypertensive should be conservative. Nonpharmacologic methods include limiting physical activity, biofeedback and other relaxation techniques, and education in home blood pressure determinations. Bedrest on the left side will increase cardiac output and increase blood flow to the kidneys and uterus, as well as lower blood pressure. A diuresis and increased fetal growth will result. Employment of these methods may reduce length of hospital stay and entire medical care costs, while improving fetal outcome. Additionally, some investigators have observed that increasing calcium in the diet will lower blood pressure among normotensive pregnant patients.[10] In nonpregnant subjects with hypertension calcium supplementation has also been found to have this blood-pressure-lowering-effect.[11] Whether, in fact, calcium supplementation will reduce the incidence of preeclampsia, remains to be determined.

Pharmacotherapy of Chronic Hypertension

A major area of controversy in therapy of chronic hypertension is whether, in fact, the treatment of chronic hypertension in pregnancy will have any beneficial pharmacologic effects with regard to fetal outcome.[12] The major concern in managing the chronic hypertensive patient is that her hypertension not become severe, placing her at risk for placental abruption or a cerebrovascular accident. In general, we do not treat mild to moderate hypertension in pregnancy with drugs, but start with bedrest on the left side. The treatment of severe hypertension in pregnancy usually involves delivery of the infant and pharmacotherapy aimed at avoiding cerebral hemorrhage. Since there is controversy with regard to whether or not to treat chronic hypertension during pregnancy, the clinician will occasionally find himself in the position of having to manage a patient's antihypertensive medication.

ALPHAMETHYLDOPA (ALDOMET)

For years alphamethyldopa has been the drug of first choice of most obstetricians choosing to treat pregnant hypertensive patients. Alphamethyldopa, also known as methyldopa, is a derivative of phenylalanine. It remains one of the most widely used antihypertensive agents in the United States, and for this reason a large body of information has been accumulated with regard to its effects and side effects. Methyldopa is converted within the central nervous system to alphamethylnorepinephrine, which is an alpha$_2$ adrenergic agonist. Experimental data have been accumulated to prove that alphamethyldopa exerts its effect centrally rather than peripherally.[13] Its major effect is to reduce peripheral resistance while minimally affecting cardiac output and heart rate. Some sedation and lethargy may occur and are usually transient, and depression, hemolytic anemia, and serious hepatic injury have been reported, as has been orthostatic hypertension. The absorption of alphamethyldopa, when given orally, is variable. Peak concentrations will occur within 2 to 3 hours and the elimination of the drug is biphasic. Approximately 60% of the drug is cleared via renal excretion. There is free transfer of alphamethyldopa across the placenta, though we have not noted any adverse fetal side effects. In one study, administration of alphamethyldopa to chronic hypertensive women during pregnancy did result in a prolongation of gestation.[14] The usual dose of alphamethyldopa is 250 mg by mouth 3 times a day. This may be increased to a maximum dose of 2 g per day in 4 divided doses. If this amount of drug is insufficient for control of blood pressure, further increase of the dose is of no benefit. It should also be noted that alphamethyldopa's antihypertensive effect may be enhanced by the concomitant administration of diuretics or general anesthesia.

CLONIDINE

Clonidine is a centrally acting alpha$_2$ adrenergic agonist. Its ability to act as agonist or partial antagonist seems to be tied to local concentrations of norepinephrine. After an initial dose of clonidine, there may be a transient rise in blood pressure followed by the exertion of its antihypertensive effect. After oral administration, there may be a reduction in heart rate and stroke volume, although this reduction in heart rate is rarely severe. Clonidine is well absorbed orally and achieves peak concentrations in 1 to 3 hours. The major half life is approximately 10 hours. Dosages will range from between 0.2 to 0.8 mg per day, with most patients requiring no more than 0.3 mg twice per day. Although there are not adequate data on the placental transfer of clonidine, it may be assumed that it is freely trnasported across the placenta to the fetal compartment. Approximately 50% of the drug is inactivated in the liver, with the remaining drug being excreted unchanged by the kidney. Sudden withdrawal of clonidine may produce a hypertensive crisis. Although clonidine has been successfully used in pregnancy, it does not seem to offer any advantage over alphamethyldopa when a centrally acting drug is required for the treatment of mild to moderate hypertension in pregnancy.

BETA-ADRENERGIC BLOCKING AGENTS

Beta-adrenergic blocking agents are the most widely used drugs for cardiovascular disease in the United States. Within the past 5 years they have become increasingly used for the management of hypertension in pregnancy. In the past, obstetricians have been reluctant to employ beta-blocking agents in the management of hypertension in pregnancy because of fears concerning their association with neonatal hypoglycemia, intrauterine growth retardation, neonatal bradycardia, respiratory depression and teratogenesis. There is no evidence of human teratogenicity of the beta-blocking agents, and the other concerns have been adequately addressed by prospective studies that would suggest that beta-blocking agents are safe when used in appropriately selected hypertensive pregnant patients.[15,16] Several specific beta-blocking agents will be discussed, but despite presumptive selectivity of the varying beta-blocking agents, no beta-blocker selectivity is absolute.

Propranolol. Propranolol is a nonselective beta-blocker that blocks the action of sympathomimetic amines in many locations. Propranolol will increase airway resistance and, although this effect is insignificant in normal individuals, it contraindicates the use of this drug in asthmatics. Propranolol reduces cardiac output and may block the release of norepinephrine from adrenergic nerve terminals. The exact antihypertensive mechanism of beta-blocking agents remains to be elucidated. Beta-blocking agents will also reduce plasma renin activity, and this may account in part for its antihypertensive activity. Although safe for most pregnant patients, propranolol should not be given to asthmatics or to patients with inadequate myocardial function. Concerns about theoretical risks regarding the possibility that propranolol administration may enhance uterine irritability seem unwarranted; propranolol seems to increase the activity of the nonpregnant human uterus much more than the pregnant uterus.[17] Propranolol is transported across the placenta and may reduce fetal heart rate reactivity. Propranolol is well absorbed after oral administration. It is almost entirely metabolized before its urinary excretion. In the treatment of mild to moderate hypertension, most patients will respond to between 120 and 240 mg per day in divided doses. Although the half life is relatively short, about 4 hours during chronic administration, when large doses of propranolol are used it can frequently be given in a single daily dose. The patient who is to be begun on beta-blocker therapy should be started slowly beginning with a dose of approximately 80 mg per day and the dose gradually increased until an adequate antihypertensive effect is achieved.

Although one study has suggested that propranolol may have contributed to fetal demise in 9 patients with severe hypertension and renal disease,[18] several studies have failed to find adverse effects of propranolol use in pregnancy.[15,19] Long term follow-up studies are not yet available.

Atenolol. Atenolol is a cardioselective beta$_1$ adrenergic blocker. The plasma half life of atenolol is approximately 8 hours, which is its major advantage over propranolol for use in treating hypertension. The mechanism of action, contraindications and side effects are similar to those for propranolol. Although considered a selective beta-blocking agent, atenolol should still only be used with extreme caution in asthmatic patients. Atenolol may be given in doses of 50 to 100 mg once a day for the control of mild to moderate hypertension in pregnancy. A prospective study examining the effects of atenolol on pregnancy-induced hypertension and neonatal outcome failed to demonstrate any deleterious effects of atenolol therapy.[16] There was an increase in neonatal bradycardia in the atenolol-treated patients, but this did not seem to be clinically significant.

Metaprolol. Metaprolol is another relatively selective beta$_1$ blocking agent. Its mechanism of action is similar to that of propranolol and atenolol and it may be substituted for either of these drugs in the management of hypertension, although there are no studies in pregnant patients. Most patients may begin on 100 mg per day in either single or divided doses, and this may be increased to a maximum of 450 mg per day. Most pregnant patients will not require greater than 100 mg per day. Metaprolol appears to be safe for use in pregnancy.[18]

Labetalol. Recently released in the United States, labetalol has been used abroad in the treatment of chronic hypertension during pregnancy.,[20] Labetalol is a combined alpha- and beta-blocking agent, and for this reason, it is less likely to reduce cardiac output and uteroplacental flow.[21] Because of this, it may turn out that labetalol will be the beta-blocking agent of choice for the treatment of hypertension in pregnancy. However, at this point in time there are insufficient data with regard to its fetal and neonatal effects. Labetalol is given at a starting dose of 100 mg 3 or 4 times a day. Occasionally, 1200 milligrams may be necessary for the control of blood pressure, although most patients will respond to doses in the range of 400 to 800 mg per day.

Of the beta-blocking agents discussed, the cost of therapy is relatively similar whether one uses propranolol, labetalol, metaprolol, or atenolol.[22]

VASODILATING AGENTS

Vasodilating agents, considered by many to be the drugs of choice for the treatment of acute hypertensive emergencies, are also occasionally used in the management of patients with chronic hypertension. The use of vasodilators among chronic hypertensive patients fell out of favor for many years due to the associated side effects of tachycardia and fluid retention. These effects have been minimized by the concurrent use of beta-blocking agents or diuretics. For these reasons, vasodilators probably have little or no place in the management of chronic hypertension during pregnancy. In the event that vasodilator therapy is necessary, hydralazine remains the drug of choice for use in pregnancy, primarily because it is the drug about which we have the most information with regard to absence of adverse effects on the mother or fetus.[23] Prazosin and minoxidil are also effective vasodilating agents, but should be avoided in pregnancy because of the absence of long-term data about the maternal, fetal or neonatal effects.

Hydralazine (Apresoline). Hydralazine causes direct relaxation of the smooth muscle of the arteriolar bed. Compensatory tachycardia and increased plasma renin activity and fluid retention occur. If the blood pressure is appropriately controlled, uteroplacental perfusion may increase in response to vasodilator therapy. Blood flow also increases to the cerebral, coronary, renal and splanchnic vascular beds unless profound hyptension occurs. Hydralazine is quickly and almost completely absorbed after oral administration. The drug is primarily metabolized by acetylation so that slow acetylators may achieve higher plasma levels than rapid acetylators since a signficant amount of the drug is metabolized in the first pass through the liver. Peak concentrations of hydralazine in the plasma after oral administration will occur within 30 minutes to 2 hours, with a mean duration of action of approximately 6 to 8 hours. Although accurate data do not exist with regard to the placental transfer of hydralazine, it may be assumed that this drug crosses the placenta. Adverse neonatal effects have not been reported.[23]

Approximately 10% of patients on hydralazine therapy will develop a lupus erythematosus-like syndrome. This syndrome will rarely occur unless duration of therapy exceeds 2 months with a daily dosage in excess of 200 mg. The mechanism of this syndrome is unknown and it appears to be completely reversible after discontinuation of the drug.

CALCIUM CHANNEL BLOCKERS

Calcium channel blocking agents have been recently approved by the U.S. Food and Drug Administration for the treatment of hypertension. The calcium channel blockers are a group of vasodilating agents for the treatment of hypertension. These agents are potent arteriolar vasodilators. Unlike hydralazine, these agents will also cause dilatation of the coronary vessels, and improved subendocardial perfusion. Nifedipine is the most potent arteriolar vasodilator of the three main calcium channel blocking agents, verapamil, nifedipine and diltiazem. We have successfully used calcium channel blocking agents to manage postpartum hypertension in patients who were refractory to other methods. At present, insufficient data exist with regard to maternal and fetal effects and placental transfer to allow for their routine use in pregnancy.

ANGIOTENSIN-CONVERTING ENZYME INHIBITORS

Vascular reactivity and angiotensin II sensitivity play key roles in the development of pregnancy-induced hypertension.[6] Thus, a drug that could inhibit the conversion of angiotensin I to angiotensin II would be an almost ideal pharmacotherapeutic agent for the treatment of pregnancy-induced hypertension. The prototype angiotensin-converting enzyme inhibitor is captopril. It is a highly specific drug. It does not seem to exert any other pharmacologic effects on the renin/angiotensin system other than the inhibition of the enzymatic conversion of angiotensin I to angiotensin II. Captopril lowers arteriolar resistance which results in a reduction of systolic and diastolic blood pressure. Paradoxically, administration of captopril results in increased renal blood flow. Captopril is rapidly absorbed after oral administration with approximately 95% of the drug being eliminated in the urine, with approximately half of it as the unchanged molecule. Captopril, being a relatively small molecule, may be assumed to cross the placenta, although adequate placental transfer studies have not been carried out. Additionally, there is no long-term information available with regard to adverse maternal, fetal or neonatal side effects. Animal studies have demonstrated that captopril may be selectively toxic to the developing fetus, possibly secondary to reduction in uteroplacental flow.[24] The mechanism of this reduction is not entirely clear, although it is thought that it involves a decrease in the synthesis of vasodilating prostaglandins.

DIURETICS

The use of diuretics in pregnancy remains controversial. Some authors suggest that diuretics may have a role in the treatment of chronic hypertension complicating pregnancy, especially for those patients who have been maintained on diuretic therapy prior to conception and whose intravascular space has already equilibrated. On the other hand, these patients may be prevented from undergoing the normal plasma volume expansion that is so necessary for proper fetal growth and development.[25] Because of these considerations, and because diuretics are generally used to treat mild hypertension, we do not usually employ diuretics in the management of patients with underlying hypertensive disease complicating pregnancy.

PREECLAMPSIA

To date, pharmacotherapy of preeclampsia has been symptomatic; the only known cure for preeclampsia is termination of the pregnancy with delivery of the infant and placenta. Magnesium sulfate remains the cornerstone of therapy in the prevention of eclampsia. Magnesium sulfate is extremely effective in preventing the development of eclampsia in patients with preeclampsia. A controversy continues as to whether magnesium sulfate has a central action or an action confined to the periphery.[26] At the periphery, magnesium sulfate acts at the myoneural junction, reducing neuromuscular transmission. A central action for magnesium sulfate has been demonstrated by some investigators and refuted by others.[27,28] The usual regimen is to utilize 4 to 6 g of magnesium sulfate by intravenous administration over 15 to 30 minutes, with a maintenance dose of magnesium sulfate of between 2 and 3 g per hour. While magnesium levels may be followed, they are no substitute for the frequent clinical assessment of the patient for signs of magnesium toxicity as evidenced by obliteration of the patellar reflex (8 to 10 mEq/L), respiratory depression (15 mEq/L), or the development of cardiac arrhythmias (20 mEq/L or greater). As magnesium sulfate freely crosses the placenta and achieves an equilibrium in the fetal compartment, clinically significant neonatal hypermagnesemia may occur if high levels of the drug are achieved. Two cases of neonatal meconium plug syndrome due to decreased bowel peristalsis have been reported at cord mg levels of 6.0 + 9.0 mEq/L.[29]

Since magnesium sulfate is excreted primarily by the renal route alterations in administration must be made for those patients with decreased renal function. Magnesium sulfate has also been reported to have tocolytic properties[30] and, in this clinical setting, may interfere with the ability to effect vaginal delivery in certain patients. A reduction in fetal heart rate variability as recorded by the electronic fetal monitor has also been reported in patients receiving magnesium sulfate therapy.[31]

Because magnesium sulfate has curare-like activity, it should be used with caution in patients receiving general anesthesia or in patients who are on aminoglycoside antimicrobial therapy. Magnesium sulfate is not an effective agent for controlling blood pressure. When preeclamptic patients require control of blood pressure as well as prophylaxis against the development of eclampsia, other antihypertensive medications should be utilized in conjunction with magnesium sulfate, as discussed in the following section.

TREATMENT OF HYPERTENSIVE EMERGENCIES

Occasionally, it is necessary to respond quickly to the development of severe hypertension in order to prevent the adverse maternal event of cerebrovascular accident. Hydralazine remains the agent of choice to treat the pregnant or postpartum patient with acute severe hypertension. Therapy is recommended for patients with persistent blood pressures in excess of 160 systolic or 110 mm Hg diastolic. A hypertensive emergency exists if the systolic blood pressure exceeds 200 mm Hg and the diastolic blood pressure exceeds 120 mm Hg.

Hydralazine

Hydralazine may be administered continuously or intermittently in severe hypertension. One method involves a 5 mg intravenous bolus followed by a 10 mg intravenous bolus in 20 minutes if there has not been an appropriate lowering of blood pressure. This 10 mg bolus may be repeated every 20 minutes until blood pressure is maintained between 140/90 and 150/100. Once this level has been achieved, a continuous intravenous infusion is begun with hydralazine 2 mg/hr and the infusion increased by 1 mg/hr every 5 minutes until a steady state blood pressure is achieved. A central venous pressure catheter may serve as a guide to fluid management during these emergencies, as hydralazine will result in fluid retention. We avoid the intramuscular use of hydralazine in these patients, since absorption is rather erratic when administered by that route. The use of hydralazine in this clinical setting will also lower blood pressure without sacrificing uteroplacental flow. No adverse effects on mother, fetus or neonate have been noted.

Beta Adrenergic Blocking Agents

Beta adrenergic blocking drugs have also been suggested for use in the treatment of acute hypertensive emergencies. In this group of drugs, labetalol may be the most efficacious since it combines both alpha- and beta-blocking properties.[32] Blood pressure may be effectively reduced without sacrificing uteroplacental flow and with a minimum of side effects. While labetalol may be an acceptable drug for the treatment of severe hypertension in pregnancy, the absence of data about adverse maternal or fetal side effects should limit its use currently.

Diazoxide

Diazoxide is a potent and efficacious antihypertensive drug. It is related to the thiazide class of diuretics and directly relaxes arteriolar smooth muscle without having any diuretic action. Significant sodium and water retention occur when diazoxide is used to treat hypertensive crises, necessitating concomitant use of diuretics. Previously, it had been recommended that diazoxide be administered by an intravenous injection of 300 mg. This dose commonly produced profound hypotension. Administering the dose by either sustained intravenous administration or giving smaller doses by intravenous bolus (50 mg at a time) has minimized this adverse effect of the drug. Diazoxide is also a tocolytic agent and is not the agent of choice in an obstetrical setting where vaginal delivery is desired. Because of these risks, diazoxide is probably best avoided for the treatment of acute hypertension during pregnancy.

Nitroprusside

Sodium nitroprusside is also an effective antihypertensive drug. Its mechanism is similar to that of organic nitrates, which cause dephosphorylation of the light chain of myosin, thus relaxing the vascular smooth muscle. Nitroprusside may be administered parenterally by continuous intravenous infusion of 0.5 to 10 μg/kg per minute. The advantages of using nitroprusside are that its onset of action is extremely rapid (1 to 2 minutes) and its duration of action is extremely short so that if discontinuation of the drug becomes necessary, its antihypertensive effect disappears quickly. The major toxicity is overdosage with profound hypotension, although other toxicities are also of concern to the obstetrician. The drug is metabolized to cyanide which is then further reduced to thiocyanate. Thiocyanate has been found to cross the placenta and may be toxic to the developing fetus.[33] Excessive concentrations of thiocyanate may also produce maternal toxic psychosis and interfere with thyroid function. For these reasons, sodium nitroprusside is best used in the obstetric patient with acute hypertension when other regimens have failed.

SUMMARY

In summary, the initial therapy for hypertension complicating pregnancy is nonpharmacologic, conservative therapy. When this type of therapy is unsuccessful, there are a number of agents available to the obstetrician. While most of these agents are safe, some of them have not been studied for long-term use in pregnancy. The treatment of mild to moderate hypertension in pregnancy remains controversial with regard to whether in fact there is an improved neonatal outcome with drug therapy. There is no question that the mother with blood pressures in excess of 160 mm Hg over 110 mm Hg needs to be treated in order to prevent the catastrophic sequelae that could occur in this situation, specifically, placental abruption and/or cerebral vascular accident.

While severe hypertension may complicate preeclampsia and result in the need for pharmacotherapy, the only definitive treament for preeclampsia is the delivery of the fetus and the placenta. Prevention of eclampsia remains the most important part of the therapy of the preeclamptic patient until her disease process starts to reverse itself. In the United States in 1986 magnesium sulfate remains the drug of choice for that purpose.

REFERENCES

1. Hodgkinson, C.P., Hodari, A.A. and Bumpus, F.M.: Experimental hypertensive disease of pregnancy. Obstet Gynecol, *30*:371, 1969.
2. Berger, M. and Cavanaugh, D.: Toxemia of pregnancy: The hypertensive effect of acute experimental placental ischemia. Am J Obstet Gynecol, *87*:293, 1963.
3. Zuspan, F.P., O'Shaughnessy, R.W., Vinsel, J., et al.: Adrenergic enervation of uterine vasculature in human term pregnancy. Am J Obstet Gynecol, *139*:678, 1981.
4. Thompson, R.H.S. and Tickner, A.: Observations on the monoamine oxidase activity of placenta and uterus. Biochem J, *45*:125, 1949.
5. Chaudhuri, S.K.: Relationship of protein caloric malnutrition with toxemia of pregnancy. Am J Obstet Gynecol, *107*:33, 1970.
6. Gant, N.F., Daley, G.L., Chand, S., et al.: A study of angiotensin II pressor response throughout primigravid pregnancy. J Clin Invest, *52*:2682, 1973.
7. Gant, N.F., Jimenez, J.M., Whalley, P.J., et al.: A prospective study of angiotensin II pressor responsiveness in pregnancies complicated by chronic essential hypertension. Am J Obstet Gynecol, *127*:369, 1977.
8. Gant, N.F. and Worley, R.J.: Hypertension in Pregnancy, Concepts and Management. Norwalk, Conn, Appleton-Century-Crofts, 1982.
9. Erne, P., Bolli, P., Burgisser, E. and Buhler, F.: Correlation of platelet calcium with blood pressure: Effect of hypertensive therapy. N Engl J Med, *310*:1084, 1984.
10. Villar, J., Belizan, J., Repke, J., et al.: The effect of calcium intake on the blood pressure of young, healthy individuals. Ann NY Acad Sci, *435*:509, 1984.
11. McCarron, D.A. and Morris, C.D.: Blood pressure response to oral calcium in persons with mild to moderate hypertension: A randomized double-blind placebo-controlled crossover trial. Ann Intern Med, *103*:825, 1985.
12. Sibai, B.M., Abdella, T.N. and Anderson, G.D.: Pregnancy outcome in 211 patients with mild chronic hypertension. Obstet Gynecol, *61*:571, 1983.
13. Langer, S.Z., Cavera, I. and Massingham, R.: Recent developments in noradrenergic neurotransmission and its relevance to the mechanism of action of certain antihypertensive agents. Hypertension, *2*:372, 1980.
14. Leather, H.M., Humphreys, D.M., Baker, P., et al.: A controlled trial of hypotensive agents in hypertension in pregnancy. Lancet, *2*:488, 1968.
15. Eliahou, H.E., Silverberg, B.S., Reisin, E., et al.: Propranol for the treatment of hypertension in pregnancy. Br J Obstet Gynecol, *85*:431, 1978
16. Rubin, P.Z., Butters, L., Clark, D.M., et al.: Placebo-controlled trial of atenolol in treatment of pregnancy-associated hypertension. Lancet, *1*:431, 1983.
17. Wansbrough, H., Nakanishi, H. and Wood, C.: The effect of adrenergic receptor-blocking drugs on the human uterus. J Obstet Gynecol Br Commonw, *75*:189, 1968.
18. Lieberman, B.A., Stirrat, G.M., Cohen, S.L., et al.: The possible adverse effect of propranolol on the fetus in pregnancies complicated by severe hypertension. Br J Obset Gynaecol, *85*:678, 1978.
19. Sandstrom, B.O.: Antihypertensive treatment with the adrenergic beta-receptor blocker metaprolol during pregnancy. Gynecol Obstet Invest, *9*:195, 1978.
20. Lardoux, H., Gerard, J., Blazquez, G., et al.: Hypertension in pregnancy: Evaluation of two beta-blockers, atenolol and labetalol. Eur Heart J, *4* (Suppl.G):35, 1983.
21. Lunell, N.O., Nylund, L., Lewander, R., et al: Acute effect of an antihypertensive drug, labetalol, on uteroplacental blood flow. Br J Obstet Gynecol, *89*:640, 1982.
22. Labetalol for hypertension. Med Lett, *26*:83, 1984.
23. Pritchard, J.A., MacDonald, P.D. and Gant, N.F.: William's Obstetrics, 17th ed., Norwalk, Conn, 1985, Appleton-Century-Crofts, p. 548–552.
24. Ferris, T.F. and Weir, E.K.: Effects of captopril on uterine blood flow and prostaglandin E synthesis in the pregnant rabbit. J Clin Invest, *71*:809, 1984.
25. Arias, F.: Expansion of intravascular volume and fetal outcome in patients with chronic hypertension in pregnancy. Am J Obstet Gynecol, *123*:610, 1975.
26. Donaldson, J.O.: Neurology in Pregnancy. Philadelphia, W.B. Saunders Co., 1978.
27. Borges, L.F. and Gucer, G.: Effect of magnesium on epileptic foci. Epilepsia, *19*:81, 1978.
28. Sibai, B.N., Spinnato, J.A., Watson, D.L., et al.: Effect of magnesium sulfate on electroencephalographic findings in preeclampsia-eclampsia. Obstet Gynecol *64*(2):261, 1984.
29. Sokol, M.M., Koenigsberger, M.R., Rose, J.S., et al.: Neonatal hypermagnesemia and the meconium-plug syndrome. N Engl J Med, *286*:823, 1972.
30. Petrie, R.H.: Tocolysis using magnesium sulfate. Seminars in Perinatol, *5*(3):266, 1981.

31. Stallworth, J.C., Eayeh, S.Y. and Petrie, R.H.: The effect of magnesium sulfate on fetal heart rate variability and uterine activity. Am J Obstet Gynecol, *140*:702, 1981.
32. Davey, D.A., Dommisse, J. and Garden, A.: The investigation of labetalol in the management of hypertension in pregnancy. Amsterdam, Excerpta Medica, 1982, p. 51.
33. Lewis, P.E., Cefalo, R.C., Naulty, J.S. and Rodkey, F.L.: Placental transfer and fetal toxicity of sodium nitroprusside. Gynecol Invest, *8*:46, 1977.

Chapter 8

The Use of Anti-Asthmatic Drugs in Pregnancy

Roberto Romero and Charles Lockwood

Asthma is a disease of hyperreactive airways resulting in intermittent and reversible airway obstruction.[1] Acute asthma, (necessitating treatment), complicates 1% of pregnancies.[2] Fortunately, an array of effective pharmacologic agents are now available for the treatment of asthma. Therefore, it is incumbent upon the obstetrician to understand the pharmacology and perinatal complications of these agents. This chapter will discuss our current understanding of the pathogenesis of asthma and its pharmacologic management in pregnancy.

PATHOGENESIS

The bronchospasm of asthma is accompanied by characteristic pulmonary pathologic changes. These include mucosal edema, desquamation of respiratory epithelium, hypersecretion of mucus and leukocytic infiltrates.[3] The majority of asthmatics (60%) appear to have a specific allergic trigger to their disorder, or extrinsic asthma.[4] Patients in whom no specific antigenic trigger can be identified often develop symptoms in response to non-specific stimuli such as cold air or exercise.[4]

Regardless of etiology, mast cell activation appears to be a critical component in the genesis of an asthma attack. Mast cells, found throughout the respiratory tract, contain specific membrane receptors for the Fc fragment of the immunoglobulin IgE.[4] The latter mediates the host's immediate hypersensitivity reaction. Antigenic binding to the FAb fragment of the IgE molecule results in a mast cell membrane pertubation.

An immediate consequence of this membrane pertubation is mast cell granule dislodgement, resulting in an immediate release of histamine. Histamine enhances bronchoconstriction directly and via reflex parasympathetic action,[5] and induces vasodilation potentiating plasma transudation and mucosal edema.[3] Degranulation also results in the release of leukocyte chemotactic factors (CF). One such factor, Eosinophil-CF, may result in eosinophil-mediated respiratory cell desquamation and account for the frequent finding of eosinophils in the sputum of asthmatics.[6]

A delayed consequence of IgE-antigen induced mast cell membrane stimulation is the production of leukotrienes.[7] Originally described as the slow-reacting substance of anaphylaxis (SRS-A), leukotrienes are biologically potent products of arachidonic acid metabolism.

It is theorized that the IgE-antigen interaction results in an influx of extracellular calcium[8] with the activation of intramembranous phospholipases. Phospholipases liberate arachidonic acid from membrane phospholipids. Mast cell lipoxygenase enzymes then convert the arachidonic acid to leukotrienes.

Leukotrienes appear to be critical factors in the pathogenesis of asthma.[9] The biologic activities of the different leukotrienes appear to account for the major pathophysiologic findings in asthma. Leukotriene C-4 and D-4 (LTC-4, LTD-4,) are extremely potent bronchoconstrictors which have rapid onset and prolonged effect.[10-12] Both substances have approximately 4000 times the potency of histamine in inducing bronchoconstriction.[13] In addition, leukotriene C-4, D-4 and E-4 promote plasma exudations from postcapillary venules, generating mucosal edema.[12] LTD-4 is also an extremely potent secretagogue, stimulating mucous glycoprotein synthesis and secretion.[13]

Leukotriene B-4 (LTB-4) is a potent stimulator of neutrophil and eosinophil chemotaxis,[14,15] contributing to the neutrophil and eosinophil infiltrates identified in the bronchial tree of asthmatics. Eosinophils may also preferentially generate leukotrienes.[16] This could suggest a contributory role in the pathogenesis of asthma.

While the activation of mast cells with resultant degranulation and leukotriene production appears to account for the bronchospasm and pathologic findings in asthma, the most prominent pathophysiologic mechanism is abnormal membrane calcium homeostasis.[17] Bronchial smooth muscle contraction is a calcium-dependent process with calcium ion flux initiating the muscle contraction.[18] Transmembrane calcium flux is also required for mast cell activation, respiratory epithelial cilial function, mucus secretion[19] and cholinergic nerve functions. Since all of the pathophysiologic processes present in asthma are calcium dependent, asthma can be characterized as a disorder of inappropriate transmembranous calcium ion activity. Indeed, virtually all current pharmacologic agents utilized in the treatment of asthma appear to impede calcium ion flux.

THEOPHYLLINE

Theophylline is a naturally occurring alkaloid of the xanthine family. It is the drug of choice for pregnant asthmatic patients who require intravenous or continuous oral bronchodilator therapy. Traditionally, its mechanism of action was ascribed to an inhibition of phosphodiesterase, the enzyme responsible for the degradation of cyclic AMP. Recent evidence suggests that minimal phosphodiesterase inhibition occurs at therapeutic tissue levels.[20] Furthermore, more potent phosphodiesterase inhibitors do not induce bronchodilation.[21] Although the precise mechanism is still unclear, inhibition of calcium ion flux may underlie the bronchodilation observed with theophylline therapy.[22,23]

In addition to relaxing bronchial smooth muscle, theophylline has a multitude of other actions. The drug has positive inotropic and chronotropic effects; causes systemic and pulmonary vasodilatation which produces mild increases in systolic pressure and decreases in diastolic pressure; and is a CNS stimulant exerting an effect at cortical, medullary and spinal levels. Theophylline sensitizes the respiratory center to CO_2, increasing both rate and depth of respiration. Diaphragmatic contractility is also improved with therapy.[24] It has been used to treat apnea in preterm infants[25] and to improve pulmonary function in chronic obstructive pulmonary disease (COPD).[26] Theophylline's efficacy in the treatment of asthma is also a consequence of enhancement in mucociliary clearance, inhibition of mucosal edema[27] and stabilization of mast cell membranes.[28]

Intravenous aminophylline decreases the intensity but not the frequency of uterine contractions;[29] its use as a tocolytic agent is limited by the cardiovascular side effects observed at doses required to elicit effective tocolysis. Experimental and indirect clinical evidence suggests that theophylline increases the synthesis of surfactant in animals and perhaps in humans.[30–32]

Theophylline crosses the placenta in humans,[33,34] with maternal and cord levels appearing identical, but heel-stick levels are slightly higher.[35] Toxicity in neonates may be present at lower peripheral blood levels than in adults; however, neonates appear to tolerate theophylline levels corresponding to maternal levels without serious adversity.[35] Toxicity is more common in preterm infants[36] in whom the drug's half-life is significantly prolonged.[37] Toxic manifestations in the neonate include vomiting, feeding difficulties, tachycardia, jitteriness, cardiac arrhythmias and transient hypoglycemia.

Theophylline is found in breast milk.[38] Peak breast milk concentrations of theophylline develop 1 to 3 hours after an oral dose at which time the infant may receive 10% of the maternal dose. In order to minimize neonatal drug exposure a nursing mother should breast feed immediately prior to taking her scheduled theophylline dose.

Theophylline appears to be mutagenic only in lower organisms which are unable to demethylate the compound.[39] Cardiac abnormalities have been reported when the drug is administered to embryonic chicks,[40] and digital malformations have been reported with parenteral administration in rats.[41] Theophylline has also been reported to induce chromosome breaks in human lymphocytes in culture.[42] The clinical significance of this finding is unclear as only one case of a chromosomal abnormality has thus far been reported in humans.[43] Of 117 women in the Collaborative Perinatal Project who took theophylline in the first trimester, no increased teratogenic risk was noted.[44]

Theophylline toxicity and side effects in the mother correlate with plasma concentrations. In general, it is rare to see symptoms of toxicity with plasma levels of less than 10 μg/ml. Anorexia, nausea, vomiting, and abdominal distention may occur, but usually improve after a slight decrease in the dose. Sinus tachycardia, atrial tachycardia, ventricular tachycardia and premature ventricular contractions can be induced by theophylline. Excitation, anxiety, insomnia, diaphoresis, tremor, lightheadedness and convulsions may occur. A generalized exfoliative dermatitis has been reported with the use of aminophylline.[45]

The mean half-life of theophylline in adults is 5.8 hours (range 2.7 to 12.8). A study of the pharmacokinetics of intravenous theophylline in pregnancy reported that the volume of distribution of theophylline in pregnant women is increased and body clearance is increased but that the half-life of the drug remains unchanged.[46] This suggests that absolute theophylline requirements may increase during pregnancy. Other authors have found that clearance rates of oral theophylline are reduced in the third trimester necessitating a decrease in the oral regimen at this time.[47]

Theophylline is partially protein bound (53 to 65%) in the plasma of healthy adults; however, it does not displace bilirubin from albumin. The drug is metabolized in the liver by the P-450 microsomal enzyme system. Clearance is reduced in patients with cardiac failure, or by concurrent erythromycin or cimetidine therapy. Elimination is enhanced in cigarette smokers. The metabolites are excreted in the urine along with the 10% of the drug in the non-metabolized form.

Theophylline can be administered orally or intravenously. Rectal suppositories are available; however, absorption is erratic, and they may produce proctitis. Because theophylline has a high pH in solution, the intramuscular route is extremely painful. Aerosol administration is ineffective. Oral administration is used for the treatment of chronic bronchospasm and is available in numerous preparations containing either theophylline itself or one of its salts. The salts (aminophylline, oxtriphylline, dyphylline, etc.) are reported to have better absorption and produce less gastric irritation than pure theophylline.

Bioavailability is improved in fasting states. Liquid preparations are absorbed rapidly and peak plasma concentrations are reached in 30 minutes to 2 hours. Forms containing microfine crystals (Slo-Phylline, Theolaire) increase solubility and absorption, thus enabling peak levels to occur in 1 hour. While regular uncoated tablets (Aminophylline, Theophyl) produce maximal levels in 2 to 3 hours, partially enteric coated tablets (Choledyl) delay the peak until 3 hours after administration. Finally, slow releasing preparations (Theo-Dur, Aminodur-Dura-Tabs) provide a constant absorption rate which avoids wide variations in theophylline blood levels and permits a decrease in the frequency of drug administration.

The oral dose of theophylline must be individualized. A recommended schedule for uncoated tablets is to start with a dose of 2.4 mg/kg/6 hours and then to increase it over 3 to 6 days to 3.0 to 3.25 mg/kg/6 hours. Serum levels should be periodically checked to allow appropriate adjustments. Peak levels are assessed 1 hour after therapy with liquids or fast-acting tablets (Slo-Phylline, Theolaire) and 4 hours after administration of a timed-release compound (Theodur). Trough levels may be obtained just prior to oral dosing. Because some evidence suggests that clearance of oral theophylline may be reduced in the third trimester, it is advisable to check peak levels frequently at this time.[47]

The intravenous route of administration is used in cases of acute asthma crisis when plasma levels must be rapidly and precisely regulated. The only preparation available for intravenous administration is aminophylline (theophylline ethylenediamine) which is equivalent to 80% anhydrous theophylline. Current intravenous dosage recommendations for healthy nonsmoking adults, not receiving oral therapy, are:[49]

(a) Loading dose: 6 mg/kg over 20 to 30 minutes
(b) Maintenance dose: 0.7 mg/kg/hr for the first 12 hours, then 0.5 mg/kg/hr in nonsmokers

If the asthma attack is refractory and the patient is without evidence of toxicity:

(a) Reload: 3 mg/kg over 20 to 30 minutes
(b) Titrate maintenance dose to serum levels.

If the patient is currently receiving an oral theophylline-containing product and develops an exacerbation in symptoms, 50% of the intravenous loading dose is given followed by the same maintenance regimen.

Steady state concentrations are reached at varying times, dependent on individual metabolism. Serum levels should be assayed after 12 hours of therapy and at regular intervals thereafter. Serum aminophylline levels should be maintained at or below 13 μg/ml as long as adequate control is achieved (46). There is a log-linear improvement in pulmonary function with increases in serum concentration from 10 to 20 μg/ml.[22] The greater the degree of initial bronchospasm, the higher the serum concentration required to elicit bronchodilation.[48] Concentrations above 20 μg/ml are associated with toxicity. Caution should be exercised in using serum levels to guide dosage adjustments, since concentrations above 20 μg/ml may be required for efficacy without evidence of toxicity, while others require less theophylline and develop side effects at lower serum levels.

ADRENERGIC AGONISTS

Ahlquist[50] classified adrenergic activity as being either alpha or beta. Alpha receptor stimulation produces smooth muscle contraction of blood vessels, the uterus and the bronchial tree. Beta adrenergic stimulation produces smooth muscle relaxation of these organs as well as gluconeogenesis and myocardial stimulation. The beta receptors were subclassified by Lands.[51] Stimulation of beta-1 receptors causes cardiac excitation while beta-2 receptor stimulation causes vasodilation, bronchodilatation and uterine relaxation.

Beta-2 adrenergic agonists bind to cell membrane receptors on respiratory tract secretory cells, bronchial smooth muscle and mast cells. Consequently, the enzyme adenylate cyclase is activated and cyclic AMP is generated. The latter enhances the re-uptake and storage of intracellular calcium.[52] The respiratory tract effects of calcium ion inhibition include bronchodilatation, enhancement of mucociliary clearance, inhibition of mucus secretion and stabilization of mast cells.[53]

The ideal adrenergic bronchodilator would be a selective beta-2 agonist which relaxes airway smooth muscle without causing cardiac side-effects. Since preferential beta-2 adrenergic agonists have only been available for the last few years, other less selective adrenergic agents have been, and continue to be, used for the therapy of bronchial asthma. These agents include epinephrine, isoproterenol and ephedrine.

Epinephrine

Epinephrine (Adrenalin, Sus-Phrine) is a naturally occurring catecholamine with both alpha- and beta-adrenergic actions. Its bronchodilator properties are due to the dominance of its beta agonist effect. However, the mild alpha-receptor stimulation is enough to cause vasoconstriction and to reduce mucosal edema of the tracheobronchial tree, thereby contributing to the therapeutic actions of epinephrine in bronchial asthma.

Epinephrine can be given subcutaneously or as an aerosol. Oral administration is ineffective because the drug is rapidly metabolized by monoamine oxidase present in the gastrointestinal tract. The drug is also available for intramuscular use in an oil base, but this route is not recommended because of erratic absorption.[54] Intravenous administration is contraindicated because it can lead to fatal cardiac arrhythmias and intracranial hemorrhage from hypertensive crisis.

For the treatment of acute asthmatic attacks, epinephrine is used in doses of 0.2 to 0.5 ml of 1:1000 solution which can be repeated every 20 to 30 minutes for a total of 3 doses. Tolerance ot the drug may develop and the presence of acidosis may lead to refractoriness. Aerosol preparations are widely used and some are available as over-the-counter medications (Primatene).

Epinephrine decreases uterine activity when administered to patients in spontaneous or induced labor; however, the cardiovascular side effects and the development of more selective agents has eliminated its use in tocolysis.[55]

Since norepinephrine and other catecholamines cross the human placenta in vitro, this is probably also true of epinephrine.[56] Enzymes responsible for the degradation of epinephrine have been identified in the human placenta, but their ability to limit access of catecholamines to the fetal compartment is not known. There is evidence of the inhibition of uteroplacental flow following the intravenous administration of epinephrine in monkeys[57] and sheep.[58] Human placental vessels appear to respond with vasoconstriction to their in vitro perfusion with epinephrine.[59] Inadvertent intravenous administration must be carefully avoided.

Abnormal fetal development has been observed in animals after maternal administration of catecholamines,[60] but the slightly increased incidence of congenital malformations found in the Collaborative Perinatal Project in the offspring of mothers who received epinephrine during pregnancy was not statistically significant.[44]

Isoproterenol

Isoproterenol (Isuprel) is the most potent of the beta adrenergic agonists. It has both beta-1 and beta-2 activity but almost no alpha effects. The major side effects are cardiac. In vitro preparations of human uterine arteries have shown that isoproterenol produces vasodilatation and crosses the human placenta in vitro.[56]

Isoproterenol induces cardiac and aortic arch anomalies in chick embryos. This effect may be mediated through beta-adrenergic stimulation, since it can be inhibited by the administration of propranolol.[61] The clinical significance of these observations for the pregnant asthmatic is not known. Thirty-one mothers in the Collaborative Perinatal Project who took isoproterenol in the first trimester of pregnancy demonstrated no teratogenic effects.[44]

Isoproterenol is used frequently as an aerosol; occasionally it is administered intravenously to treat respiratory failure in childhood status asthmaticus.[62] It is not administered orally because it is inactivated in the intestinal mucosa and the liver. Sublingual absorption is erratic.

Isoproterenol is commercially available in a variety of aerosolized solutions and metered dose inhalers. Dosage depends upon the concentration of the solution and the quantity delivered by each puff. The weaker solution (1:200) should be used first in a dose of 5 to 15 inhalations up to 5 times/day; in the absence of clinical response or side effects, the higher concentration (1:100) can be used in a dose of 3 to 7 inhalations up to 5 times/day.[51] The dose of metered inhalers is between 125 and 250 mg/dose up to 5 times/day. When given as an aerosol the bronchodilator effect starts in 2 to 5 minutes, reaches its peak in 15 to 30 minutes and lasts 1 to 3 hours.

Ephedrine

Ephedrine causes the release of catecholamines from sympathetic nerve endings and consequently has alpha, beta-1 and beta-2 effects. The newer beta-2 specific agonists have greater potencies with fewer side effects and therefore should be used in place of ephedrine.[63]

Beta-2 Adrenergic Agents

Selective beta-2 adrenergic agents currently available in the United States include metaproterenol, terbutaline and isoetharine. Other preparations used abroad include salbutamol, carbuterol and fenoterol.

TERBUTALINE

Terbutaline (Brethine, Bricanyl) is a preferential beta-2 agonist exerting its effect on the adrenergic receptors of the tracheobronchial tree, blood vessels and skeletal muscle. Stimulation of receptors on skeletal muscle is responsible for the muscle tremor seen in approximately 25% of patients taking a dose of 5 mg every 6 hours. Since it also has mild beta-1 adrenergic activity, other side effects include tachycardia, palpitations and hyperglycemia.

There is extensive experience with terbutaline in pregnancy because of its efficacy as a tocolytic.[64-66] Uterine blood flow in pregnant ewes is not decreased at doses required to inhibit preterm labor.[67] There has, however, been one report of paradoxical uterine hypertonus following the intravenous administration of terbutaline.[68]

Antenatal administration may be associated with a decreased incidence of Respiratory Distress Syndrome in preterm neonates.[69] Prolonged infusion of terbutaline caused a release of fetal pulmonary surfactant in pregnant rabbits; however, subsequent depletion of stored intracellular surfactant may occur.[70,71] Teratogenesis has not been reported with the administration of the drug during pregnancy, and it is not known if it is secreted in breast milk.[72]

Terbutaline is available for oral and subcutaneous use in this country. When given orally, 33 to 50% of the drug is absorbed; the onset of action occurs 45 minutes to 1 hour after administration; peak changes in FEV-1 are achieved in 2 to 3 hours; and the duration of action is usually 4 to 6 hours. The dose is 2.5 to 5 mg every 6 to 8 hours. If the dose is increased to 7.5 mg, the incidence of side effects increases.

Subcutaneous terbutaline 0.25 mg has been calculated to be equivalent to 2.5 to 5 mg of the oral drug. When administered subcutaneously, the onset of action is 10 minutes. Maximum effect is seen in 45 minutes and the duration of action is 3.5 to 4 hours. If no clinical improvement is apparent 30 minutes after the first dose of subcutaneous terbutaline, a second dose of 0.25 mg may be administered. No more than two doses should be given by this route.

The drug is metabolized in the liver to an inactive sulfate conjugate. Most of the absorbed drug is excreted in the urine. Excretion of the drug and its metabolites is essentially complete 72 to 90 hours after a single parenteral or oral dose.[73]

The use of subcutaneous terbutaline is preferable to that of epinephrine in the pregnant patient. Terbutaline has a faster onset and longer duration of action. The incidence of side effects is similar with both drugs, and they seem to be equally potent bronchodilators.[74]

METAPROTERENOL

Metaproterenol (Alpent, Metaprel) can be administered by mouth in the form of tablets or as an aerosol. When administered orally, the dose is 20 mg every 6 to 8 hours. The onset of action takes place in approximately 15 to 30 minutes with peak effect 2 hours after administration and a mean duration of 4 hours. The aerosol form has the advantage of being the longest acting preparation of this type marketed in the United States. The dose is one to three 0.65 mg puffs every 4 hours. Onset occurs within 5 minutes with peak effect in 30 to 60 minutes and the duration of action up to 5 hours.

Side effects occur in 5 to 8% of patients following aerosol administration and in 17% of patients following oral administration.[54] Side effects include tachycardia, hypertension, palpitation, tremor, nausea and vomiting.[75]

ISOETHARINE

Isoetharine is a selective beta-2 adrenergic agent available in combination with phenylephrine (Bronkosol, Bronkometer) as an aerosol. The onset of action is 5 minutes, duration of action is 1.5 to 3 hours and the peak effect is observed beteen 15 to 60 minutes after administration. Each puff of Bronkometer delivers 0.34 mg of isoetharine and the dose is 1 to 2 puffs/every 3 to 4 hours. No information is available about transplacental transfer or teratogenesis in the human or secretion in breast milk.

CORTICOSTEROIDS

The use of corticosteroids is a well established adjunctive therapy in the treatment of refractory asthma. Possible mechanisms of action include direct relaxation of bronchial smooth muscle and indirect effects secondary to increased beta-adrenergic receptor production.[76] Corticosteroids also inhibit leukotriene production, improve mucociliary clearance and decrease mucus formation.[76]

Complications of steroid use during pregnancy include maternal and fetal adrenal insufficiency, steroid induced maternal hyperglycemia, psychosis and hypertension.

There is evidence that cortisol,[77,78] prednisone,[79] prednisolone,[79] bethamethasone[80] and dexamethasone[81,82] all cross the placenta. No information is available about transplacental transfer of beclomethasone.[83] In vivo measurements indicate that when prednisone or prednisolone is administered to pregnant patients, the concentration of active compound in fetal blood is close to 10% of that in the mother. The feto-maternal gradient of betamethasone, on the other hand, is estimated to be 1:3, while concentrations of dexamethasone are similar in both fetal and maternal compartments. Based on this information, it appears reasonable to use either prednisone or prednisolone if steroids are required to treat pregnant asthmatic patients.[84]

Although animal studies have demonstrated an increased incidence of cleft palate in the offspring of mothers given steroids during pregnancy, this association has not been found in human studies. Gestational administration of steroids is associated with decreased placental weight in monkeys, rats and rabbits, and increased incidence of stillbirth in rodents.[85] Triamcinolone acetonide has been shown to retard fetal rhesus monkeys' body growth and lung septa development, when administrered early in development.[86]

In 145 infants exposed to corticosteroids in the first trimester, no increase in abnormalities was noted.[44] Schatz et al. reported their experience with 70 pregnancies in 55 asthmatic patients receiving an average dose of 8.2 mg of prednisone daily. They found no increased risk of spontaneous abortion, congenital malformations, stillbirth, neonatal death, toxemia or bleeding. They did find an increased incidence of prematurity, but felt that this was not necessarily attributable to the use of steroids.[87] Snyder and Snyder have found no maternal or fetal complications in a retrospective evaluation of 36 patients receiving steroid therapy during pregnancy.[88]

Concern exists about the effect that prenatal administration of steroids may have on fetal brain development and on the immunologic status of the neonate. No studies to date, however, have demonstrated that these systems are adversely affected.

Prednisone is secreted in breast milk but doses of less than 30 mg/day are unlikely to create any problems for the infant.[89]

Intravenous glucocorticoids are utilized in status asthmaticus. There are, however, conflicting reports on the efficacy of corticosteroid therapy in this acute setting.[72] Should intravenous therapy be employed, one recommended program is the use of hydrocortisone (Solucortef) or equivalent quantities of methylprednisolone (Solu-medrol) in doses of 200 mg every 1 to 2 hours until the patient is no longer in the critical phase of respiratory distress. Doses as high as 4 g of hydrocortisone or its equivalent may be needed during the first 24 hours. The dose of parenteral glucocorticoids should be doubled if the patient has been on chronic steroid therapy and presents with status asthmaticus. With clinical improvement, the corticosteroids should be switched to the oral route of prednisone 5 to 10 mg every 4 to 6 hours, and then quickly tapered.[90]

Parenteral steroids are indicated in the pregnant patient with steroid-dependent asthma during stressful situations such as labor or surgical procedures. Two hours prior to surgery, 100 mg of hydrocortisone can be given intravenously. This dose is repeated every 6 hours for 24 to 48 hours; thereafter the patient can resume her usual maintenance dose.

Maintenance oral corticosteroid therapy may be required in asthmatics refractory to bronchodilator therapy. The lowest dose of prednisone which elicits clinical improvement should be utilized. Alternate day therapy with short acting agents (prednisone, prednisolone, methylprednisolone) has multiple advantages including less pituitary-adrenal axis suppression and less inhibition of the febrile response.[66] An initial 3- to 4-fold increase in dose is required when changing from a daily to alternate day regimen.

The optimal mode of steroid therapy appears to be broncho-inhalant. Beclomethasone diproprionate is a corticosteroid aerosol which dramatically lowers systemic steroid exposure while providing similar efficacy.[77] When given to pregnant rats at a dose of 100 μg/kg via inhalation, there were no reported teratogenic effects.[91] Its use in human pregnancy has been evaluated, and it appears to be both safe and effective.[91,92] Oral candidiasis is a frequent complication of long term therapy; however, its incidence may be minimized by mouthwashing after each treatment.

Beclomethasone is administered by a metered dose aerosol unit which deposits it in the nasopharynx, oropharynx and bronchial tree. The dose is two inhalations (50 μg each) every 6 to 8 hours. The dose may be increased up to a maximum of 1000 μg in 24 hours. An aerosol bronchodilator can be used 5 minutes prior to taking beclomethasone in order to increase its dispersion to the distal airways.

Patients with steroid-dependent asthma should be clinically stable before being switched to beclomethasone. The aerosol should be used simultaneously with oral steroid therapy for 2 weeks prior to tapering therapy at a rate of 2.5 mg/week. Attention must be paid to signs of adrenal insufficiency. If they appear, the dose of oral steroids should be increased and later tapered at a slower rate.

CROMOLYN SODIUM

Cromolyn Sodium (Intal, Aarane) has been increasingly employed in the treatment of asthma. It appears comparable in efficacy to theophylline[93,94] and is now utilized as a first line therapy.

The exact mechanism of cromolyn sodium action is unknown. It is a potent inhibitor of bronchospasm caused by both antigenic and non-specific stimuli. Cromolyn appears to stabilize mast cell membranes by inhibiting calcium ion flux.[95] It may also inhibit pulmonary parasympathetic activity.[96] The drug does not have a direct bronchodilator, antihistaminic or anti-inflammatory effect. Its pharmacologic actions after inhalation of the usual dose are limited to the respiratory tract.

There are multiple reports of the safety and efficacy of cromolyn sodium therapy in pregnancy;[72] however, the manufacturer does not recommend its use in this setting. No increase in the incidence of congenital anomalies has been reported in the offspring of human asthmatic mothers on chronic cromolyn suppression.[97] High parenteral doses, sufficient to produce maternal toxicity, inhibit fetal growth and increase stillbirth rates in pregnant rabbits, mice and rats. Congenital anomalies, however, have not been observed in experimental animals receiving high doses during pregnancy. No information is available on transplacental passage or breast milk secretion.

The drug is marketed in gelatin capsules and is administered with a special inhaler. Only 10 to 20% of each 20 mg capsule reaches the alveoli. The remainder is retained in the trachea and oropharynx and subsequently swallowed. Only 8% of the drug is absorbed into the systemic circulation. The plasma half-life is 60 to 90 minutes. Maximal benefit from the drug is achieved 10 to 30 minutes after administration, and clinical effects last approximately 6 hours. The absorbed drug is excreted by the kidney and the liver without undergoing metabolic inactivation.[98,99]

The usual oral dose of the drug is 20 mg every 6 hours, but this can be reduced to the lowest dosage necessary to control symptoms. Response to the medication is generally observed within 3 to 5 days but may take as long as 1 month. In the face of an acute asthma attack, the drug should be discontinued because it may cause additional bronchial irritation and worsen the bronchospasm. When used prophylactically against induced bronchospasm, the protective effect is virtually non-existent 2 hours after administration.

Side effects include sore throat, nasal congestion, cough, urticaria, maculopapular rash, angioedema, anaphylaxis, fever, nausea, vomiting, pulmonary infiltrates, muscular weakness and pericarditis.

IMMUNOTHERAPY

Immunotherapy (desensitization or hyposensitization) consists of the administration of gradually increasing doses of the allergens responsible for a given allergic reaction in order to blunt the immunologic response ordinarily activated after exposure to the antigen.

The mechanisms of action of immunotherapy include[100]:

(a) Induction of the synthesis of IgG (blocking) antibodies which combine with the offending allergen before it reacts with sensitized mast cells.

(b) Blunting of the anamnestic response of IgE present after seasonal exposure to the allergen.

(c) Decreased release of histamine secretion after stimulation of sensitized mast cells with allergens. This phenomenon is at least partially dependent on the concentration of IgE attached to the mast cell.

Immunotherapy has been effective in the treatment of ragweed and grass hay fever, but its role in the therapy of allergic asthma is less clear. Its use should probably be limited to the patient with proven extrinsic asthma and a poor response to conventional treatment.

The limited available literature concerning the use of immunotherapy during pregnancy indicates that the incidence of abortion, prematurity, toxemia and neonatal death is similar to that in the general population.[101] The main danger of immunotherapy during pregnancy seems to be the development of maternal anaphylactic reactions. Some authors have recommended the use of baseline concentrations of allergen rather than increasing dosage schedules in order to decrease the risk of anaphylaxis.

The incidence of allergic disease in the offspring of mothers treated with immunotherapy appears to be no different from that in atopic families studied as controls.

AGENTS TO BE AVOIDED IN PREGNANCY

Iodine is occasionally administered to non-pregnant asthmatics as an expectorant. Preparations which contain iodine are contraindicated during pregnancy and lactation because of the risk of producing congenital goiter and hypothyroidism in the newborn infant.

Iodines

Iodine crosses the placenta and may interfere with the fetal synthesis of thyroid hormones. Reduced circulating levels of thyroid hormones in the fetus may cause hypothyroidism and increased secretion of TSH. This, in turn, stimulates the growth of the thyroid gland and may produce goiter.[102,103] Congenital goiter has been responsibile for fatal upper airway obstruction in the neonatal period.[103–106] Iodine is also secreted in breast milk and may cause goiter and hypothyroidism in the nursing infant.

The clinician should be aware of the fact that some over-the-counter anti-asthmatic preparations contain iodine and its presence may not be suggested by the brand names (106).

Combination Agents

Theophylline has been used for many years in combinations with ephedrine, phenobarbital and hydroxyzine in commercially available oral anti-asthmatic preparations (Tedral, Marax, Bronkotabs). These combinations should be avoided in the therapy of pregnant asthmatic patients because they unnecessarily expose the infant to pharmacologic agents which are of unproven benefit for the mother. The addition of ephedrine increases theophylline toxicity without significant improvement of bronchodilation. Phenobarbital, in the doses present in these preparations, is not effective in eliminating the central nervous system side effects of theophylline.

RECOMMENDATIONS

Patients who have mild and infrequent episodes of asthma and are asymptomatic during the intervening periods can be treated with any of the adrenergic aerosol bronchodilators (metaproterenol, isoetharine, isoproterenol, or epinephrine). Metaproterenol and isoetharine are selective beta-2 agonists with a lower incidence of cardiac side effects than isoproterenol. Furthermore, their use has not been generally associated with the paradoxical bronchoconstriction which is occasionally seen with isoproterenol. It should be noted that some patients may only respond to one specific adrenergic aerosol.

If symptoms persist after the use of these aerosols, the patient should be given a systemic bronchodilator. Oral theophylline is the drug of choice because of the wide experience with its use during pregnancy. Serum levels of the drug can be obtained allowing for adjustment of the dose to produce maximal bronchodilatation with minimal side effects. The availability of long acting preparations permits the drug to be administered twice daily. If the pattern of the disease is one of prolonged remissions after an acute attack, theophylline can be discontinued after a short course of 4 to 5 days. Measurement of FEV-1 and MMFR (forced expiratory volume in 1 second and maximum end expiratory flow rate) is helpful in detecting subclinical bronchospasm. This can provide objective criteria on which to base a decision to discontinue the drug.

If symptoms persist despite theophylline therapy, the addition of an oral beta-2 adrenergic agonist (terbutaline or metaproterenol) is indicated. Terbutaline is preferred because of the wide experience amassed with its use during pregnancy as a tocolytic agent.

When a non-pregnant patient continues to be symptomatic despite maximal doses of systemic bronchodilators, a successful trial of cromolyn sodium may avoid the necessity of using glucocorticoids. Since experience with this drug during pregnancy is limited and the manufacturer does not recommend its use in the gravid patient, caution should be exercised and informed consent obtained prior to its use.

The administration of inhaled steroids (beclomethasone) may obviate the use of systemic medication in patients requiring long-term corticosteroid therapy. This aerosol preparation should not be used in the treatment of an acute bronchospastic attack because it may aggravate the severity of airway obstruction. Inhaled steroids may be unable to produce symptomatic relief, or the disease pattern may be such that a patient would benefit more from short courses of oral therapy. Prednisone is the oral glucocorticoid preparation of choice for the pregnant patient. When clinical improvement occurs, an attempt should be made to wean the patient from this medication.

If a pregnant patient has acute and severe bronchospasm, treatment with subcutaneous terbutaline is preferred over subcutaneous epinephrine. Terbutaline has a faster onset of action, longer duration of action and the same incidence of side effects and bronchodilator potency as epinephrine. Furthermore, it has none of the theoretical adverse effects of epinephrine on the uteroplacental circulation. Intravenous theophylline should be used in cases where subcutaneous terbutaline is unsuccessful in achieving therapeutic objectives. Persistence of severe bronchospasm for more than 60 minutes following the initiation of this regimen indicates that the patient is in status asthmaticus. This requires admission to the hospital and a combination of aggressive pharmacologic and respiratory care, which includes the use of intravenous corticosteroids.

REFERENCES

1. Kaliner, M.A.: Mast cell-derived mediators and bronchial asthma. In: Hargreave, FE, ed, Airway reactivity Mississauga, Ontario, Canada. Astra Pharmaceuticals, 1980, p. 178–187.
2. Hernandez, E., Angell, C.C. and Johnson, J.W.: Asthma in pregnancy: Current Concepts. Obstet Gynecol, *55*:739, 1980.
3. Kaliner, M.: Mast cell mediators and asthma. Chest, *87*:2S, 1985.
4. Ford, R.M.: Etiology and asthma: A continuing review (8071 cases seen from 1970–1980). Annal Allergy, *50*:47, 1983.
5. Rosenthal, R.R., Norman, P.S., Summer, W.R., et al.: Role of the parasympathetic system in antigen-induced bronchospasm. J Appl Physiol, *42*:600, 1977.
6. Frigas, E., Loegering, D.A., Solley G.O., et al.: Elevated levels of eosinophil granules major basic protein in the sputa of patients with bronchial asthma. Mayo Clin Proc, *56*:345, 1981.
7. Votava, Z.: Are the leukotrienes involved in the bronchial asthma? Biomed Biochem Acta, *43*:434, 1984.
8. Ishizako, T., Hirata, F., Ishizaka, K., Axelrod, J.: Stimulation of phospholipid methylation, $Ca-++$ influx and histamine release by bridging of IgE receptors on rat mast cells. Proc Natl Acad Sci, *77*:1903, 1980.
9. Weissman, C.: The Eicosanolds of asthma (editorial). N Engl J Med, *308*(18):454, 1983.
10. Griffin, M., Weiss, J., Leitch, A., et al.: Effects of leukotriene D on the airways in asthma. N Engl J Med, *308*:436, 1983.
11. Smith, L., Greenberger, P., Patterson, R., et al.: the effect of inhaled leukotriene D-4 in humans. Am Rev Respir Dis, *131*:368, 1985.
12. Hedqvist, P. and Dahlen, S.: Pulmonary and vascular effects of leukotrienes imply involvement in asthma and inflammation. Adv Prostaglandins, Thromboxane and Leukotriene Research, *11*:27, 1983.
13. Lewis, R: Leukotrienes and other lipid mediators of asthma. Chest, *87*:5S, 1983.
14. Ford-Hutchinson, A., Bray, M., Doig, M., et al.: Leukotriene B, a potent chemokinetic and aggregating substance released from polymorphonuclear leukocytes. Nature, *286*:264, 1980.
15. Goetzl, E. and Pickett, W.: The human polymorphonuclear leukocyte chemotactic activity of complex hydroxy-eicosetetraenoic acids (HETE's). J Immunol, *125*:1789, 1980.
16. Weller, P., Lee, C., Foster, D., et al.: Generation and metabolism of 5- lipoxygenase pathway leukotrienes by human eosinophiles. A predominant production of leukotriene C-4. Proc Natl Acad Sci (USA), *80*:7626, 1983.
17. Triggle, D.J.: Calcium, the control of smooth muscle function and bronchial hyperreactivity. Allergy, *38*:1, 1983.
18. Middleton, E. Jr.: Anti asthmatic drug therapy and calcium ions: Review of pathogenesis and role of calcium. J Pharm Sci, *69*:243, 1980.
19. Middleton, E. Jr.: Newer drugs in management, calcium antagonists. Chest, *87*:79S, 1985.
20. Polson, J.B., Krzanowski, J., Goldman, A., et al: Inhibition of human pulmonary phosphodiesterase activity by therapeutic levels of theophylline. Clin Exp Pharmacol Physiol, *5*:536, 1978.
21. Ruffin, R. and Newhouse, M.: Dipyridamole is it a bronchodilator? Eur J Respir Dis, *62*:123, 1981.
22. Robertson, C. and Levison, H.: Bronchodilators in asthma. Chest, *87*:64S, 1985.
23. Middleton, E. Jr.: Airway smooth muscle, asthma, and calcium ions. J Allergy Clin Immunol, *73*:643, 1984.
24. Aubier, M., Detroyer, A., Sampson, M., et al: Aminophylline improves diaphragmatic contractility. N Engl J Med, *305*:249, 1982.
25. Lurey, J.F.: The xanthine treatment of apnea of prematurity. Pediatrics, *55*:584, 1975.
26. Ingram, R. Jr.: Chronic bronchitis, emphysema and airways obstruction. In: Harrison's Principles of Internal Medicine. Eds. R. Petersdorf, R. Adams, E. Braunwald, et al. New York, McGraw-Hill, 1983, p. 1550.
27. Pederson, C.: Some pharmacological aspects of xanthines in asthma. Eur J Respir Dis, *61*:7S, 1980.
28. Perrson, C., Erjetalt, I. and Karlsson, T.: Adenosine antagonism, a less desirable characteristic of xanthine-asthma drugs? Acta Pharmacol Toxicol, *49*:317, 1981.
29. Lipshitz, J.: Uterine and cardiovascular effects of aminophylline. Am J Obstet Gynecol, *131*:716–6, 1978.

30. Soyka, L.F.: Effects of methylxanthines on the fetus. Clin Perinatol, *6*:137, 1979.
31. Hadjigeoriou, E., Kitsiou, S., Psaroudakis, A., et al: Antepartum aminophylline treatment for prevention of the respiratory distress syndrome in premature infants. Am J Obstet Gynecol, *135*:257, 1979.
32. Karotin, E.H., Kido, M., Cashore, W.J., et al.: Acceleration of fetal lung maturation by aminophylline in pregnant rabbits. Pediatr Res, *10*:722, 1976.
33. Yeh, T.F. and Pildes, R.S.: Transplacental aminophyllin toxicity in a neonate. Lancet, *1*:910, 1977.
34. Arwood, L.L., Dasta, J.F. and Friedman, C.: Placental transfer of theophylline: two case reports. Pediatrics, *63*:844, 1979.
35. Labovitz, E., and Spector, S.: Placental theophylline transfer in pregnant asthmatics. JAMA, *247*:786, 1982.
36. Shannon, D., Gotay, F., Stein, I., et al.: Prevention of apnea and bradycardia in low birthweight infants. Pediatrics, *55*:589, 1975.
37. Aranda, J., Sitar, D. and Parsons, W.: Pharmokinetic aspects of theophylline in premature newborns. N Engl J Med, *295*:413, 1976.
38. Yurchak, A. and Jusko, J.: Theophylline secretion into breast milk. Pediatrics, *57*:518, 1976.
39. Timson, J.: Theobromine and theophylline. Mutation Res, *32*:169, 1975.
40. Ishikawa, S., Gilbert, E.F., Bryyere, H.J. Jr., et al.: Aortic aneurysms associated with cardiac defects in theophylline stimulated chick embryos. Teratol, *18*:23, 1978.
41. Georges, A. and Denef, J.: Les Anomalies digitales manifestations terogeniques des derives xanthiques chez le rat. Arch Int Pharmacodyn Ther, *172*:219, 1968.
42. Weinstein, D.I., Mauer, M., Katz, L., et al.: The effect of methylxanthines on chromosomes of human lymphocytes in culture. Mutation Res, *31*:57, 1975.
43. Halbrecht, I., Komlos, L., Shabtay, F., et al.: Triploidy 69XXX in a stillborn girl. Clin Genet, *4*:210, 1973.
44. Heinonen, O.P., Slone, D. and Shapiro, S.: Birth Defects and Drugs in Pregnancy. Littleton, Mass, Publishing Sciences Group, 1977.
45. Van Dellen, R.G.: Theophylline practical application of new knowledge. Mayo Clin Proc, *54*:733, 1979.
46. Romero, R., Kadar, N., Govea, F.G., et al.: Pharmacokinetics of intravenous theophylline in pregnant patients at term. Am J Perinatol, *1*:31, 1983.
47. Carter, B.L., Driscoll, C.E. and Smith, G.D.: Theophylline clearance during pregnancy. Obstet Gynecol, *68*:555, 1986.
48. Karlsson, J.A. and Perrson, C.G.: Influence of tracheal contraction on relaxant effects in vitro of theophylline and isoprenaline. Br J Pharmacol, *74*:73, 1981.
49. IV dosage guidelines for theophylline products. FDA Drug Bull, *10*:4, 1980.
50. Ahlquist, R.P.: A study of the adrenotopic receptors. Am J Physiol, *153*:586, 1948.
51. Lands, A.M., Arnold, A., McAuliff, J.P., et al.: Differentiation of receptor systems activated by sympathomimetic amines. Nature, *214*:597, 1967.
52. Bourne, H., Lichtenstein, L., Henney, C., et al.: Modulation of inflammation and immunity by cyclic AMP. Science, *184*:19, 1974.
53. Schneid, C., Honeyman, T. and Fay, F.: Mechanisms of beta-adrenergic relaxation of smooth muscle. Nature, *277*:32, 1979.
54. Webb-Johnson, D.C. and Andrews, J.L.: Bronchodilator therapy. N Engl J Med, *297*:476, 1977.
55. Pose, S.V., Cibils, L.A. and Zuspan, F.: Effect of L-epinephrine infusion on uterine contractility and cardiovascular system. Am J Obstet Gynecol, *84*:297, 1962.
56. Morgan, C.D., Sandler, M. and Panigel, M.: Placental transfer of catecholamines in vitro and in vivo. Am J Obstet Gynecol, *112*:1068, 1972.
57. Misenhimer, H.R. and Margulies, S.I., Panigelm, P., et al: Effect of vasoconstrictive drugs on the placental circulation of the rhesus monkey. Invest Radiol, *7*:496, 1972
58. Rosenfield, C.R., Barton, M.D. and Mescha, G.: Effects of epinephrine on distribution of blood flow in the pregnant ewe. Am J Obstet Gynecol, *124*:156,1976.
59. Euler, U.S.: Action of adrenaline, acetylcholine and other substances on nerve free vessels (Human placenta). J Physiol, *93*:129, 1938.
60. Cliff, M.M. and Reynolds, S.R.: A dose-stress response to adrenaline affecting fetuses at critical time in pregnant rabbits. Anat Rec, *134*:379, 1959.
61. Hodach, R.J., Hodach, A.E., Fallon, J.F., et al.: The role of beta-adrenergic activity in the production of cardiac and aortic anomalies in chick embryos. Teratol, *12*:33, 1975.
62. Wood, D.W., Downes, J.J., Scheinkopf, H., et al.: Intravenous isoproterenol in the management of respiratory failure in childhood status asthmatics. J Allergy Clin Immunol, *50*:75, 1972.
63. Galant, S.: Current status of beta-adrenergic agonists in bronchial asthma. Ped Clin North Am, *30*:931–942, 1983.
64. Ingemarsson, I.: Effect of terbutaline on premature labor. Am J Obstet Gynec, *125*:520, 1976.

65. Wallace, R.L., Caldwell, D.L., Ansbacher, R. and Otterson, W.N.: Inhibition of premature labor by terbutaline. Obstet Gynecol, *51*:387, 1978.
66. Caritis, S., Toig, G., Heddinger, L.A. and Ashmead, G.: A double-blind study comparing ritodrine and terbutaline in the treatment of preterm labor. Am J Obstet Gynecol, *150*:7, 1984.
67. Caritis, S., Mueller-Heubach, E., Morishima, H.O., et al.: Effect of terbutaline on cardiovascular state and uterine blood flow in pregnant ewes. Obstet Gynecol, *50*:603, 1977.
68. Bhat, N., Seifer, D. and Hensleigh, P.: Paradoxical response to intravenous terbutaline. Am J Obstet Gynecol, *153*:310, 1985.
69. Bergman, B. and Hedner, T.: Antepartum administration of terbutaline and the incidence of hyaline membrane disease in preterm infants. Acta Obstet Gynecol Scan, *57*:217, 1978.
70. Ekelund, L., Burgoyne, R. and Enhorning, G.: Pulmonary surfactant release in fetal rabbits: immediate and delayed response to terbutaline. Am J Obstet Gynecol, *147*:437, 1983.
71. Ekelund, L. and Enhorning, G.: Glucocorticoids and beta-adrenegeric-receptor agonists: their combined effect on fetal rabbit lung surfactant, *152*:1063, 1985.
72. Spection, S.: The treatment of the asthmatic mother during pregnancy and lactation. Ann Allergy, *51*:173, 1983.
73. Nilsson, H.T., et al.: The metabolism of terbutaline in man. Xenobiotica, *2*:363, 1972.
74. Johansen, S.: Clinical comparison of intramuscular terbutaline and subcutaneous adrenalin in bronchial asthma. Eur J Clin Pharmacol, *7*:163, 1974.
75. Hurst, A.: Metaproterenol a potent and safe bronchodilator. Ann Allergy, *31*:460, 1973.
76. Spector, S.: the use of corticosteroids in the treatment of asthma. Chest, *87*:73S, 1985.
77. Beitins, I.Z., Bayard, F., Ances, I.G., et al.: The metabolic clearance rate, blood production, interconversion and transplacental passage of cortisol and cortisone in pregnancy near term. Pediatr Res, *7*:509, 1973.
78. Pasqualini, J.R., Nguyen, B.L., Uhrich, F., et al.: Cortisol and cortisone metabolism in the human foeto-placental unit at midgestation. J Steroid Biochem, *1*:209, 1970.
79. Beitins, I.Z., Bayard, F., Ances, I.G., et al.: The transplacental passage of prednisone and prednisolone at term. J Pediatr, *81*:936, 1976.
80. Ballard, P.L., Grandberg, P. and Ballard, R.A.: Glucocorticoid levels in maternal and cord serum after prenatal betamethasone therapy to prevent respiratory distress syndrome. J Clin Invest, *56*:1548, 1975.
81. Osathanondh, A., Tulchinsky, D., Kamali, H., et al.: Dexamethasone levels in treated pregnant women and newborn infants. J Pediatr, *90*:617, 1977.
82. Funkhouser, J.D., Peevy, K.J., Mockridge, P.B., et al.: Distribution of dexamethasone between mother and fetus after maternal administration. Pediatr Res, *12*:1053, 1978.
83. Greenberger, P. and Patterson, R.: Beclomethasone diproprionate for severe asthma during pregnancy. Ann Intern Med, *98*:478, 1983.
84. Davies, I.J.: The fetal adrenal. In: Maternal Fetal Endocrinology. Tulchinsky, D., and Ryan, K.J. (eds). Philadelphia, W.B. Saunders Co., 1980.
85. Taeusch, H.W. Jr.: Glucocorticoid prophylaxis for respiratory distress syndrome: A review of potential toxicity. J Pediatr, *87*:617, 1975.
86. Bunton, T.E. and Plopper, G.C.: Triamcinolone-induced structural alterations in the development of the lung of the fetal rhesus macague. Am J Obstet Gynecol, *148*:203, 1984.
87. Schatz, M., Patterson, R., Zeitz, S., et al.: Corticosteroid therapy for the pregnant asthmatic patient. JAMA, *223*:804, 1975.
88. Snyder, R.D. and Snyder, D.: Corticosteroid for asthma during pregnancy. Ann Allergy, *41*:340, 1978.
89. Katz, F.H. and Duncan, B.R.: Entry of prednisone into human breast milk. N Engl J Med, *293*:1154, 1975.
90. Thorn, G.W. and Lauler, D.P.: Treatment schedules with steroids. In: Bronchial Asthma Mechanism and Therapeutics. Weiss, E.B. and Segal, M.S. (eds). Boston, Little, Brown & Co., 1976.
91. Greenberger, P.A., and Patterson, R.: Beclomethasone diproprionate for severe asthma during pregnancy. Ann Intern Med, *98*:478, 1983.
92. Morrow-Brown, H. and Storey, G.: Beclomethasone diproprionate aerosol in long term treatment of perennial and seasonal asthma in children and adults. A report of five and half years experience in 600 asthmatic patients. Br J Clin Pharm, *4*:259, 1977.
93. Edmunds, A., Carswell, F., Robinson, P. and Hughes, A.: Controlled trial of cromoglycate and slow-release aminophylline in perennial childhood asthma. Br Med J, *281*:842, 1980.
94. Hambleton, G., Weinberger, M., Taylor, J., et al.: Comparison of cromoglycate (cromolyn) and theophylline in controlling symptoms of chronic asthma: a collaborative study. Lancet, *1*:381, 1977.
95. Mazurek, N., Berger, G. and Pecht, I.: A binding site on mast cells and basophils for the anti-allergic drug cromolyn. Nature, *286*:722, 1980.
96. Richards, I.: Humoral and neural modes of action of sodium cromoglycate. International Con-

ference on Bronchial Hyperreactivity. Oxford, The Medicine Publishing Foundation, 1982, p. 29.

97. Wilson, J.: Utilisation en cromoglycate de sodium au cours de la grossesse. Acta Ther, *8*:45, 1982.

98. Falliers, C.J.: Cromolyn sodium (disodium cromoglycate) prophylaxis. Pediatr Clin North Am, *22*:2:141, 1975.

99. Bernstein, I.L., Johnson, C.L. and Ted Tse, C.S.: Therapy with cromolyn sodium. Ann Intern Med, *89*:228, 1978.

100. Rosenthal, R.R. and Lichtenstein, L.W.: The status of immunotherapy in asthma. In: Bronchial Asthma Mechanisms and Therapeutics. Weiss, E.B. and Segal, M.S. (eds). Boston, Little Brown & Co., 1976.

101. Metzger, W.J., Turner, E. and Patterson, R.: The safety of immunotherapy during pregnancy. J Allergy Clin Immunol, *61*:268, 1978.

102. Martin, M.M. and Rento, R.D: Iodine goiter with hypothyroidism in two newborn infants. J Pediatr, *61*:94, 1962.

103. Carswell, F., Kerr, M.M. and Hutchinson, J.H.: Congenital goiter and hypothyroidism produced by maternal ingestion of iodines. Lancet, *1*:1241, 1970.

104. Galina, M.P., Avent, N.L. and Einhor, A.: Iodines during pregnancy, an apparent cause of neonatal death. N Engl J Med, *267*:1124, 1962.

105. Miyagewa, N.: An autopsy case of congenital goiter. Acta Pathol Jpn, *23*:531, 1973.

106. American Academy of Pediatrics. Committee on drugs. Adverse reactions to iodine therapy of asthma and other pulmonary diseases. Pediatrics, *57*:272, 1976.

Chapter 9

Anticoagulants in Pregnancy

Edward Goldberg

Since the advent of anticoagulant therapy, death from thromboembolic disease has been markedly reduced. In antepartum patients with thromboembolic disease, a mortality rate as high as 13% has been reported, yet the use of anticoagulants can reduce this rate to less than 1%.[1] While thromboembolic disease is more common in pregnancy than in the non-pregnant state, its incidence in pregnancy has been reported to range from 0.2 to 0.4%. Although the number of affected patients is therefore low, the therapeutic success of anticoagulation requires its clinical use in patients with thromboembolic disease as well as patients with cardiac valve prostheses who are highly prone to thrombotic disease.

Thrombus formation occurs as a result of damage to the intima of the blood vessel, venous stasis, "hypercoagulability" as described by Virchow in 1846, and adherence of platelets to the area of intimal damage.[2] The purpose of anticoagulant therapy is to interfere with the clotting process to prevent the enlargement of existing thrombi, prevent the embolization of such thrombi, and to prevent the occurrence of new thrombi.

HEPARIN

Heparin is the anticoagulant of choice in the treatment of acute thromboembolic disease. It is a complex mucopolysaccharide consisting of glucuronic acid, glucosamine and sulfuric ester groups and has a molecular weight of approximately 12,000. It also has a strong negative charge, and for this reason as well as the large size of the molecule, it does not cross the placenta. It is found naturally in the mast cells in both humans and animals, and while it has been synthesized, its clinical source is as an extract from the gut and lungs of cattle.

Heparin has several actions which contribute to its anticoagulant properties.[3] It is an antithromboplastin, combining with a cofactor to inactivate thromboplastin. Secondly, it appears to activate an antithrombin in the blood, and thirdly, it tends to decrease the adhesiveness of platelets. Its strong negative charge enables it to combine with a variety of proteins involved in the clotting process and further interfere with clot formation.

The major problems with heparin use are a tendency to spontaneous bleeding (usually with overdosage), hemorrhage when surgical procedures are performed during heparin therapy, and the considerable inconvenience caused by its route of administration, which must be either intravenous or subcutaneous. Its duration of action, however, is short and its anticoagulant effects can be quickly reversed by cessation of therapy, and if necessary, administration of protamine sulfate. Potential bleeding may therefore be promptly prevented in the event that a surgical procedure or labor and delivery are imminent. As it does not cross the placenta, there is subsequently no risk of either teratogenicity or fetal hemorrhage, an obvious and major advantage to the obstetric patient.

COUMARIN DERIVATIVES (WARFARIN SODIUM)

The coumarin derivatives are in extremely wide usage as long-term anticoagulants because of their principal advantages: oral administration and relative ease of control. They are regularly used on an outpatient basis after initial acute therapy with heparin, or for chronic preventative therapy in susceptible patients, such as those with cardiac valve prostheses.

Warfarin and its related compounds are vitamin K antagonists, interfering with the formation of certain clotting factors, namely prothrombin, factor VII, factor IX and factor X, all of which are formed in the liver and all of which require vitamin K for synthesis to occur. Warfarin has a delayed onset of action and long duration of action, making it more difficult to reverse in the event of spontaneous hemorrhage or imminent emergency surgical procedures. Since warfarin is of low molecular weight, it crosses the placenta, creating concern of possible teratogenicity and fetal hemorrhagic disorders.

CLINICAL USE OF ANTICOAGULANTS IN PREGNANCY

Because of the marked reduction in maternal mortality when anticoagulants are used in the treatment of acute thromboembolic disease, there is absolutely no question about the propriety of their use once a diagnosis has been established. The only controversy revolves around the choice of drug. In the acute phase of therapy, there is little question that heparin, either intravenously or subcutaneously, is the drug of choice, as has been pointed out by Villa Santa,[1] Beller,[4] and numerous other authors. Beller described a technique of intermittent intravenous therapy for the acute phase, followed by longer term treatment with a coumarin derivative. When thrombophlebitis occurred at or near term, heparin alone was used and the heparin was discontinued at the time of labor. Other authors prefer continuous intravenous heparin, maintaining a Lee-White clotting time at 2 to 3 times normal or the partial thromboplastin time (PTT) at 1 1/2 times normal for the acute phase of therapy. First a bolus of 5,000 to 10,000 units is given I.V., followed by 1000 to 1200 units per hour by continuous infusion. The controversy begins after the acute phase, when one considers long-term anticoagulation in pregnancy.

Long-term anticoagulation may be indicated when acute thromboembolic disease occurs in early pregnancy, or when the patient has a need for continuous therapy, such as in patients with cardiac valve prostheses. Indeed, these latter patients will be on oral anticoagulants prior to and at the time of conception and during the early weeks of pregnancy. Only patients with porcine valves do not require anticoagulation, a particular advantage for women of reproductive age. Indeed, the results of pregnancies in patients with mechanical valve prostheses is notoriously bad. Salazar et al.[5] studied pregnancies in 156 women. In 68 pregnancies treated only with antiplatelet agents (such as aspirin), there were 3 deaths, 7.4% stillbirths and 29% with cerebral thromboembolism. In patients treated with coumarin, they found 7.9% coumarin embryopathy, 7.1% stillbirths and 2.3% neonatal death from cerebral hemorrhage. On the other hand, in 15 pregnancies with porcine valves, there was 1 stillbirth, 1 patient died of a calcified valve and there were 13 normal pregnancies. Deviri et al.[6] and Javares et al.[7] showed similar advantages of the biologic valves in pregnancy. Patients who have a prior history of thromboembolic disease seem to be at greater risk when pregnant[8] and are considered by some as candidates for prophylactic therapy. The risks of anticoagulation, however, probably outweigh the potential recurrence of thrombosis, and most authors support Howie's view that therapy should be withheld in these patients until a definite recurrence has been documented.[9] In addition, one has to wonder if such prophylactic therapy is indicated in the first place. Making the diagnosis of thrombophlebitis in pregnancy is not at all easy and the supposed "prior episode" may have been an incorrect diagnosis. This inconsistency of diagnosis was shown by Kierkegaard[10] who found that only 2 of 17 pregnant women with the diagnosis of thromboembolic disease actually had the diagnosis confirmed by venogram. (The clinical diagnoses were more accurate in puerperal patients). Even if the original diagnosis was correct, recurrence may not be all that frequent. Howell et al.[11] followed 40 patients with a previous history of deep vein thrombosis during pregnancy; half were treated with heparin, 20,000 units subcutaneously daily and half were not treated. One control patient developed another episode of thrombosis, while one heparin treated patient developed severe osteopenia.

Whereas heparin is generally considered the drug of choice for acute therapy, the coumarin derivatives, principally warfarin, have been universally accepted, at least in the absence of pregnancy, for long-term therapy. This use must be re-examined in the pregnant patient because of the known ability of the coumarin derivatives to cross the placenta, unlike heparin which cannot. In fact, a variety of fetal effects of the coumarin derivatives have been reported.

DiSaia[12] reported the first case of teratogenicity due to warfarin. The infant showed nasal hypoplasia, bilateral optic atrophy and mental retardation, a syndrome that has become known as the fetal warfarin syndrome (similar in appearance to chondrodysplasia punctata). Shaul and Hall[13] and Hall et al.[14] in 1980 reviewed the cases of fetal warfarin syndrome known to them. In these 24 patients, the most common findings were nasal hypoplasia and stippled epiphyses. In all cases coumarin drugs were used in the first trimester of pregnancy. Hill and Stern[15] suggested the more disconcerting possibility that while the chondrodysplasia punctata-like syndrome occurs with first trimester exposure, even when warfarin is used only in the second and third trimester, the ophthalmic abnormalities and mental retardation may still occur. The inescapable conclusion is that there may be considerable teratogenic risk with the use of warfarin in the first trimester, and that even beyond the first trimester teratogenicity might occur. As Bonnar[16] pointed out, only about 2/3 of pregnancies in which warfarin has been used will be normal.

The other major fetal concern regarding warfarin therapy is the possibility of fetal hemorrhage if delivery occurs while the mother is on warfarin, especially since reversal attempts with vitamin K frequently may not be sufficiently prompt. Tejani[17] reported a fetal wastage of 14 out of 46 fetuses in mothers with cardiac valve prostheses on oral anticoagulants. This wastage included 2 spontaneous abortions, 5 stillbirths and 4 neonatal deaths, with massive hemorrhage being found in all those coming to autopsy. This concern has led a number of authors to advocate using heparin in the first trimester, warfarin in the second trimester, and switching back to heparin at 37 weeks, so that when delivery occurs, the fetus will no longer be affected by the warfarin.[3,18,19,20] The hazards of such a protocol are two: the possibility of premature delivery before stopping warfarin at 37 weeks and the possibility of second and third trimester teratogenicity. The risk of oral anticoagulants in pregnancy is well demonstrated not only in the work of Tejani quoted above, but also in a study of 55 pregnancies in women with cardiac valve prostheses reviewed by Harrison and Roschke.[21] There were only 32 normal outcomes in these 55 pregnancies.

However, another reasonable, effective approach is the exclusive use of heparin, both for short-term and long-term anticoagulation. Spearing et al.[22] successfully treated 22 patients with subcutaneous heparin on an outpatient basis, and showed this protocol to be both safe and effective. Doses were given every 12 hours, using between 10,000 and 30,000 units daily. It would seem logical and practical that if patients can be taught to self-administer insulin, similar use of heparin is realistic. The major drawback to long-term heparin usage is, however, the possible development of osteoporosis. Griffith et al.[23] reported, in 1965, the first case of heparin-induced osteoporosis. In 1980, Wise and Hall[24] reported a case of multiple vertebral compression fractures in a woman receiving heparin through her pregnancy. De Swiet et al.[25] specifically evaluated 20 women, showing signficantly increased demineralization in patients treated with heparin for 25 weeks or more as compared to patients treated for 7 weeks or less. Whether this trend is reversible is unclear.

Low-dose heparin has been advocated as prophylaxis against venous thrombosis in non-pregnant circumstances with favorable results.[2,26,27] Generally, heparin in doses of 5,000 units subcutaneously is given every 12 hours and can be given for protracted periods with little risk. In pregnant women with artificial heart valves, heparin 5000 units q12 hr is not enough to prevent valve thrombosis.[28] Of 60 patients treated with this regimen, 3 had massive thrombosis of a Bjorh-Shiley mitral valve. Two cases occurred during the first trimester, with one death and another patient died postpartum. In this study, the incidence of coumadin embryopathy in patients on continuous coumadin was 28.6%[28] Though no large studies evaluating low-dose heparin in pregnancy exist, the safety and efficacy of this method warrant its careful consideration for certain high risk obstetric patients. Bell and Zuidema[29] suggested some risk factors that might warrant low-dose heparin therapy (Table 9-1).

ANTICOAGULANTS DURING LACTATION

In general, mothers requiring anticoagulation may continue to nurse their infants without problems. Heparin does not pass into the milk[30] and is not effective orally in any case and so does not hurt the infant.

In 7 patients taking a maternal dose of warfarin (Coumadin) of 5 to 12 mg/

Table 9–1.   Risk Factors For Thromboembolism

Past history of thromboembolism
Severe chronic lower extremity venous stasis
Chronic pulmonary disease
Obesity
Lower extremity paralysis
Congestive heart failure
Protracted bed rest

day (maternal plasma concentrations of 0.5 to 2.6 μg/ml), no warfarin is detectable in breast milk or in infant plasma at a sensitivity of 0.025 μg/ml.[31] Thus, 1 liter of milk would contain 20 μg of the drug at maximum, not significant in amount to have an anticoagulant effect. Another report[32] confirmed that warfarin appeared only in insignificant quantities in breast milk in 4 additional patients, and all infant prothrombin times were normal. Thus, with careful monitoring of maternal prothrombin time so that the dosage is minimized, warfarin may be safely administered to nursing mothers.

The oral anticoagulant bishydroxycoumarin (Dicumerol) has been given to 125 nursing mothers with no effect on the infants' prothrombin times and no hemorrhages.[33] This safety does not apply to all oral anticoagulants, however. In one case in which phenindione was being taken by a nursing mother, the infant underwent surgical repair of an inguinal hernia at 5 weeks of age. He developed a large hematoma and his prothrombin time was elevated.[34]

RECOMMENDATIONS

Until such time as safer methods of anticoagulation evolve, patients who certainly require anticoagulation, such as those with cardiac valve prostheses, should be informed of the risks of pregnancy. These patients and those with established diagnoses of thromboembolic disease should be anticoagulated during pregnancy, but it is evident that one cannot undertake antcoagulant therapy in pregnancy without considerable risk. When acute thromboembolic disease occurs in pregnancy, however, therapy is mandatory, and can best be accomplished with continuous intravenous infusion of heparin. In those cases occurring late enough in pregnancy, heparin may well be the only drug necessary. When the disease occurs early in pregnancy, or when other illness (i.e., cardiac valve prosthesis) coexists with pregnancy, the previously mentioned protocol of full dose heparin, then warfarin, then heparin again at 37 weeks may be considered. This plan of management carries the risk of fetal warfarin syndrome and the possibility of premature labor occurring during the warfarin phase of therapy.

However, the use of only heparin through pregnancy, with subcutaneous heparin used after the acute phase of intravenous therapy has been completed, may be safest for mother and infant. If labor ensues, reversal of the anticoagulant effect can be accomplished quickly, but the risk of osteoporosis must always be considered. Low-dose heparin therapy may also have a place in prophylaxis for certain high-risk patients, but long-term full dose heparin or warfarin use in pregnant patients with previous thromboembolic disease is probably not indicated due to the considerable risk of such treatment.

REFERENCES

1. Villa Santa, U.: Thromboembolic disease in pregnancy. Am J Obstet Gynecol, *93*:142, 1965.
2. Clagett, G.P. and Salzman, E.W.: Prevention of venous thromboembolism in surgical patients. N Engl J Med, *290*:93, 1974.
3. Bloomfield, D.K.: Fetal deaths and malformations associated with the use of coumarin derivatives in pregnancy. Am J Obstet Gynecol, *107*:883, 1970.
4. Beller, F.K.: Thromboembolic disease in pregnancy. Clin Obstet Gynecol, *11*:290, 1968.
5. Salazar, E., Zajarias, A., Gutierrez, N. and Iturbe, I.: The problem of cardiac valve prostheses, anticoagulants, and pregnancy. Circ *70*(Suppl.I):169, 1984.
6. Deviri, E., Levinsky, L., Yechezkel, M. and Levy, M.J.: Pregnancy after valve replacement with porcine xenograft prosthesis. Surg Gynecol & Obstet, *160*:437, 1985.

7. Jarvares, T., Coto, E.O., Maiques, V., et al.: Pregnancy after heart valve replacment. Int J Cardiol, *5*:731, 1984.
8. Badaracco, M.A. and Vessey, M.P.: Recurrence of venous thromboembolic disease and use of oral contraceptives. Br Med J, *1*:215, 1974.
9. Howie, P.W.: Thromboembolism. Clin Obstet Gynecol, *4*:397, 1977.
10. Kierkegaard, A.: Incidence and diagnosis of deep vein thrombosis associated with pregnancy. Acta Obstet Gynecol Scan, *62*:239, 1983.
11. Howell, R., Fidler, J., Letsky, E. and DeSwiet, M.: The risks of antenatal subcutaneous heparin prophylaxis: a controlled trial. Br J Obstet Gynaec, *90*:1124, 1983.
12. DiSaia, P.J.: Pregnancy and delivery of a patient with a Starr-Edwards mitral valve prosthesis. Obstet Gynecol, *28*:469, 1966.
13. Shaul, W.L. and Hall, J.G.: Multiple congenital anomalies associated with oral anticoagulants. Am J Obstet Gynecol, *127*:191, 1977.
14. Hall, J.G., Pauli, R.M. and Wilson, K.M.: Maternal and fetal sequelae of anticoagulation during pregnancy. Am J Med, *68*:122, 1980.
15. Hill, R.M. and Stern, L.: Drugs in pregnancy: effects on the fetus and newborn. Drugs, *17*:182, 1979.
16. Bonnar, J.: Venous thromboembolism and pregnancy. Clin Obst Gynec, *8*:455, 1981
17. Tejani, N.: Anticoagulant therapy with cardiac valve prostheses during pregnancy. Obstet Gynecol, *42*:785, 1973.
18. Hirsh, J., Cade, J.F. and O'Sullivan, E.E.: Clinical experience with anticoagulant therapy during pregnancy. Br Med J, *1*:270, 1970.
19. Pridmore, B.R., Murray, K.H. and McAllen, P.M.: The management of anticoagulant therapy during and after pregnancy. Br J Obst Gynaecol, *82*:740, 1975.
20. Ramsay, D.M.: Thromboembolism in pregnancy. Obstet Gynecol, *45*:129, 1975.
21. Harrison, E.C. and Roschke, E.J.: Pregnancy in patients with cardiac valve prostheses. Clin Obstet Gynecol, *1*, 18:107, 1975.
22. Spearing, G., Fraser, I., Turner, G., et al.: Long-term self-administered subcutaneous heparin in pregnancy. Br Med J, *1*:1457, 1978.
23. Griffith, G.C., Nichols, G., Asher, J.D. and Hanagan, B.: Heparin osteoporosis. JAMA, *193*:91, 1965.
24. Wise, P.H. and Hall, A.J.: Heparin-induced osteopenia in pregnancy. Br Med J, *1*:110, 1980.
25. De Swiet, M., Ward, P.D., Fidler, J., et al.: Prolonged heparin therapy in pregnancy causes demineralizaton. Brit J Obstet Gynaecol, *90*:1129, 1983.
26. Gallus, A.S., Hirsh, J., Tuttle, R.J., et al.: Small subcutaneous doses of heparin in prevention of venous thrombosis. N Engl J Med, *288*:545, 1973.
27. Verstraete, M.: The prevention of postoperative deep vein thrombosis and pulmonary embolism with low-dose subcutaneous heparin and dextran. Surg Gynecol Obstet, *143*:981, 1976.
28. Iturbe-Alessio, I., del Carmen Fonseca, M., Mutchinik, O., et al.: Risks of anticoagulant therapy in pregnant women with artificial heart valves. N Engl J Med, *315*:1390, 1986.
29. Bell, W.R. and Zuidema, G.D.: Low-dose heparin-concern and perspectives. Surgery, *85*:469, 1979.
30. Gilman, A., et al. (eds.): The Pharmacological Basis of Therapeutics, 7th ed., New York, Macmillan, 1985.
31. Orme, M.E., Lewis, P.J. and deSwiet, M., et al: May mothers given warfarin breast-feed their infants? Br Med J, *1*:1564, 1977.
32. deSwiet, M. and Lewis, P.J.: Excretion of anticoagulants in human milk. N Engl J Med, *297*:1471, 1977.
33. Brambel, C.E. and Hunter, R.: Effect of dicumarol on the nursing infant. Am J Obstet Gynecol, *59*:1153, 1950.
34. Eckstein, H.B. and Jack, B.: Breastfeeding and anticoagulant therapy. Lancet, *1*:672, 1970.

Chapter 10

Antineoplastic Drugs and Pregnancy

Joseph Buscema, Jeffrey L. Stern and Timothy R.B. Johnson

The advent of successful anticancer agents permits us to treat malignancies, many of which preferentially strike women of reproductive age. Balancing the benefits of antineoplastic drugs, often of low therapeutic index, against side effects, is especially difficult in the pregnant woman. In addition to drug effects on mother and fetus, the question of teratogenicity has been raised when males receive antineoplastic agents, further extending the responsibility of the concerned physician.

Approximately 3,500 cancer-related deaths occurred in women aged 15 to 34 years in 1976,[1] and the reported incidence of pregnancy complicated by cancer is approximately 1 in 1,100.[2] In addition, pregnancy occurs in 25 to 33% of women with Hodgkin's disease and in 3% of women with breast cancer.[3] However, only 3 of the 50,282 pregnant women studied in the Collaborative Perinatal Project received cytotoxic agents.[4] Recently, indications for chemotherapeutic agents have expanded to include non-neoplastic diseases such as systemic lupus erythematosus, nephrotic syndrome, psoriasis, and renal transplantation.

The literature on the older antineoplastic agents remains scant with substantially less reference information available on recently introduced drugs and combination chemotherapy regimens. This chapter reviews documented adverse effects of antineoplastic agents when administered at the time of conception and during pregnancy.

Most antineoplastic drugs affect nucleic acid and protein synthesis. As a result, rapidly proliferating normal and malignant cells are often susceptible targets. Experimentally, adverse cytotoxic drug effects can be influenced by the stage of gestation, dose and duration of therapy, and the species and strain of the animals studied. A broad spectrum of drug effects may be seen, but the untoward effects in animal models are not necessarily directly applicable to man. In fact, most of the commonly used antineoplastic drugs are embryolethal or teratogenic in animals, whereas human conceptuses seem to be less susceptible to these ill effects (Chapter 1).

ALKYLATING AGENTS (TABLE 10–1)

Nitrogen Mustard (HN$_2$)

A wide variety of malformations (skeletal, limbs, CNS, palate) have been observed in the offspring of animals treated with nitrogen mustard.[5-7] In humans, 2 women have had normal children after treatment with nitrogen mustard in

Table 10–1. Pregnancy Outcome After Administration of Alkylating Agents

Drug	Animal Malformations	Trimester (humans)	Single Agents (humans)	Given with Other Cytotoxic Drugs
Nitrogen Mustard	skeletal limb CNS cleft palate embryolethal	First	3-spontaneous abortions 1-induced abortion- normal 2-normal	1-spontaneous abortion- normal 1-normal 1-IUGR, preterm 1-digit, limb, ear abnormalities 1-Renal anomaly, IUGR
		Beyond first	4-normal	4-normal 1-normal, preterm
Cyclophosphamide	skeletal limb CNS cleft palate ocular defects IUGR embryolethal	First	1-small hemangioma 1-induced abortion- absent digits 1-multiple anomalies 1-absent toes, single coronary artery	1-normal
		First and after	1-normal	2-normal 1-IUGR, pancytopenia
		Beyond first	3-normal	9-normal 2-IUGR
Chlorambucil	skeletal limb CNS cleft palate ocular urogenital	First	1-normal 1-spontaneous abortion 1-induced abortion- absent left kidney and ureter	—
		Beyond first	1-normal	3-normal
Busulfan	skeletal limb cleft palate IUGR sterility	First	1-induced abortion- normal 1-induced abortion- malformed 1-spontaneous abortion 20-normal 1-anomalous 1-preterm normal	1-normal 1-cleft palate, microphthalmus
		First and after	1-normal 1-IUGR 1-Trisomy 21 Microcephaly	—
		Beyond first	8-normal 1-hypertrophic pyloric stenosis 2-Renal agenesis hydronephrosis	2-normal (SGA)
Thiotepa	skeletal limb CNS	First	—	—
		Beyond first	1-normal	—
Triethylene Melamine	skeletal limb CNS	First	2-normal 2-spontaneous abortions	—
		Beyond first	5-normal	—
Uracil Mustard	skeletal CNS	—	—	—
		—	—	—
Mitomycin C	skeletal CNS cleft palate	—	—	—
		—	—	—
Alkeran (L-PAM)	—	—	—	—

the first trimester,[8,9] 3 had spontanoeous abortions,[10] and 1 had an induced abortion in which the fetus was normal.[11] Of the 4 woman treated with nitrogen mustard after the first trimester, no birth defects were noted.[10]

Nitrogen mustard used in combination with other cytotoxic agents during the first trimester of pregnancy resulted in one normal infant,[12] one normal preterm infant with intrauterine growth retardation (IUGR), [13] one infant with digital, ear, and lower extremity anomalies,[14] one pregnancy termination in which the fetus demonstrated renal anomalies,[15] and one spontaneous abortion with an apparently normal fetus. Five normal infants have been delivered exposed to nitrogen mustard in combination with other agents after the first trimester, without obvious effect, one of which was preterm.[10,12,16–18]

Cyclophosphamide (Cytoxan)

Cytoxan is highly teratogenic in experimental animals.[5,19,20] In mice, the palate closes on day 14 to 15 of gestation. Gibson[21] showed that a cleft palate could be induced in mice with administration of cyclophosphamide on day 9 to 12, but not on day 13 to 14 of gestation. He concluded that cyclophosphamide produces its effect at a time remote to closure of the palate, but has no effect when given at the time of closure. The drug's effects are species specific, since it does not interfere with palate closure in rats, although Scott demonstrated that administraton to pregnant rats resulted in IUGR and abnormal growth and development.[20]

Of the women who received Cytoxan as a single agent in the first trimester, one child had only a small hemangioma,[22] another had multiple anomalies of the toes and extremities, as well as palatine grooves and hernias,[23] and a third had absent toes and single coronary artery.[24] In one induced abortion, absent digits were noted. A normal infant resulted following single agent cyclophosphamide exposure in all three trimesters.[25] In two cases, cyclophosphamide used in combination with other antineoplastic drugs beginning in the first trimester resulted in entirely normal outcomes;[26,27] one additional infant manifested IUGR.[27] Beyond the first trimester, single agent cyclophosphamide use led to normal outcome in three cases.[28–30] Nine women received cyclophosphamide in combination with other cytotoxic drugs after the first trimester, without untoward effects;[10,16,31–37] in two additional cases, IUGR was noted.[38,39]

Chlorambucil

Chlorambucil has been associated with a variety of animal malformations, including defects in the urogenital system.[3,5,40]

Three women were treated with chlorambucil in the first trimester; in one a normal outcome was documented,[41] whereas one spontaneous abortion occurred[10] and in a therapeutic abortion performed at 18 weeks, absent left kidney and ureter were noted.[10,42] A normal infant was born to a woman who was treated with chlorambucil after the first trimester of pregnancy.[10] In addition, three normal infants were born to women who received chlorambucil, as well as other cytotoxic agents, after the first trimester.[17]

Busulfan

Busulfan, given to pregnant animals, results in skeletal and limb defects, as well as cleft palate, growth retardation, and sterility.[5,6]

Reports describe 28 human fetuses exposed to busulfan as a single agent in the first trimester. One spontaneous abortion occurred and 2 therapeutic abortions were performed; 1 of these infants was malformed.[10] Twenty-three normal infants and 2 anomalous infants were delivered, and among the latter was a Mongoloid infant with trisomy 21 and microcephaly.[10,43–47] An infant with a cleft palate and microphthalmia was exposed to busulfan, 6-mercaptopurine, and radiation in the first trimester,[48] but a normal infant was delivered after first trimester exposure to busulfan, 6-mercaptopurine, and aminopterin.[10]

Eleven women received busulfan as a single agent after the first trimester. Eight normal infants were delivered.[10,49] One infant had pyloric stenosis and two had right renal agenesis and hydronephrosis.[10,50] Two received multiple agents including busulfan after the first trimester, and had growth retarded but otherwise normal infants.

Only 2 of the 13 infants exposed to busulfan beyond the first trimester had appropriate weight for gestational age.[10,49,51]

Thio-Tepa

Thio-Tepa has been shown to be teratogenic in experimental animals.[6,51] It has been used only once in humans during the third trimester, with a good outcome.[10]

Miscellaneous Alkylating Agents

Use of uracil mustard and mitomycin C, known teratogens in rodents,[5,51] has not been reported in pregnant women. Trimethylene melamine, no longer used therapeutically, is teratogenic in animals.[5,52,53] It reportedly has been used in all three trimesters without recognizable defects.[10,11,54,55] Interestingly, Alkeran (melphalan), widely used to treat ovarian cancer, has not been evaluated experimentally and its use has not been reported in pregnant women.

ANTIMETABOLITES (Table 10–2)

Aminopterin

Aminopterin is highly teratogenic in rats and chicks.[56–58] It has been taken by 53 women in the first trimester of pregnancy,[10,59,60] in some cases as an abortifacient, and spontaneous abortions occurred in 34. In 13 cases in which the state of the fetus was described, 11 had congenital anomalies, and 2 were phenotypically and karyotypically normal. In the 25 cases in which the drug was used as an abortifacient, 5 abnormal fetuses were described, 3 with neural tube and 2 with craniofacial defects.[10,60,61] In the other 28 first trimester administrations, 6 abnormal fetuses were described with craniofacial anomalies, cleft palate, hydrocephalus, limb, digital, and ocular anomalies.[10,61] Two were specifically reported as normal and also had normal karyotypes.[10]

One patient received aminopterin as a single agent after the first trimester of pregnancy with delivery of a normal child.[10] When aminopterin was given with other agents beyond the first trimester, one normal infant and one spontaneous abortion were described. In the latter, the fetus was phenotypically normal.[10]

Table 10–2. Pregnancy Outcome After Administration of Antimetabolites

Drug	Animal Malformations	Trimester (humans)	Single Agents (humans)	Given with Other Cytotoxic Drugs
Aminopterin 2-4 diamino-pyrimidine	skeletal limb CNS cleft palate ocular craniofacial cardiac embryolethal	First	25-used as abortifacient 5 abnormal fetuses 1) meningoencephalocele 2) hydrocephalus 1) cleft palate 1) anencephaly 1) craniofacial 28-also 1st. trimester 6 abnormal fetuses craniofacial cleft palate hydrocephalus limb and digital ocular 2-normal phenotypes and karotypes	—
		Beyond first	1-normal	1-normal 1-normal spontaneous abortion
Methotrexate	skeletal limb embryolethal	First	2-abnormal 1-cranial and extremity anomalies 1-cranial anomalies	—
		First and after		4-normal 1-IUGR, pancytopenia
		Beyond first	6-normal	10-normal 1-leukopenia
Azothioprine	skeletal limb cleft palate IUGR	First only	1-spontaneous abortion 1-ectopic 1-normal	—
	small thymus embryolethal	First and after	42 39 without malformations (5 spontaneous abortions) (5 induced abortions) (3 premature) 3 abnormal	—
		Unspecified	8-no malformations	
Cytosine Arabinoside	skeletal CNS hypoplasia cleft palate facial anomalies	First	—	1-induced abortion-normal phenotype and genotype 2-normal without IUGR and normal neonatal growth 1-induced abortion-normal phenotype 19 weeks

Table 10–2. *Continued*

Drug	Animal Malformations	Trimester (humans)	Single Agents (humans)	Given with Other Cytotoxic Drugs
		First and after	—	1-normal 1-IUGR 1-digital anomalies-feet, absent phalanges-hands, genotype normal
		Beyond first	—	22-normal 2-IUGR 2-toxemia 2-premature, normal 1-normal, spontaneous abortion 1-induced abortion, Trisomy, group C
6-Thioguanine	skeletal limb digital IUGR embryolethal	First	—	1-induced abortion at 20 weeks with normal phenotype and genotype 1-normal
		First and after	—	1-digits foot, phalanges hand (absent) genotype normal
		Beyond first	—	2-normal with IUGR 10-normal 2-normal premature 1-normal phenotype with group C Trisomy-induced abortion 1-normal induced abortion 1-premature, IUGR 1-toxemia, death, phenotype normal 1-toxemia, death, genotype normal
6-Mercaptopurine	limb CNS cleft palate ocular IUGR embryolethal	First	3-spontaneous abortions 1-premature 2-died undelivered	2-spontaneous abortions 1-normal
		First and after	3-spontaneous abortions 8-live births 1-microophthalmia, cleft palate, corneal opacities	3-normal 1-IUGR, pancytopenia
		Beyond first	1-spontaneous abortion 1-stillborn (premature)-normal 19-live births-normal 3-died undelivered	12-normal 1-normal, leukopenia
5-Fluorouracil	skeletal	First	1-multiple anomalies	—
	CNS cleft palate embryolethal	Beyond first	1-normal with 5FU intoxication	—

Methotrexate

Methotrexate has been implicated in skeletal and limb defects and at high doses is embryolethal in animals.[5,57,62] When methotrexate is given simultaneously with citrovorum factor, death is prevented, as are malformations.

Two women received methotrexate in the first trimester, both of whom had infants with multiple congenital anomalies including cranial defects, malformed extremities, as well as intrauterine growth retardation and poor neonatal growth.[10,59] In 5 women who received methotrexate in combination with other agents in the first trimester and after, normal infants were delivered except for pancytopenia and IUGR in one.[27,63]

When methotrexate was employed as a single agent beyond the first trimester, 6 normal outcomes have been documented.[65] Beyond the first trimester, combination regimens with methotrexate have resulted in 10 normal infants and 1 with leukopenia.[27,37,65–67]

In general, the potential risks of cytotoxic agents would outweigh the benefits of continuing nursing if these were required. However, after oral administration to a lactating patient with choriocarcinoma, methotrexate was found in milk in low but readily detectable levels (0.26 µg/dl). Most patients would elect to avoid any exposure to the infant of this drug. However, in environments in which bottle feeding is rarely practiced and presents practical and cultural difficulties, therapy with this drug would not in itself appear to constitute a contraindication to breast feeding.[68]

Azathioprine (Imuran)

Azathioprine, a purine analogue, works via its metabolite, 6-mercaptopurine. The teratogenicity in laboratory animals exposed to azathioprine is well documented.[12,69]

The majority of women receiving azathioprine during pregnancy had either renal transplants or systemic lupus erythematosus. Of the three women treated in the first trimester, only one had a normal outcome,[10] one had a spontaneous abortion, and the third an ectopic pregnancy. Forty-two women have been treated with azathioprine through pregnancy.[17,70] Thirty-nine infants were without gross anomalies, although 5 spontaneous abortions and 3 premature births occurred.[70] Five patients had induced abortions. Of the 3 infants who were abnormal, 2 had leukopenia and adrenal cortical insufficiency. The third abnormal infant, though phenotypically normal, had genotypic derangements as well as IUGR.[71] In an additional 8 patients treated at unspecified times during pregnancy, no malformations were observed[22].

Cytosine Arabinoside (ARA-C)

A variety of congenital anomalies have been reported in laboratory animals exposed to ARA-C in utero including skeletal, CNS, palate and facial abnormalities.[5,72–74]

ARA-C in combination with other cytotoxic drugs was given to 4 patients with exposure restricted to the first trimester. Two phenotypically normal fetuses were aborted[75,76] and two normal infants were delivered[26,77] who had normal neonatal growth.

Three infants have been described when ARA-C was used in combination in the first trimester and after; anomalies of hands and feet occurred in one with normal genotype,[77] whereas in two other pregnancies, a normal infant and one with IUGR resulted.[27]

Beyond the first trimester, 30 pregnancies have been reported with ARA-C in combination regimens. Twenty-two normal infants at term have resulted.[27,63,65,66,76,78–88] Two infants with IUGR and two premature normal births also occurred.[89,90] In two pregnancies, fetal death was associated with severe toxemia, but infants were phenotypically normal.[83,88] One woman reportedly received ARA-C and 6-thioguanine at 20 weeks, had a therapeutic abortion at 24 weeks, and delivered an abortus with trisomy C;[91] another patient receiving the same drugs had a normal infant.[65] In addition, one spontaneous abortus was normal.

6-Thioguanine (6-TG)

6-Thioguanine has been demonstrated to cause multiple anomalies in the offspring of rats including limb anomalies and growth retardation.[5,52]

No single agent 6-TG exposure in pregnancy has been reported. Among exposures to multi-agent regimens containing 6-TG confined to the first trimester, one normal pregnancy and one genotypically and phenotypically normal 20 week abortus have been reported.[75,77] A term infant with absent phalanges of the foot and hand, but normal genotype, has been described in an exposure beginning in the first trimester and after.[77]

Nineteen pregnancies comprise the experience with 6-TG beyond the first trimester. Ten normal infants at term, two premature though normal neonates, and two with IUGR resulted. An additional premature infant manifested IUGR. Two gestations complicated by toxemia eventuated in two in utero fetal demises. In two pregnancy terminations, two normal phenotypes were observed, but in one, a group C trisomy was noted.[65,66,78,80,83,86–91]

6-Mercaptopurine (6-MP)

A variety of congenital malformations have been reported in offspring of experimental laboratory animals who were exposed to 6-MP in utero, including limb, palatal closure, ocular and CNS defects.

Spontaneous abortion has been a frequent complication in pregnancy with first trimester 6-MP exposure. Among 25 first trimester exposures (single and multi-agent regimens), 8 spontaneous abortions were observed and in 2 additional cases, in utero fetal demise occurred.[10,48] In other first trimester exposures, 8 normal pregnancies in a single agent setting and 4 normal outcomes in multi-agent use were observed;[10,27,63] multiple anomalies including microphthalmia, cleft palate and corneal opacity resulted in one single agent 6-MP exposure, whereas IUGR with pancytopenia was observed once in a multi-agent setting.[27,48]

Beyond the first trimester, single agent 6-MP exposure was not associated with malformation, however, pregnancy wastage occurred in 5 of 24 gestations. Nineteen normal outcomes have been reported. In multi-agent use, 13 normal outcomes resulted except for leukopenia in one.[27–37,64–67]

5-Fluorouracil (5-FU)

5-fluorouracil has been associated with skeletal defects, CNS anomalies, cleft palate and fetal death in utero in animal models.[5,92] One fetus with multiple anomalies was aborted after first trimester use of 5-FU.[93] A phenotypically normal infant was delivered to a woman treated with 5-FU in the second trimester, but the infant suffered reversible 5-FU toxicity in the neonatal period.

ANTIBIOTICS (TABLE 10–3)

Daunorubicin and Doxorubicin

In certain animal models, cardiac, CNS, ocular and renal anomalies have been observed with doxorubicin and daunorubicin exposure. Embryolethality has also been noted.[7,94,95] Conversely, in rat models, no malformations have been reported.[5]

Human experience with these agents has been confined to multi-drug settings. For first trimester exposure, four normal outcomes have been reported, one complicated by prematurity.[26,27,96,97] An induced abortion at 19 weeks resulted in a phenotypically normal fetus.[76]

Beyond the first trimester, 29 pregnancies with daunorubicin or doxorubicin

Table 10–3. Pregnancy Outcome After Administration of Antineoplastic Antibiotics

Drug	Animal Malformations	Trimester (humans)	Single Agents (humans)	Given with Other Cytotoxic Drugs
Daunorubicin	CNS	First	—	1-normal without IUGR
Doxorubicin	cardiac ocular renal embryolethal	First	—	1-normal 1-premature, normal 1-induced abortion-pheno- type normal (19 weeks)
		First and after	—	1-normal
		Beyond first	—	18-normal 1-normal, leukopenia 2-toxemia, death, pheno- type normal* 4-premature, normal* 1-stillborn, autopsy neg *(Pt. received daunorubicin) 1-normal phenotype and genotype-20 weeks in- duced abortion 1-normal induced abortion 1-normal premature with IUGR and poor neonatal growth
Actinomycin D	CNS optic nerve	First	—	—
		First and after	—	—
		Beyond first	—	1-normal twins 1-normal premature 2-normal
Bleomycin	—	First	—	—
		First and after	—	—
		Beyond first	—	2-normal 1-IUGR, genotype normal
Mithromycin	—	—	—	—

exposure have been catalogued. No malformations occurred. Prematurity complicated five, and in one, IUGR was also noted. Toxemia and in utero fetal demise manifested in two, stillbirth was the result in one, and abortion was induced in two others, the fetuses being phenotypically unremarkable. Nineteen normal outcomes were described, one with documented leukopenia.[26,33,35,37,63.66,75,76,78,79,83–85,88,90,98–100] It has been suggested that doxorubicin does not cross the placenta.[101]

Actinomycin D

Actinomycin D has been reported to cause CNS malformations and optic nerve damage in laboratory animals.[102,103] No first trimester human exposures have been reported. Four infants exposed to actinomycin D in combination regimens after the first trimester were phenotypically normal, one of which was delivered preterm.[10,31,35,36]

Bleomycin

Bleomycin has not been studied in experimental animals. It has been used in combination with other cytotoxic drugs in three gestations after the first trimester. Two normal outcomes and one neonate (genotype normal) with IUGR are documented.[16,36,39]

Mithramycin

Mithramycin has not been studied in animals and its use has not been reported in human pregnancy.

VINCA ALKALOIDS (TABLE 10–4)

Vincristine and Vinblastine

Teratogenic potential of the Vinca alkaloids in animal models is sustained by observation of CNS, ocular, and skeletal malformations.[104–106] In infants exposed to single agent chemotherapy, 14 neonatal outcomes are available. In 12 first

Table 10–4. Pregnancy Outcome After Administration of Vinca Alkaloids

Drug	Animal Malformations	Trimester (humans)	Single Agents (humans)	Given with Other Cytotoxic Drugs
Vincristine	skeletal	First	12-normal	3-normal
Vinblastine	CNS ocular			1-normal premature with IUGR 1-skeletal and digital and ear anomalies 1-induced abortion with renal malformation 1-induced abortion, phenotype normal (19 weeks)
		First and after	—	—
		Beyond first	1-premature, normal 1-normal	24-normal 5-premature, normal 4-IUGR, normal 1-IUGR, premature 1-IUGR, pancytopenia 1-normal, leukopenia 1-normal, induced abortion

trimester exposures, normal outcomes are documented.[107–110] Beyond the first trimester, two normal neonates have been reported, one of which was premature.[10,111] Combination regimens containing the Vinca alkaloids in first trimester exposures are reported to involve 7 pregnancies. Three normal neonates and one premature neonate with IUGR resulted. Conversely, in one gestation, skeletal, digital and ear anomalies occurred and in one induced abortion, renal malformation was observed. A phenotypically normal fetus resulted from a 19-week induced abortion.[14,15,27,75,112]

Beyond the first trimester, Vinca alkaloids used in combination regimens were not associated with malformations in 37 pregnancies. IUGR was observed in 6, prematurity in one, and pancytopenia in one. Prematurity complicated 5 additional pregnancies. Twenty-four normal neonatal outcomes have been reported. One additional normal neonate manifested leukopenia. An induced abortion resulted in a phenotypically normal fetus.[10,12,16,18,26,27,31,33–39,63,65–67,76,80,82,85,90,98,108]

MISCELLANEOUS AGENTS (TABLE 10–5)

Procarbazine

Procarbazine is a known teratogen and carcinogen in animals.[5,113,114] In humans, it has been used once as a single agent in the first trimester of pregnancy without apparent adverse effect.[114] It has been used in combination with other agents in the first trimester in 5 women. Two had a normal outcome,[115,116] one delivered a preterm and growth retarded infant,[13] and one infant had skeletal, digital, and ear anomalies.[14] An induced abortion produced a fetus with renal malformations.[15]

Beyond the first trimester, exposure to procarbazine has occurred in combination regimens in 6 pregnancies. Three were normal, prematurity complicated two, and IUGR was observed in one.[12,18,38,108]

Hydroxyurea

Hydroxyurea is reported to be teratogenic in animals.[5,117–119] It has been used twice in pregnant women, both in combination after the first trimester. One normal fetus was aborted and one preterm, growth retarded, but otherwise normal infant was delivered.[66]

Urethane

Urethane is teratogenic in animals.[5,118] It has been used as a single agent in 8 women; 3 in the first trimester and 5 after the first trimester. In seven cases, the neonatal outcomes were reported as normal.[10,118]

Cis Platinum

The murine model has provided the majority of animal data regarding teratogenicity of cisplatinum. Cleft palate, CNS anomalies, and skeletal defects are documented. Embryolethality and IUGR are also associated with this agent.[120–123]

In one human pregnant exposure, an induced abortion at 10-weeks gestation resulted in a phenotypically normal fetus.[124]

Table 10–5. Pregnancy Outcome After Administration of Miscellaneous Agents

Drug	Animal Malformations	Trimester (humans)	Single Agents (humans)	Given with Other Cytotoxic Drugs
Procarbazine	skeletal limb cleft palate ocular	First	1-normal	1-normal 1-normal premature with IUGR 1-skeletal and digital and ear abnormalities 1-induced abortion renal malformation
		First and after	—	1-normal
		Beyond first	—	3-normal 1-IUGR, normal 2-premature, normal
Hydroxyurea	skeletal limb	First	—	—
	cleft palate CNS	Beyond first	—	1-normal induced abortion 1-normal premature with IUGR
Urethane	+	First	3-	} state of fetus recorded in 7-all normal	—
		Beyond first	5-		—
cis-Platinum	Murine Model IUGR skeletal defects cleft palate CNS anomalies embryolethal	First	1-pregnancy termination 10 weeks-phenotype normal	—
Ethylnitrosourea	skeletal CNS ocular	—	—	—
		First and after	1-normal-genotype & phenotype	—
Methylnitrosourea	CNS	— —	— —	— —
Asparaginase	skeletal pulmonary renal intestinal	— —	— —	— —
		Beyond first	—	1-normal 1-normal-leukopenia
5-Bromo 2'-deoxyuridine	limb digital CNS cleft palate	— — —	— — —	— — —
5-Iodo 2'-deoxyuridine	limb digital cleft palate CNS	— — —	— — —	— — —
Dibromomannitol	—	First and after	1-normal	—
Methylchlorethamine	—	Beyond first	—	1-premature, normal
Cyclosporin A	— —	First and after	1-IUGR, premature 1-normal	—

Nitrosourea

Ethylnitrosourea and methylnitrosourea have been associated with CNS, skeletal and ocular teratogenicity in animal models.[5,115,125–129] Only one human pregnant exposure involving ethylnitrosourea in the first trimester has been reported and this neonate was genotypically and phenotypically normal.[116]

Asparaginase

The potential of Asparaginase as a teratogen in animal models has been demonstrated to show intestinal, pulmonary, renal, and skeletal anomalies.[5,115,125–129] Two exposures to Asparaginase in multi-agent regimens have been documented beyond the first trimester. Normal neonatal outcomes except for leukopenia are reported.[37,100]

Dibromomannitol

Dibromomannitol has been used in one human pregnancy beginning in the first trimester. This single agent application resulted in a normal outcome.[130]

Methylchlorethamine

This agent has been used in one human pregnancy beyond the first trimester in a multi-agent application. A normal neonate, albeit premature resulted.[90]

Cyclosporin A

This cyclic fungal peptide is an immunosuppressive drug with selective T cell activity. With increasing utilization in human transplantation, it has interfaced in recent years with human pregnancy.

In animal studies, embryo and fetotoxicity have been observed; however, no cases of teratogenic effects are documented with Cyclosporin A.[131]

In two human pregnancies, the use of Cyclosporin A beginning in the first trimester resulted in a normal neonate and a premature outcome with IUGR.[132,133]

5-Bromo 2'-deoxyuridine, 5-iodo 2'-deoxyuridine

These two agents have demonstrated teratogenic activity in animals. Cleft palate, CNS anomalies, digital, and other skeletal malformations are documented.[5,115,125–129]

RECOMMENDATIONS

The diverse spectrum of antineoplastic drugs outlined in this chapter is held together by the common property of teratogenic potential in animals. Every agent in which an animal model has been used to investigate teratogenesis, has demonstrated potential for malformation with the exception of Cyclosporin A, which is an immunosuppressive, not an antineoplastic drug. Fortunately, this penchant for developmental anomalies is not observed as dramatically with the human fetus. It should be appreciated, however, that the methodologic approaches in demonstrating teratogenic potential in animal models are substantially different from the exposures to these agents in human pregnancy (see Chapter 1).

The majority of malformations observed in human hosts exposed to chemotherapeutic agents are noted in the first trimester exposures. Exposure to single agents in the first trimester resulted in 13% malformed infants, 11% spontaneous abortions, and 76% ostensibly normal offspring. Combination chemotherapy regimens produced 18% malformed infants, 6% spontaneous abortions, and 76% normal offspring for first trimester exposures.

Chemotherapeutic agents administered after the first trimester resulted in substantially fewer anomalous outcomes. Single agents administered beyond the first trimester resulted in 4.3% malformed, 1.4% spontaneous abortions, and 94.2% normal outcomes. Multi-agent therapy beyond the first trimester led to only 1.1% malformations, 1.6% spontaneous losses, and 97% normal outcomes.

If the chemotherapy preceded the pregnancy, there does not seem to be a teratogenic risk. In 13 women who became pregnant after receiving combination chemotherapy for Hodgkin's disease, 17 pregnancies resulted. Thirteen infants were normal including one set of twins, and three therapeutic abortions were performed. One infant was of low birth weight.[134]

Determining the responsible drug when a multi-agent regimen is associated with an adverse outcome is of course difficult. The distribution of malformations in single agent exposure prevents implicating any one drug class, much less, one agent. In addition, the possible contribution of the neoplastic disease process itself to anomalous development should not be overlooked. Derangements in metabolism and altered nutritional states may result from the malignancy and/or the post therapy condition, and have an unknown impact on the developing fetus.

Recent reports[135] have raised the possibility that chronic exposure by nurses to antineoplastic drugs, specifically cyclophosphamide and daunorubicin might increase the incidence of miscarriage and pregnancy loss. Care in the handling of these substances by those in the reproductive age group should be emphasized.[136]

In animal models, antineoplastic agents have been associated with runting or IUGR. Such effects on the fetus are purportedly dose-dependent phenomena with an impact that extends to alter neonatal growth.[20] The data reviewed herein suggest a 3.9% incidence of IUGR observed with a single agent chemotherapy, and 9.6% with multi-agent exposure. The incidence of prematurity was also 3.9% for the group receiving single agent therapy and 11.4% for multi-agent chemotherapy. IUGR and prematurity appear to function independently for the majority of reported cases; the latter is increased at least with multi-agent exposure.

In both animals and humans, the antineoplastic drug appears to be the cause of IUGR rather than the underlying disease process. Nicholson reported an incidence of IUGR of 40% in 49 women exposed to antineoplastic drugs who delivered after the 28th week of pregnancy. This was compared to 14% in women not receiving drug therapy.[10] The experience reported by Boros with busulfan (only 1 of 11 exposures in the third trimester of appropriate weight for gestational age) further supports this belief.[50]

The management of women with neoplasia in pregnancy poses special clinical challenges largely mandated by concern for the welfare of the developing fetus. The requirement for chemotherapy administration in this setting adds further complication. Fortunately, the observed incidence of fetal malformation associated with first trimester human exposure is less ominous than the animal experience.

For chemotherapy exposure beyond the first trimester, anomalous outcomes are not observed to be greater than the rate in the general population; concerns for IUGR and/or prematurity, however, are appropriate especially for the fetus exposed to multi-agent regimens. Although intervention to prevent these outcomes may not be possible, the increased awareness of potential for inhibited fetal growth should prompt increased fetal surveillance with antepartum electronic monitoring and ultrasound. In addition, since experience with many agents in pregnancy remains limited, every effort should be made to document outcome in pregnancies with chemotherapy exposure. This should include phenotypic as well as genotypic data on neonates and abortuses, as well as long term neonatal outcome when feasible.

ANTINEOPLASTIC DRUGS AND MALE REPRODUCTIVE PEFORMANCE

There are few reports of men successfully fathering offspring while on antineoplastic therapy. This is due in large part to the well-known inhibitory effects of these drugs on testicular function and sperm production.[137–147] Return of spermatogenesis, sometimes 2 to 4 years later, has been shown in a number of studies and successful pregnancies have been reported with normal outcome in men treated with these agents.[85,88,91–93,142,145,148–152] In the rat, chronic cyclophosphamide therapy is reported to cause a high frequency of fetal death with malformations and growth retardation in the surviving fetuses.[153] Congenitally abnormal infants born to two fathers after treatment with ARA-C and daunomycin have been reported.[154] One infant had syndactyly and tetralogy of Fallot and the second had anencephaly. Given the paucity of reports and experimental data, no estimate can be made of the risk of this occurrence. Amniocentesis can permit detection of karyotypic abnormalities, and other biochemical (AFP) and ultrasonic modalities for prenatal diagnosis might be usefully employed.

In the one case[155] of an infant conceived during paternal chemotherapy with 6-mercaptopurine, methotrexate, vincristine, and prednisone for acute lymphoblastic leukemia, pregnancy was uneventful, except for a preterm delivery, and the infant was normal. A previous pregnancy conceived while the father was on the same regimen had aborted spontaneously, and was also karyotypically normal.

Given the sterility induced by the chemotherapeutic agents mentioned and, despite its potential reversibility, sperm storage prior to introduction of therapy should be kept in mind, especiallly if immediate pregnancy is desired. In the event that therapy is unsuccessful or results in permanent sterilization, insemination could be carried out at a later date.

Generally, little is known about the mutagenic effect of antineoplastic agents on spermatogenesis; as more long-term survivors become fathers, our clinical experience will undoubtedly expand.

REFERENCES

1. National Cancer Institute Surveillance, Epidemiology and End Results (SEER) Program (1973–1976). New York, American Cancer Society.
2. Rothman, L.A., Cohen, C.J. and Astriola, J.: Placental and fetal involvement by maternal malignancy. Am J Obstet Gynecol, *116*:1023, 1973.
3. Stutzman, L. and Sohal, J.: Use of anticancer drugs in pregnancy. Clin Obstet Gynecol, *11*:416, 1968.

4. Heinonen, O.P., Slone, D. and Shapiro, L.: Birth Defects and Drugs and Pregnancy. Littleton, Mass., Publishing Sciences Group, Inc., 1977.

5. Chaube, S. and Murphy, M.L.: The teratogenic effects of the recent drugs active in cancer chemotherapy. Adv Teratol, 3:181, 1968.

6. Murphy, M.L., Del Moro, A. and Lacon, C.: The comparative effects of five polyfunctional alkylating agents on the rat fetus with additional notes on the chicken embryo. Ann NY Acad Sci, 68:762, 1958

7. Kalter, H.: Teratology of the Central Nervous System, Chicago, Uiversity of Chicago Press, 1968, pp. 139–140.

8. Barry, R.M., Diamond, H.D. and Craven, L.F.: Influence of pregnancy on the course of Hodgkin's disease. Am J Obstet Gynecol, 84:445, 1962.

9. Zoet, A.G.: Pregnancy complicating Hodgkin's disease. Northwest Med, 49:373, 1950.

10. Nicholson, H.O.: Cytotoxic drugs in pregnancy. J Obstet Gynecol Br Cwlth, 75:307, 1968.

11. Boland, J.: Reticularis: clinical experience with nitrogen mustard in Hodgkin's disease. Br J Radiol, 24:513, 1951.

12. Jones, R.T. and Weinerman, B.H.: MOPP (nitrogen mustard, vincristine, procarbazine, and prednisone) given during pregnancy. Obstet Gynecol, 54:477, 1979.

13. Thomas, P.R.M. and Peckham, M.J.: The investigation and management of Hodgkin's disease in the pregnant patient. Cancer, 38:1433, 1976.

14. Garrett, M.J.: Teratogenic effects of combination chemotherapy. Ann Intern Med, 80:667, 1974.

15. Mennuti, M.T., Shepard, T.H. and Mellman, W.J.: Fetal renal malformation following treatment of Hodgkin's disease during pregnancy. Obstet Gynecol, 46:194, 1975.

16. Oretga, J.: Multiple agents chemotherapy including bleomycin of non- Hodgkins lymphoma during pregnancy. Cancer, 40:1829, 1977.

17. Schein, P.S. and Winokur, S.H.: Immunosuppressive and cytotoxic chemotherapy: long-term complications. Ann Intern Med, 82:84, 1975.

18. Johnson, I.R. and Filshie, G.M: Hodgkin's disease diagnosed in pregnancy. Br J Obstet Gynecol, 84:791, 1977.

19. Chaube, S., Kury, G and Murphy, M.L.: Teratogenic effects of cyclophosphamide in the rat. Cancer Chemother. Rep., 51:363, 1967.

20. Scott, J.R.: Fetal growth retardation associated with maternal administration of immunosuppressive drugs. Am J Obstet Gynecol, 128:668, 1977.

21. Gibson, J.E. and Becker, B.A.: The teratogenicity of cyclophosphamide in mice. Cancer Res, 28:475, 1968.

22. Symington, G.R., Mackay, I.R. and Lambert, R.P.: Cancer and teratogenesis: infrequent occurrence after medical use of immunosuppressive drugs. Aust NZ J Med, 7:368, 1977.

23. Greenberg, L.H. and Tanaka, K.R.: Congenital anomalies probably induced by cyclophosphamide. JAMA, 188:423, 1964.

24. Toledo, T.M., Harper, R.C. and Moser, R.H.: Fetal effects during cyclophosphamide and irradiation therapy. Ann Intern Med, 74:87, 1971.

25. Lergier, J.E., Jimenez, E., Maldonado, N., et al.: Normal pregnancy in multiple myeloma treated with cyclophosphamide. Cancer, 34:1018, 1974.

26. Sears, H.F. and Reid, J.: Granulocytic sarcoma. Cancer, 37:1808, 1976.

27. Pizzuto, J., Aviles, A., N. J., et al.: Treatment of acute leukemia during pregnancy: presentation of nine cases. Cancer Treat Rep, 64:679, 1980.

28. Hardin, J.: Cyclophosphamide treatment of lymphoma during third trimester of pregnancy. Obstet Gynecol, 39:850, 1972.

29. Durodola, J.: Administration of cyclophosphamide during late pregnancy and early lactation: a case report. J Nat Med Assoc, 71:165, 1979.

30. Mehta, A. and Vakil, R.M.: Use of endoxan in case of lymphosarcoma with pregnancy during third trimester. A Case Report Ind J Cancer, 3: 198, 1966.

31. Weed, J.C., Poh, R.A. and Mendenhall, H.W.: Recurrent endodermal sinus tumor during pregnancy. Obstet Gynecol, 54:653, 1979.

32. Krueger, J.A., Davis, R.B. and Field, C.: Multiple drug chemotherapy in the management of acute lymphocytic leukemia during pregnancy. Obstet Gynecol, 48:324, 1976.

33. Abhimanyu, G. and Kochupillai, V.: Non-Hodgkin's lymphoma in pregnancy. So Med J, 78:1263, 1985.

34. Lacher, M.J. and Geller, W.: Cyclophosphamide and vinblastine sulfate in Hodgkin's disease during pregnancy. JAMA, 195:486, 1966.

35. Gililland, J. and Weinstein, L.: The effects of cancer chemotherapeutic agents on the developing fetus. Obstet Gynecol Surv, 38:6, 1983.

36. Haerr, R.W. and Pratt, A.T.: Multiagent chemotherapy for sarcoma diagnosed during pregnancy. Cancer, 56:1028, 1985.

37. Khurshid, M. and Saleem, M.: Acute leukemia in pregnancy. Lancet, 2:534, 1978.

38. Daly, H., McCann, S.R., Hanratty, T.D., et al.: Successful pregnancy during combination chemotherapy for Hodgkin's disease. Acta Haemat, *64*:154, 1980.
39. Falkson, H.C., Simson, I.W. and Falkson, G.: Non-Hodgkin's lymphoma in pregnancy. Cancer, *45*:1679, 1980.
40. Monie, I.W.: Chlorambucil-induced abnormalities on the urogenital system of fetuses. Anat Rec, *139*:145, 1961.
41. Jacobs, C., Donaldson, S.S., Rosenberg, S.A., et al.: Management of the pregnant patient with Hodgkin's disease. Ann Intern Med, *95*:669, 1981.
42. Shotton, D. and Monie, L.W.: Possible teratogenic effect of chlorambucil on a human fetus. JAMA, *186*:74, 1963.
43. Williams, D.W.: Busulfan in early pregnancy. Obstet Gynecol, *27*:738, 1966.
44. Nolan, G.H., Marks, R. and Perez, C.: Busulfan treatment of leukemia during pregnancy. Obstet Gynecol, *38*:136, 1971.
45. Uhl, N., Eberle, P., Quellhorst, E., et al.: Busulfan treatment in pregnancy. A case report with chromosome studies. Ger Med Mon, *14*:383, 1969.
46. Dugdale, M. and Fort., A.T.: Busulfan treatment of leukemia during pregnancy. Case report and review of the literature. JAMA, *199*:131, 1967.
47. Bhisey, A.N., Advani, S.H. and Khare, A.G.: Cytogenetic anomalies in a child born to a mother receiving busulfan for chronic myeloid leukaemia. Ind J Cancer, *19*:272, 1982.
48. Diamond, I., Anderson, M.M. and McCreadie, S.R.: Transplacemental transmission of busulfan in a mother with leukemia: production of fetal malformation and cytomegaly. Pediatrics, *25*:85, 1960.
49. Kadowaki, J., Moghissi, K.S. and Loomus, G.N.: Granulocytic leukemia in pregnancy. Mich Med, *69*:297, 1970.
50. Boros, S.J. and Reynolds, J.W.: Intrauterine growth retardation following third trimester exposure to busulfan. Am J Obstet Gynecol, *129*:111, 1977.
51. Tanimura, T.: Developmental disturbances in the offspring induced by administration of mitomycin C to mice during pregnancy. Acta Anat Nippon, *36*:354, 1961.
52. Thiersch, J.B.: Effect of 2, 4, 6 triamino-"S"-triazine, 2, 4, 6 "Tris" (ethyleneimino)-"S"-Trizine and N, N, N triethylenephosphoramide (TEPA) on rat litter in utero. Proc Soc Exp Biol Med, *94*:36, 1957.
53. Jurand, A.: Action of triethanomelamine on early and later stages of mouse embryos. J Embryol Exp Morphol, *7*:526, 1959.
54. Smith, R.B.W., Sheehy, T.V. and Rothberg, H.: Hodgkins disease and pregnancy. Arch Intern Med, *102*:777, 1958.
55. Wright, J.C., Prigot, A., Logan, M., et al.: The effect of trimethylene melamine and of trimethylene phosphoramide in human neoplastic diseases. Int J Cancer, *11*:220, 1955.
56. Thiersch, J.B.: Effects of certain 2-4 diaminopyrimidine antagonists of folic acid on pregnancy and rat fetus. Proc Soc Exp Biol Med, *87*:571, 1954.
57. Thiersch, J.B. and Philips, F.S.: Effect of 4-animo-pterolyglutamic acid (Aminopterin) on early pregnancy. Proc Soc Exp Biol Med, *74*:204, 1950.
58. Karnofsky, D.A., Poltenar, P.A. and Ridgeway, L.P.: Effects of folic acid, "4-amino" folic acids and related substances on growth of chicken embryo. Proc Soc Exp Biol Med, *71*:447, 1949.
59. Milunsky, A., Graef, J.W. and Gaynor, M.F., Jr.: Methotrexate-induced congenital malformations. J Pediatr, *72*:790, 1968.
60. Shaw, E.B. and Steinbach, H.L.: Aminopterin induced fetal malformation. Am J Dis Child, *115*:477, 1968.
61. Thiersch, J.B.: The control of reproduction in rats with the aid of antimetabolites and early experiences with antimetabolites as abortifacient agents in man. Acta Endocrinol (Suppl) (Kbh), *28*:37, 1956.
62. Adams, C.E., Hay, M.F. and Lutwach,-Mann, C.: The action of various agents upon the rabbit embryo. J Embryol Exp Morphol, *9*:468, 1961.
63. Dara, P, Slater, LM and Arementrout, SA: Successful pregnancy during chemotherapy for acute leukemia. Cancer, *47*:845, 1981.
64. Rubaltelli, F.F., Mittiga, S. and Solito, P.: Growth and development of children born to mothers treated with cytotoxic drugs during pregnancy (letter). Helv Paediatr Acta, *37*:599, 1982.
65. Raich, P.C. and Curet, L.B.: Treatment of acute leukemia during pregnancy. Cancer, *36*:861, 1975.
66. Doney, K.C., Kraemer, F.G. and Shepard, T.H.: Combination chemotherapy for acute myelocytic leukemia during pregnancy: Three case reports. Cancer Treat Rev, *63*:369, 1979.
67. Coopland, A.T, Friesen, W.J. and Galbraith, P.A.: Acute leukemia in pregnancy. Am J Obstet Gynecol, *105*:1288, 1969.
68. Johns, B.G., Rutherford, C.D., Laighton, R.C., et al.: Secretion of methotrexate into human milk. Am J Obstet Gynecol, *112*:978, 1972.

69. Tuchmann-Dulplessis, T. and Mercier-Parot, L.: Production experimentale de malformations des membres. Union Med Can, *97*:283, 1968.
70. Golby, M.: Fertility after renal transplantation. Transplantation, *10*:201, 1970.
71. Leb, D.E., Weisskopf, B. and Kanovitz, B.S.: Chromosome aberrations in the child of a transplant recipient. Arch Intern Med, *128*:441, 1971.
72. Chaube, S. and Murphy, L.S.: The teratogenic effects of cytosine arabinoside on the rat fetus. Proc Am Assoc Cancer Res, *6*:11, 1965.
73. Karnofsky, D.A. and Lacon, C.R.: The effects of 1- -D arabinofuranosyl cytosine on the developing chicken embryo. Biochem Pharmacol, *15*:1435, 1966.
74. Fischer, D.A. and Jones, A.M.: Cerebellar hypoplasia resulting from cytosine arabinoside treatment in the neonatal hamster. Clin Res, *13*:540, 1965.
75. Lilleyman, J.S., Hill, A.S. and Anderson, K.J.: Consequences of acute myelogenous leukemia in early pregnancy. Cancer, *40*:1300, 1977.
76. Fassas, A., Kartalis, G., Klearchou, N., et al.: Chemotherapy for acute leukemia during pregnancy. Five case reports. Nouv Rev Fr Hematol, *26*:19, 1984.
77. Schafer, A.I.: Teratogenic effects of antileukemic chemotherapy. Arch Intern Med, *141*:514, 1981.
78. Hamer, J.W., Beard, M.E.J. and Duff, G.B.: Pregnancy complicated by acute myeloid leukemia. NZ Med J, *89*:212, 1979.
79. Gokal, R., Durrant, J., Baum, J.D., et al.: Successful pregnancy in acute monocytic leukemia. Br J Cancer, *34*:299, 1976.
80. Durie, B.G.M. and Giles, H.R.: Successful treatment of acute leukemia in pregnancy. Arch Intern Med, *137*:90, 1973.
81. Lowenthal, R., Marsden, K.A., Newmann, W.M., et al: Normal infant after treatment of acute myeloid leukemia in pregnancy with daunorubicin. Aust NZ J Med, *8*:431, 1978.
82. Pawliger, D.F., McLean, F.W. and Noyes, W.D.: Normal fetus after cytosine arabinoside therapy. Ann Intern Med, *74*:1012, 1971.
83. O'Donnell, R., Costigan, C. and O'Connell, L.G.: Two cases of acute leukaemia in pregnancy. Acta Haemat, *61*:298, 1979.
84. Cantini, E. and Yanes, B.: Acute myelogenous leukemia in pregnancy. So Med J, *77*: 1050, 1984.
85. Newcomb, M., Balducci, L., Thigpen, J.T., et al.: Acute leukemia in pregnancy. Successful delivery after cytarabine and doxorubicin. JAMA, *239*:2691, 1978.
86. Manoharan, A. and Leyden, M.J.: Acute non-lymphocytic leukaemia in the third trimester of pregnancy. Aust NZ J Med, *9*:71, 1979.
87. Au-Yong, R., Collins, P. and Young, J.A.: Acute myeloblastic leukaemia during pregnancy. Br Med J, *4*:493, 1972.
88. O'Donnell, R., Costigan, C. and O'Connell, L.G.: Two cases of acute leukaemia in prgenancy. Acta Haematol, *61*:298, 1979.
89. Taylor, G. and Blom, J.: Acute leukemia during pregnancy. So Med J, *73*:1314, 1980.
90. Tobias, J.S. and Bloom, H.J.G.: Doxorubicin in pregnancy. Lancet, 776, 1980.
91. Maurer, L.H., Forcier, R.J., McIntyre, O.R., et al.: Fetal group C trisomy after cytosine arabinoside and thioguanine. Ann Intern Med, *75*:809, 1971.
92. Dagg, C.P.: Sensitive stages for the production of developmental abnormalities in mice with 5-fluorouracil. Am J Anat, *106*:89, 1960.
93. Stephens, J.D., Golbus, M.S. and Miller, T.R.: Multiple congenital anomalies in a fetus exposed to 5-fluorouracil during the first trimester. Am J Obstet Gynecol, *137*:747, 1980.
94. Muller, H.: Does nitrogen mustard affect the foetus directly or secondarily by its effect on the mother? Experientia, *22*:247, 1966.
95. Roux, J. and Taillemite, J.L.: Action teratogene de la inibidomycine chez le rat. CR Soc Biol (Paris), *163*:1299, 1969.
96. Sanz, M.A. and Rafecas, F.J: Successful pregnancy during chemotherapy for acute promyelocytic leukemia (letter). N Engl J Med, *306*:939, 1982.
97. Alegre, A., Chunchurreta, R., Rodriguez-Alarcon, J., et al: Successful pregnancy in acute promyelocytic leukemia. Cancer, *49*:152, 1982.
98. Ho, M., Bear, R.A. and Garvey, M.B.: Symptomatic hypophosphatemia secondary to 5-azacytidine therapy of acute non-lymphocytic leukemia. Cancer Treat Rev, *60*:1400, 1976.
99. Karp, G.I., Von Oeyen, P., Valone, F., et al.: Doxorubicin in pregnancy: possible transplacental passage. Cancer Treat Rep, *67*:773, 1983.
100. Awidi, A.S., Tarawneh, M.S., Shubair, K.S., et al.: Acute leukemia in pregnancy: report of five cases treated with a combination which included a low dose of adriamicin. Eur J Cancer Clin Oncol, *19*:881, 1983.
101. Roboz, J., Gleicher, N., Wu, K., et al: Does doxorubicin cross the placenta? Lancet, *2*:1382, 1979.

102. Wilson, J.G.: Effects of acute and chronic treatment with actinomycin D on pregnancy and the fetus in the rat. Harper Hosp Bull, *24*:109, 1966.
103. Wilson, J.G.: Teratogenic interaction of chemical agents in the rat. J Pharmacol Exp Ther, *144*:429, 1964.
104. Cohlan, S.Q. and Kitay, D.: The teratogenic effect of vincaleukoblastine in the pregnant rat. J Pediatr, *66*:541, 1965.
105. Ferm, V.H.: Congenital malformations in hamster embryos after treatment with vinblastine and vincristine. Science, *141*:426, 1963.
106. DeMyer, W.: Cleft lip and jaw induced in fetal rats by vincristine. Arch Anat Histol Embryol (Strasb), *48*:179, 1965.
107. Goguel, A.: Etude de l'influence de la grossesse sur le pronostic et le traitement de la maladie de Hodgkin. La Presse Medicale, *78*:1507, 1970.
108. McCann, S.R., Daley, H., Hanratty, T.D., et al.: Hodgkin's disease and pregnancy. Acta Haematol, *66*:67, 1981.
109. Rosenzweig, A.I., Crews, Q.E., Jr. and Hopwood, H.G.: Vinblastine sulfate in Hodgkin's disease in pregnancy. Ann Intern Med, *61*:108, 1964.
110. Armstrong, J.E., Dyke, R.W., Fouts, P.I., et al.: Delivery of a normal infant during the course of oral vinblastine sulfate therapy for Hodgkin's disease. Ann Intern Med, *61*:106, 1964.
111. Nordlund, J.J., DeVita, V.T. and Gabbone, P.P.: Severe vinblastine-induced leukopenia during late pregnancy with delivery of a normal infant. Ann Intern Med, *69*:581, 1968.
112. Cramblett, H.G., Friedman, J.L. and Najjar, S.: Leukemia in an infant born of a mother with leukemia. N Eng J Med, *259*:727, 1958.
113. Chaube, S. and Murphy, M.L.: The teratogenic effects of 1-methyl-2 para (isopropylcarbamoyl) benzyl hydrazine. Proc Am Assoc Cancer Res, *5*:11, 1964.
114. Wells, J.H., Marshall, J.R. and Carbone, P.P.: Procarbazine therapy for Hodgkin's disease in early pregnancy. JAMA, *205*:935, 1968.
115. Chaube, S. and Swinyard, C.A.: Cellular and biochemical aspects of growth retardation in rat fetuses induced by maternal administration of selected anti-cancer agents. Teratol, *21*:259, 1975.
116. Schapira, D.V. and Chudley, A.E.: Successful pregnancy following continuous treatment with combination chemotherapy before conception and throughout pregnancy. Cancer, *54*:800, 1984.
117. Ferm, V.H.: Teratogenic activity of hydroxyurea. Lancet, *1*:1339, 1965.
118. Ferm, V.H.: Severe development malformations induced by urethane and hydroxyurea in the hamster. Arch Pathol, *81*:174, 1966.
119. Chaube, S. and Murphy, M.L.: The effects of hydroxyurea and related compounds on the rat fetus. Cancer Res, *26*:1448, 1966.
120. Kopf-Maier, P.: Stage of pregnancy-dependent transplacental passage of 195 m Pt after cis-Platinum treatment. Eur J Cancer & Clin Oncol, *19*:533, 1983.
121. Kopf-Maier, P.: Erkenswick, P. and Merker, J.J.: Lack of severe malformations versus occurrence of marked embryotoxic effects after treatment of pregnant mice with cis-Plastinum. Toxicol, *34*:321, 1985.
122. Lazar, R., Conran, P.C. and Damjanov, I.: Embryotoxicity and teratogenicity of Cis-diamminedichloroplatinum. Experentia, *35*:647, 1979.
123. Keller, K.A. and Aggarwal, S.K: Embryotoxicity of cisplatin in rats and mice. Toxicol & Appl Pharmacol, *69*:245, 1983.
124. Jacobs, A.J. Marchevsky, A., Gordon, R.E., et al: Oat cell carcinoma of the uterine cervix in a pregnant woman treated with Cis-diamminedichloroplatinum. Gyn Oncol, *9*:405, 1980.
125. Lazar, R., Conran, P.C. and Damjanov, I.: Embryotoxicity and teratogenicity of CIS-diamminedichloroplatinum. Experientia, *35*:647, 1979.
126. Druchery, H., Ivankovic, S. and Preussmann, R.: Teratogenic and carcinogenic effects in the offspring after a single injection of ethylintrosurea to pregnant rats. Nature, *210*:1378, 1966.
127. Alexandrov, V.A. and Janisch, W.: Die teratogene wirkung von Athylharnstoff und nitrit bei ratten. Experientia, *27*:538, 1970.
128. Koyama, T., Handa, J., Handa, H., et al.: Methylnitrosourea-induced malformations. Arch Neurol, *22*:342, 1970.
129. Adamson, R.H., Fabro, S., Hahn, M.A., et al.: Evaluation of the embryotoxic activity of L-Asparaginase. Arch Int Pharmacodyn Ther, *186*:310, 1970.
130. Bruder, M.L., Prager, D. and Renninger, C.W.: Dibromomannitol therapy of chronic myelogenous leukemia during pregnancy. Obstet Gynecol, *43*:54, 1974.
131. Ryffel, B.: Experimental toxicological studies with cyclosporin A. *In* Cyclosporin A, (ed.) White, D.J.G., Amsterdam, Elsevier, 1982, p.45.
132. Klinntmalm, G., Althoff, P., Appleby, G., et al.: Renal function in a newborn baby delivered in a renal transplant patient taking cyclosporine. Transplantation, *38*:198, 1984.
133. Lewis, G.J., Lamont, C.A.R., Lee, H.A., et al.: Successful pregnancy in a renal transplant recipient taking cyclosporin A. Br Med J, *286*:603, 1983.
134. Horning, S.J., Hoppe, R.T., Kaplan, H.S., et al.: Female reproductive potential after treatment for Hodgkin's disease. N Engl J Med, *304*:1377, 1981.

135. Selevan, S.G., Lindbohm, M.L. Hornung, R.W., et al.: A study of occupational exposure to antineoplastic drugs and fetal loss in nurses. N Engl J Med, *313*:1173, 1985.

136. Antineoplastic drugs and spontaneous abortion in nurses. (Letter) N Engl J Med, *314*:1048, 1986.

137. Richter, P., Claamera, J.C., Morgenfeod, M.C., et al.: Effect of chlorambucil on spermatogenesis in the human with malignant lymphoma. Cancer, *25*:1026, 1970.

138. Jackson, H.: Antispermatogenic agents. Br Med Bull, *26*:79, 1970.

139. Miller, D.G.: Alkylating agents and human spermatogenesis. JAMA, *217*:1662, 1971.

140. Fairley, K.F., Barrie, J.U. and Johnson, W.: Sterility and testicular atrophy related to cyclophosphamide therapy. Lancet, *1*:568, 1972.

141. Kumar, R., McEvoy, J., Biggard, J.D., et al: Cyclophosphamide and reproductive function. Lancet, *1*:1212, 1972.

142. Hinkes, E. and Plotkin, D.: Reversible drug induced sterility in a patient with acute leukemia. JAMA, *223*:1490, 1973.

143. Shering, R.J. and Devita, V.T.: Effect of drug treatment for lymphoma on male reproductive capacity: studies of men in remission after therapy. Ann Intern Med, *79*:216, 1973.

144. Asbjornsen, G., Molne, K., Klepp, O., et al.: Testicular function after combination chemotherapy for Hodgkin's disease. Scand J Haematol, *16*:66, 1976.

145. Blake, D.A., Heller, R.H., Hsu, S.H., et al.: Return of fertility in a patient with cyclophosphamide-induced azoospermia. Johns Hopkins Med J, *139*:20, 1978.

146. Roeser, H.P., Stocks, A.E. and Smith, A.J.: Testicular damage due to cytotoxic drugs and recovery after cessation of therapy. Aust NZ J Med, *8*:250, 1978.

147. Lenden, M., Plamer, M.K., Hann, M., et al.: Testicular histology after combination chemotherapy in childhood for acute lymphoblastic leukemia. Lancet, *2*:439, 1978.

148. Lilleyman, J.S.: Male fertility after successful chemotherapy for lymphoblastic leukemia. Lancet, *2*:1125, 1979. (letter)

149. Shani, A., Talpaz, M., Chemke, J., et al.: Absence of chromosomal changes in fetus after paternal chemotherapy. Lancet, *2*:637, 1979. (letter)

150. Li, F.P. and Jaffe, N.: Progeny of childhood cancer survivors. Lancet, *2*:707, 1974.

151. Rubery, E.D.: Return of fertility after curative chemotherapy for disseminated teratoma of testis. Lancet *1*:186, 1983.

152. Damewood, M.D. and Grochow, L.B.: Prospects for fertility after chemotherapy or radiation for neoplastic disease. Fertil Steril, *45*:443, 1986.

153. Trasler, J.M., Hales, B.F. and Robaire, B.: Paternal cyclophosphamide treatment of malformations without affecting male fertility. Nature, *316*:144, 1985.

154. Russell, J.A., Powles, R.L. and Oliver, R.T.D.: Conception and congenital abnormalities after chemotherapy of acute myelogenous leukaemia in two men. Br Med J, *1*:1508, 1976.

155. Kroner, T.H. and Tschuma, A.: Conception of a normal child during chemotherapy of acute lymphoblastic leukaemia in the father. Br Med J, *1*:1322, 1977.

Chapter 11

Progestins in Pregnancy

John W.C. Johnson

Progesterone is generally referred to as the "hormone of pregnancy," and many animal investigations do demonstrate that its principal effect is to maintain pregnancy and to prolong it. It has been more than a half century since Corner and Allen[1] first isolated progesterone, and more than a quarter century since the potent analogues, hydroxyprogesterone acetate and 17-alpha-hydroxyprogesterone caproate, were synthesized.[2] Despite the fact that progesterone and a number of other synthetic progestins are presently available, their clincal use to treat problems in pregnancy remains highly debatable. In fact, few pregnant women are treated with progestins. Conversely, nonpregnant women probably receive greater quantities of progestins than any other administered hormone. These circumstances seem all the more confusing in view of the fact that the data from a number of studies strongly suggest that progestins do have therapeutic uses in a number of cirumstances in human pregnancy. Widespread use of these agents in the United States has undoubtedly been curtailed by the FDA refusal to approve the use of these agents in early pregnancy and concerns about teratogenicity. In this chapter, we will discuss the physiology and pharmacology of progestins, their utilizaton in pregnancy, and the current information regarding possible adverse effects.

PROGESTINS

Although progestins are defined as hormones capable of inducing secretory change in estrogen-primed endometria, their primary biologic function appears to be the maintenance of pregnancy.[3] Studies in animal species have demonstrated that progestogens can maintain pregnancy after oophorectomy, and can delay the onset of labor or delivery.[3]

The synthesis of progesterone takes place in the adrenal gland, the testes, and the ovarian follicle, where it functions primarily as an intermediate for other steroids. It also is a major steroid product of the corpus luteum and placenta.[4] It is possible that the fetal membranes may also engage in progesterone synthesis. Gant and co-workers have reported that a microsomal fraction prepared from the chorion may produce progesterone.[5] Schwarz et al. have identified a protein in human amnion and chorion that appears to bind progesterone.[6] It has been hypothesized that increased concentrations of this specific binding protein could result in a "progesterone withdrawal" in close proximity to the myometrium, without detectable changes being evident in the peripheral plasma.

Although all of these tissues can synthesize progesterone from acetate, it is generally derived from circulating chlolesterol. During the follicular phase of the cycle, the production rate of progesterone is about 2.6 mg per 24 hours, whereas in the secretory phase it reaches 22 mg per 24 hours.[7] At the halfway point in pregnancy, production is about 75 mg per day, with the majority coming form the placenta and about one third coming from extraplacental sites including the maternal ovaries. Near the end of pregnancy, the placenta may produce progesterone at the rate of 250 to 300 mg per 24 hours. Most of the progesterone is secreted into the uterine venous blood, whereas 10% is transported to the fetus.[8]

In assessing the teratogenic risks for the fetus, it is important to review the normal metabolic relationships between progesterone and the fetus. The available evidence suggests that progesterone produced by the placenta is metabolized primarily by the fetal adrenal glands to form corticosteroids and the fetal liver to form pregnanetriol and pregnanediol.[3] Studies utilizing tritiated pregnanediol have demonstrated that the fetal liver, spinal cord, and brain are the area that display the highest concentrations. Similar findings have been noted with progesterone. Apparently, there is no conjugation or metabolism of progesterone in nervous tissue. Fetal neural tissue appears to be saturated with progesterone, and probably does not have the capacity for additional progesterone uptake.[9]

Csapo and Pulkkinen[10] demonstrated that removal of the corpus luteum of human pregnancy prior to 7 weeks resulted in abortion. However, if the corpus luteum was not removed until 9 weeks of pregnancy, abortion did not occur because of the placental production of progesterone. A progesterone antagonist, RU-486, has been shown to bind to progesterone receptors, displacing progesterone. This antagonist has an affinity for progesterone receptors reported to be eight-fold that of progesterone itself. It has been demonstrated to be an effective abortifacient when used early in pregnancy.[11]

Interestingly, most of the known progesterone effects that occur in late pregnancy are achieved by much smaller quantities of progesterone than are ordinarily secreted by the human placenta. Why such large amounts are produced in pregnancy is not understood.

Animal studies indicate that progesterone inhibits the onset of labor in a number of ways: there is an inhibition of the effect of oxytocin; there is a reduction in prostaglandin F2-alpha synthesis, a reduction in the myometrial sensitivity to prostaglandin F2-alpha, a reduction in alpha-adrenergic effects, and a decrease in the formation of intercellular gap junctions.[12]

Although it is generally believed that progesterone does play a significant role in human parturition, efforts to demonstrate decreases in serum progesterone (or relative increases in serum estradiol) in association with labor have yielded opposite results. Whereas a number of authors have found a reduction in peripheral plasma values in conjunction with term or preterm labor,[13,14,15,16] others have not been able to demonstrate such changes.[17] The wide fluctuations in plasma steroid values might account for these changes. Urine or saliva steroid assays may serve to integrate these moment-to-moment variations in plasma concentrations. Hercz[8] has demonstrated an increase in the estradiol to progesterone ratio in the urine samples of patients in preterm labor, and Lachelin[18] has found an increase in the same ratio in the saliva of patients prior to human labor.

PHARMACOLOGY

Progesterone preparations are available for oral, sublingual, nasal, vaginal, rectal and intramuscular administration.[19] Previously, oral progesterone had not been found to be effective because of its poor absorption and relatively short half-life. Recently, it has been determined that micronized progesterone can be taken orally with effective absorption and detectable plasma progesterone changes.[20] Although assay methods vary, a review of the literature by Steege et al.[19] suggests that progesterone bioavailability may not vary linearly with larger doses but asymptomatically, reaching a plateau even with increasing doses.

Several decades ago, when it was thought that the oral route was not an effective means of administering this hormone, synthetic analogues were developed which could be given intramuscularly and which had prolonged half-lives. Two such preparations which continue to be used today are medroxyprogesterone acetate and 17-alpha-hydroxyprogesterone caproate (17-OHPC). These or similar synthetics may be the only convenient means of achieving higher plasma and end organ levels. Progesterone effects on the estrogen primed endometrium are readily attained with these compounds. These synthetic progestins may have reduced affinity for myometrial progesterone receptors and therefore less than optimal effects on this end organ, unless high dosages are utilized.

The pharmaceutical company that originally marketed 17-OHPC, no longer does so, since their patent expired. They no longer find it profitable to manufacture this preparation. However, at least ten generic preparations are available through other companies, such as Prodrox (Arizona), Hyrex Pharmaceuticals (Memphis, TN), Hauck Pharmaceuticals (Georgia), Keene Pharmaceuticals (Texas), Vortech Pharmaceuticals (Dearborne, MI), and O'Neal Pharmaceuticals (Missouri).

CLINICAL USE OF PROGESTINS IN PREGNANCY

Use of Progestins in the First Half of Pregnancy

Progesterone vaginal suppositories, as well as progesterone in oil, are used by a number of investigators to treat the luteal phase defect, which is thought to be etiologic in some repeated spontaneous abortions.[12,21] 17-OHPC may also be used for this purpose, and is utilized extensively in patients undergoing in vitro fertilization and embryo transfer.[3,22] Although there is a large number of physicians who feel strongly that these agents have therapeutic efficacy, there are no prospective controlled studies to substantiate these claims.[23]

Use of Progestins in the Last Half of Pregnancy

Studies of the efficacy of progestins in disorders of pregnancy have been difficult to undertake. It may require 24 to 48 hours for steroids to produce their effects, and it may be difficult to identify obstetric problems far enough in advance to facilitate timely utilization. Once premature labor is imminent or has begun, there may not be enough time remaining for supplemental progestins to have a beneficial effect. Progesterone has a short half-life, and large dosages might have to be administered over a prolonged period of time in order for sufficient plasma or target organ concentrations to be achieved. Last but not least, although teratogenic risks appear to be very low, these cannot be completely disregarded on the basis of our current information. Even remote possibilities of fetal teratogenic risks understandably concern physicians and patients.

A number of investigators in past years have not been able to effectively inhibit labor in human patients by administering progesterone intravascularly.[24] These negative results could be explained by the fact that too little medication was given too late. There have been more recent studies where the progestins were given earlier, that indicate these agents may be helpful in certain pregnancy circumstances.

The prevention of preterm labor with 17-OHPC has met with modest success. Both Reifenstein[25] and Sherman[26] presented preliminary evidence that this agent seemed effective in preventing preterm labor in certain high-risk pregnancies. Johnson and his co-workers reported in a pilot study that patients with a history of previous preterm deliveries and/or spontaneous abortions benefited from the utilization of this agent.[27] In their prospective double-blind study, they found that 250 mg of 17-OHPC once weekly was associated with a statistically significant increase in the mean duration of pregnancy and mean birth weight, as well as a significant reduction in the incidence of prematurity and perinatal mortality. Additional patients were reported by this group of investigators in 1979, with similar but less dramatic results.[15]

Yemini et al.[28] recently reported that 17-OHPC administered to patients at high risk for preterm labor experienced a longer duration of pregnancy and a lower incidence of preterm delivery than placebo-treated controls. Kauppila et al.[29] reported that 17-OHPC and corticosteroids were more effective than beta agonists in prolonging the duration of pregnancy in patients in preterm labor. A number of French studies are alleged to have shown efficacy in the case of 17-OHPC in preventing preterm labor.[30,3,31,32] More recently, Erny and co-workers[33] reported that oral micronized progesterone effectively inhibits preterm labor.

Berkowitz and co-workers[34] reported the outcomes of pregnancies complicated by early gestational bleeding with and without hormonal treatment. In this retrospective study, and using a logistic regresson model, they reported that pregnant women treated with progestins had significantly less risk of preterm delivery and low birth weight than those not treated with hormones. Although there are serious limitations to this study, it does represent one of the largest regarding the efficacy of hormonal treatment in early pregnancy.

In another controlled study, Hartikainen-Sorri[35] found the prophylactic use of 17-OHPC in twin pregnancies was ineffective in prolonging the duration of pregnancy, although treatment was started late. Hauth and his co-workers found that 250 mgm of 17-OHPC, given twice weekly, did not reduce the incidence of preterm delivery in an obstetric population at low risk for prematurity.[36] Their results could be criticized on the basis of a Type 2 statistical error, since the number of patients was insufficient to discount a beneficial effect on the incidence of prematurity.

Another proposed indication for the use of progestins in pregnancy has been to reduce the incidence of premature delivery associated with pelvic surgery. Kaltreider and Kohl[37] reported that patients with appendicitis were at threefold increased risk of preterm delivery. It has been suggested that surgical manipulation or the stress of the surgical procedure might trigger labor under such circumstances and that supplemental progesterone might reduce the frequency of this problem. There have been few prospective studies to evaluate such an effect. Hill and his co-workers[38] reviewed retrospectively their experience in regard to the efficacy of 17-OHPC in pregnant patients undergoing abdominal surgery. In this case-controlled study, they found no statistically significant difference in pregnancy wastage between patients treated with 17-OHPC and controls. However, of the two preterm deliveries in the treated patient group, one occurred 14 weeks after the surgery in association with abruptio placentae, and the other occurred 10 days after a surgical procedure for ruptured appendicitis. The dosage regimens were not provided from this study. If one excludes the preterm delivery occurring 3 months after surgery in the 17-OHPC treated population, the preterm delivery rates tend to be in favor of progesterone prophylaxis (2.8% versus 8.6%)

ADVERSE EFFECTS OF PROGESTINS

The adverse side effects and potential teratogenic risks must be considered in assessing the use of these medications. Possible maternal side effects include drug sensitivity,[39] hypercalcemia, cholestatic jaundice, postpartum hemorrhage, postpartum amenorrhea, lactation abnormalities, and impaired gallbladder function.[40] Such adverse reactions must be extremely uncommon, however. Aside from occasional bruising at the site of the injection, Johnson et al. reported no untoward reactions in their patients who received 17-OHPC.[15]

Studies in rats have failed to show that progesterone at high dosages has any effects on the mother or the fetus.[41] 17-alpha-Hydroxyprogesterone (17-OHP) is produced in substantial amounts by the corpus luteum of early pregnancy.[42] It seems unlikely that this compound could be teratogenic. However, 17-OHPC, which is derived from 17-OHP, is a much more potent and long acting progestin. Previous laboratory[43] and clinical experience tends to refute the possibility that 17-OHPC is a teratogen. Reifenstein reviewed a number of pregnancies in which 17-OHPC was administered early in pregnancy and no increase in anomalies was noted.[44] Johnson reported the same findings.[15] Recent evidence has suggested that 17-OHPC, given prior to the sixteenth week, might be associated with hypospadias in the newborn,[45] but other investigators have not been able to confirm this concern.[46]

There have been several retrospective case control studies linking progestational and estrogenic agents (alone or in combination) to cardiovascular abnormalities, central nervous system defects, limb reduction defects, and multiple congenital anomalies (VACTERL).[47] Very few of these previous studies have made an effort to distinguish between the various sex steroids, their dosages, and the time in pregnancy that they were taken. Other studies that have attempted to control for these variables have not found these same associations. More recent studies by Check,[48] Smith,[49] Wilson,[50] Wiseman,[51] Katz,[52] Rock,[53] Resseguie,[54] and Michaelis[55] tend to refute the hypothesis that progesterone, 17-OHPC, or medroxyprogesterone acetate are teratogenic.

Although these studies are encouraging in regard to short-term adverse effects, no systematic investigation has been undertaken to determine what the long-term adverse effects of the progestational agents might be. There is no statistical evidence that progesterone or 17-OHPC administered in the early weeks of pregnancy is associated with vaginal or cervical lesions such as those described after prenatal exposure to diethylstilbestrol.[56] Reinisch[57] has reported that prenatal progestin treatment may have long-term effects on the infant's personality. Dalton[58,59] concluded from her studies that prenatally administered progesterone not only accelerated childhood development, but enhanced academic performance. However, Lynch et al. could not confirm these effects.[9] It is obvious from these conflicting studies that until the teratogenic risks of each progestational agent have been clearly identified, these agents should be used with caution in pregnancy.

SUMMARY

An increasing number of studies tend to support the hypothesis that progestational agents are useful in maintaining the duration of human pregnancies. Although the risks of progestational treatment appear to be minimal, their exact extent has not been clearly delineated.

The Food and Drug Administration (FDA) first issued their warning in 1975 that all progestational agents might be teratogenic and therefore should be withheld during the early months of pregnancy. Although this warning was based on a number of retrospective studies in which the types, quantities, and timing of sex hormone therapy in early pregnancy were not clearly defined, the FDA has not lifted its ban. This is despite the fact that the Obstetrics and Gynecology Advisory Committee to the FDA recommended that their ban on the use of progesterone and 17-OHPC in early pregnancy be lifted. Additional clinical studies are needed to identify the benefits and risks of these hormonal agents. In the meantime, physicians who elect to use these agents should provide to their patients the package insert recommended by the FDA and should obtain an informed consent in writing from the patient.

REFERENCES

1. Corner, G.W. and Allen, W.M.: Physiology of the corpus luteum; production of special uterine reaction (progestational proliferation) by extracts of corpus luteum. Am J Physiol, *88*:326, 1929.
2. Cohen, M.R., Frank R. and Dresner, M.H.: The use of a new long-acting progestational steroid (17-alpha-hydroxyprogesterone caproate) in the therapy of secondary amenorrhea: A preliminary report. Am J Obstet Gynecol, *72*:1103, 1956.
3. Johnson, J.W.C. and Dubin, N.H.: Progestins in the Prevention of Preterm Birth, in Fuchs, F., and Stubblefield, P.G. (eds): Preterm Birth: Causes, Prevention, and Management. New York, Macmillan Publishing Co. 1984, pp. 197–206.
4. Mauvais-Jarvis, P.: Progesterone and Progestins: A General Overview, in Bardin, C.W., Milgrom, E. and Mauvais-Jarvis, P. (eds): Progesterone and Progestins. New York, Raven Press, 1983, pp. 1-16.
5. Gant, N.F., Milewich, L., Calvert, M.E., et al.: Steroid sulfatase activity in human fetal membranes. J Clin Endocrinol Metab, *45*:965, 1977.
6. Schwarz, B.E., Milewich, L, Johnston, J.M., et al: Intiation of human parturition: V. Progesterone binding substance in fetal membranes. Obstet Gynecol, *48*:685, 1976.
7. Landau, R.L., Bergenstal, D.M., Lugibihl, K, et al: The metabolic effects of progesterone in man. J Clin Endocrinol Metab, *15*:1194, 1955.
8. Hercz, P.: Quantitative changes in steroid and peptide hormones in the maternal-fetoplacental system between the 28th-40th weeks of pregnancy. Acta Med Hung, *42*:29, 1985.
9. Lynch, A. and Mychalkiw, W.: Prenatal progesterone II. Its role in the treatment of pre-eclamptic toxaemia and its effect on the offspring's intelligence: A reappraisal. Early Hum Dev, *2*:323, 1978.
10. Csapo, A.I. and Pulkkinen, M.: Indispensability of the human corpus luteum in the maintenance of early pregnancy; luteectomy evidence. Obstet Gynecol Surv, *33*:69, 1978.
11. Vervest, H.A.M. and Haspels, A.A.: Preliminary results with the antiprogestational compound RU-486 (mifepristone) for interruption of early pregnancy. Fertil Steril, *44*:627, 1985.
12. Fainstat, T. and Bhat, N.: Recurrent Abortion and Progesterone Therapy, in Bardin, C.W.,

Milgrom, E. and Mauvais-Jarvis, P. (eds): Progesterone and Progestins. New York, Raven Press, 1983, pp. 259–276.

13. Cousins, L.M., Hobel, C.J, Chang, R.J., et al.: Serum progesterone and estradiol-17 beta levels in premature and term labor. Am J Obstet Gynecol, *127*:612, 1977.

14. Dubin, N.H., Moszkowski, E.F., Kavoussi, K.M., et al.: Serum progesterone and estradiol in pregnant women selected for progestagen treatment. Int J Fertil, *24*:86, 1979.

15. Johnson, J.W.C., Lee, P.A., Zachary, A.S., et al.: High-risk prematurity—progestin treatment and steroid studies. Obstet Gynecol, *54*:412, 1979.

16. TambyRaja, R.L., Anderson, A.B. and Turnbull, A.C.: Endocrine changes in premature labour. Br Med J, *4*:67, 1974.

17. Block, B.S.B., Liggins, G.C. and Creasy, R.K.: Preterm delivery is not predicted by serial plasma estradiol or progesterone concentration measurements. Am J Obstet Gynecol, *150*:716, 1984.

18. Lachelin, G.C.L. and McGarrigle, H.H.G.: Increasing saliva (free) estriol (E3)/ progesterone (P) ratio before onset of human labor. Abstract #241. Program Scientific Sessions, 1985, p. 137.

19. Steege, J.F., Rupp, S.L., Stout, A.L., et al.: Bioavailability of nasally administered progesterone. Fertil Steril, *46*:727, 1986.

20. Ferre, F., Uzan, M., Janssens, Y., et al.: Oral administration of micronized natural progesterone in late human pregnancy. Am J Obstet Gynecol, *148*:26, 1984.

21. Wentz, A.C., Herbert, C.M., Maxson, W.S., Garner C.H.: Outcome of progesterone treatment in luteal phase inadequacy. Fertil Steril, *41*:856, 1984.

22. Ng, S.C. and Ratnam, S.S.: Endometrial reaction after embryo replacement: A report of two cases. J Reprod Med, *30*:621, 1985.

23. Andrews, W.C.: Luteal phase defects. Fertil Steril, *32*:501, 1979.

24. Johnson, J.W.C.: 17-Alpha-Hydroxprogesterone Caproate in Pregnancy, in Niebyl JR: Drug Use in Pregnancy. Philadelphia, Lea & Febiger, 1982, pp. 91–102.

25. Reifenstein, E.C.: Clinical use of 17-alpha-hydroxyprogesterone 17-n-caproate in habitual abortion. Ann NY Acad Sci, *71*:762, 1958.

26. Sherman, A.I.: Hormonal therapy for control of the incompetent os of pregnancy. Obstet Gynecol, *28*:198, 1966.

27. Johnson, J.W.C., Austin, K, Jones, G.S., et al.: Efficacy of 17-alpha-hydroxyprogesterone caproate in the prevention of premature labor. N Engl J Med, *293*:675, 1975.

28. Yemini, M.., Borenstein, R., Dreazen, E., et al.: Prevention of premature labor by 17-alpha-hydroxyprogesterone caproate. Am J Obstet Gynecol, *151*:574, 1985.

29. Kauppila, A., Hartikainen-Sorri, A., Janne, O., et al.: Suppression of threatened premature labor by administration of cortisol and 17-alpha-hydroxyprogesterone caproate: A comparison with ritodrine. Am J Obstet Gynecol, *138*:404, 1980.

30. Breart, G., Lanfranchi, M., Chavigny, C., et al: A comparative study of the efficiency of hydroxyprogesterone caproate and of chlormadinone acetate in the prevention of premature labor. Int J Obstet Gynecol, *16*:381, 1979.

31. Lepage, F., Sureau, C. and Guillaume, M.F.: La prevention de l'accouchement premature par l'acetate de chlormadinone. Bull Fe Soc Gyn Obst LF *22*, No 5 Bis, 404, 1970.

32. Sureau, C., Germain, G., Ferre, F., et al.: Therapeutic Use of Progesterone During the Last Two Trimesters of Pregnancy, in Bardin, C.W., Milgrom, E., and Mauvais-Jarvis, P. (eds): Progesterone and Progestins. New York, Raven Press, 1983, pp. 247–258.

33. Erny, R., Pigne, A., Prouvost, C.: The effects of oral administration of progesterone for premature labor. Am J Obstet Gynecol, *154*:525, 1986.

34. Berkowitz, G.S., Harlap, S., Beck, G.J., et al: Early gestational bleeding and pregnancy outcome: A multivariable analysis. Int J Epidemiol, *12*:165, 1983.

35. Hartikainen-Sorri, A., Kauppila, A., and Tuimaia, R.: Inefficacy of 17-alpha-hydroxyprogesterone caproate in the prevention of prematurity in twin pregnancy. Obstet Gynecol, *56*:692, 1980.

36. Hauth, J.C., Gilstrap, L.C., Brekken, A.L., et al: The effect of 17-alpha-hydroxyprogesterone caproate on pregnancy outcome in an active-duty military population. Am J Obstet Gynecol, *146*:187, 1983.

37. Kaltreider, D.F. and Kohl, S.: Epidemiology of Preterm Delivery, in Johnson, J.W.C. (ed): Obstetric Aspects of Preterm Delivery, Clinical Obstetrics and Gynecology. Hagerstown, Maryland, Harper and Row, 1980, p. 17.

38. Hill, L.M., Johnson, C.E. and Lee, R.A.: Prophylactic use of hydroxyprogesterone caproate in abdominal surgery during pregnancy: A retrospective evaluation. Obstet Gynecol, *46*:287, 1975.

39. Meggs, W.J., Pescovitz, O.H., Metcalfe, D., et al.: Progesterone sensitivity as a cause of recurrent anaphylaxis. N Engl J Med, *311*:1236, 1984.

40. Shaffer, E.A., Taylor, P.J., Logan, K., et al: The effect of a progestin on gallbladder function in young men. Am J Obstet Gynecol, *148*:504, 1984.

41. Coyle, I.R., Ankers, R. and Cragg, B.: Behavioral, biochemical, and histological effects of prenatal administration of progesterone in the rat. Pharmacol Biochem Behav, *5*:587, 1976.

42. Yoshimi, T., Strott, C.A. and Marshall, J.R.: Corpus luteum function in early pregnancy. J Clin Endocrinol Metab, *29*:225, 1969.
43. Seegmiller, R.E., Nelson, G.W. and Johnson, C.K.: Evaluation of the teratogenic potential of Delalutin (17-alpha-hydroxyprogesterone caproate) in mice. Teratology, *28*:201, 1983.
44. Reifenstein, E.C., Jr: Introduction of marked as well as prolonged biologic activity by esterification: 17-alpha-hydroxyprogesterone caproate, a unique progestational compound. Fertil Steril, *8*:50, 1957.
45. Aarskog, D.: Maternal progestins as a possible cause of hypospadias. N Engl J Med, *300*:75, 1979.
46. Avellan, L.: On aetiological factors in hypospadias. Scand J Plast Reconstr Surg, *11*:115, 1977.
47. Nora, J.J., Nora, A.H. and Wexler, P.: How teratogenic are the sex steroids? Contemp OB/GYN, Feb 1983, p. 39.
48. Check, J.H. Rankin A. and Teichman, M: The risk of fetal anomalies as a result of progesterone therapy during pregnancy. Fertil Steril, *45*:575, 1986.
49. Smith, E.S.O., Dafoe, C.S. and Miller, J.R.: An epidemiologic study of congenital limb reduction deformities of the limbs. Br J Prev Soc Med, *31*:39, 1977.
50. Wilson, J.G. and Brent, R.L.: Are female sex hormones teratogenic? Am J Obstet Gynecol, *141*:567, 1981.
51. Wiseman, R.A. and Dodds-Smith, I.C.: Cardiovascular birth defects and antenatal exposure to female sex hormones: A reevaluation of some base data. Teratology, *30*:359, 1984.
52. Katz, Z., Lancet. M., Skornik, J., et al.: Teratogenicity of progestogens given during the first trimester of pregnancy. Obstet Gynecol, *65*:775, 1985.
53. Rock, J.A., Wentz, A.C., Cole, K.A., et al.: Fetal malformations following progesterone therapy during pregnancy: A preliminary report. Fertil Steril, *44*:17, 1985.
54. Resseguie, L.J., Hick, J.F., Bruen, J.A., et al.: Congenital malformation among offspring exposed in utero to progestins, Olmsted County, Minnesota, 1936–1974. Fertil Steril, *43*:514, 1985.
55. Michaelis, J., Michaelis, H., Gluck, E., et al.: Prospective study of suspected associations between certain drugs administered during early pregnancy and congenital malformations. Teratology, *27*:57, 1983.
56. Scully, R.E., Robboy, S.J. and Welch, W.R.: Pathology and Pathogenesis of Diethylstilbestrol-related Disorders of the Female Genital Tract, in Herbst, A.L.: Intrauterine Exposure to Diethylstilbestrol in the Human. Chicago, The American College of Obstetricians and Gynecologists. 1978.
57. Reinisch, J.M.: Prenatal exposure of human foetuses to synthetic progestin and oestrogen affects personality. Nature, *226*:561, 1977.
58. Dalton, K.: Antenatal progesterone and intelligence. Br J Psychiatry, *114*:1377, 1968.
59. Dalton, K.: Prenatal progesterone and educational attainment. Br J Psychiatry, *129*:438, 1976.
60. Acosta, Anibal A.: Personal communication. February 26, 1986.

Chapter 12

Corticosteroid Therapy in the Prevention of Respiratory Distress Syndrome

Ronald L. Thomas

All practicing obstetricians are well aware of the tremendous strides which have been made in neonatology over the last two decades. The age of presumed and possible viability has been markedly lowered; survival for the premature infant at early gestational ages has been tremendously increased. The seventeenth edition (1985) of *William's Obstetrics* notes a survival of 60% for infants weighing 900 to 999 g.[1] This compares to <20 to 40% for the same weight category published in the twelfth edition (1961).[2] New stresses are being placed on the obstetrician/perinatologist in deciding not only on route of delivery, but on the safety of delaying delivery, and on antenatal pharmacologic intervention. With a lowering of the point of "viability," the numbers of patients requiring in depth assessment for premature labor, premature rupture of membranes, and premature delivery are expanding. The preterm delivery rate in the United States has remained stable at approximately 8 to 9%.[3,4] An estimated 40,000 infants per year will be diagnosed with respiratory distress syndrome (RDS).[3] This represents an incidence of RDS of approximately 14% amongst infants with birth weights less than 2500 g.[5,6] The respiratory distress which occurs secondary to hyaline membrane disease (HMD) has a high mortality rate ranging from 20 to 95%.[7,8] Farrell and Avery[9] reported a mortality of 28% based on early numbers tabulated by the National Center for Health Statistics.[3] Long-term morbidity may include both neurologic and pulmonary sequelae; several extensive reviews of RDS/HMD address these.[3,9] Fortunately, these long-term sequelae may be decreasing as neonatal therapeutic advances are made. Programs to prevent premature delivery showing success in other countries[10,11] have in their first formal testing in this country in black inner-city women failed to reduce preterm delivery.[12] Whether future studies will prove successful in other populations or with a more prolonged application of this program remains to be seen. Emphasis must therefore be placed on the antepartum and intrapartum management of preterm infants which provides the best possible physiologic preparation for extrauterine survival. This will involve identifying factors influencing the development of RDS and subsequently making a judgment as to whether antepartum management might alter outcome (Table 12–1).

Since the initial observations of Avery and Mead[25] correlating hyaline membrane disease and decreased surfactant, there has been an effort to alter prog-

Table 12–1.

Factors Favoring RDS Development	Factors Favoring Pulmonary Maturation
Prematurity[13]	IUGR[17]
Diabetes mellitus[13]	PROM[17,23]
Cesarean section without labor[14]	Pre-eclampsia[18]
Male sex[15,21]	Heroin addiction[19]
Low amniotic fluid L/S ratio[16,21]	Abnormal antepartum testing[22]
Genetic predisposition[20]	Vaginal bleeding for more than 24 hours prior to delivery[22]
	Amnionitis[21]
	Tocolytics used[24]
	Corticosteroids (see text for studies)

nosis in infants at risk for RDS through pharmacologic manipulation. Although there are some early studies evaluating the efficacy of introducing human surfactant into the airways of premature infants,[26–30] only early data are available. Both therapeutic and prophylactic modalities are currently being tested.

The pharmacologic approach for which there is the greatest experience and accumulated data to date is the antepartum use of corticosteroids. A rationale for this approach is based on:

1. Association of hyaline membrane disease and decreased airway surfactant.[25]
2. Identification of Type II alveolar cells as the producers of pulmonary surfactant.[9]
3. Animal models demonstrating increased pulmonary maturation with antepartum steroid administration.[31,32]

It requires an in depth analysis of patients to identify appropriate candidates for therapy and to define efficacy. This chapter will review clinical studies in humans comparing information available more than a decade ago to studies more recently completed. The studies considered will be limited to those with double blind, prospective design. Following an analysis of the major studies available, a brief look at future therapies will be presented.

The largest single study available for review is from the Collaborative Group on Antenatal Steroid Therapy.[33] The original study reported in 1981 was updated in the fall of 1985.[34] From 1977 to 1980, 696 patients were enrolled and follow-up for 36 months was planned.

The questions addressed by the study included:

1. Does antepartum intramuscular administration of dexamethasone to mothers at risk for premature delivery reduce the incidence of RDS amongst the offspring?
2. Are there adverse short term sequelae?
3. Are there long-term (18 and 36 months) sequelae for the infants?

The study answered these questions but raised some new ones. Several unexpected correlations and observations were made. As with any well-controlled study seeking to answer specific and limited questions, exclusion criteria were stringent; in this case, 7,893 patients were screened with only 696 study candidates enrolled. Many patients were excluded when it was anticipated that they would deliver in less than 24 hours, when in fact they did not do so.

The study design included patients between 26 and 37 weeks at risk for premature delivery. The major exclusion categories were cervix dilated to more than 5 cm; delivery expected in less than 24 hours or after more than 7 days; signs of intrauterine infection; and patients already receiving corticosteroids or in which corticosteroids would be contraindicated. Intervention consisted of intramuscular injection of dexamethasone phosphate 1.25 ml (4 mg/ml) every 12 hours for a maximum of 4 doses. In some cases, when not contraindicated, tocolysis was attempted to postpone delivery for 48 hours or more.

The patient groups (treatment/placebo) were similar in regard to race, sex of infant, gestational age at entry, incidence of chronic hypertension or pre-eclampsia, premature rupture of membranes, and use of tocolytics. The incidence of RDS was established by standardized criteria and categorized as mild, moderate, or severe. Long-term assessment included examination at 9, 18, and 36 months. A baseline examination was performed at 40 weeks of corrected gestational age and included a Prechtl examination and the visual components of the Brazelton test. A Bayley examination with neurologic and general pediatric evaluation was performed at 9 and 18 months. At 36 months, a McCarthy test was conducted in conjunction with other routine assessments.

The conclusions of the study addressing the original three questions included the following:

1. Mortality rate (fetal and neonatal) was not altered by steroid therapy nor was the severity of RDS. The incidence of mothers with at least one RDS infant was decreased in the treatment group (12.6 vs 18%; $p = 0.05$). From a neonatal standpoint, the improvement in singleton pregnancies was also significant (10.1 vs 16.1%; $p = 0.03$). This improvement was not seen when multiple gestations were evaluated. In assessing untoward events, no association was found between treatment and postpartum infections, hypertension, or neonatal infections. Total hospitalization was reduced in infants of steroid-treated mothers.

2. The Prechtl examination did not show a significant difference but suggested a trend for improved results in the steroid-treated group.

3. Long-term sequelae were not identified.

Analysis of the Collaborative Study data led to the following recommendations, observations, and qualifiers: Antepartum therapy with dexamethasone does reduce the overall incidence of RDS. This effect does not extend to patients with multiple gestations or premature rupture of membranes. The question of steroid use with multiple gestations will not be completely closed until larger numbers are available to adjust for confounding variables. Although no significant benefit of steroids was identified for male fetuses, the existence of other studies implying advantage was felt to warrant further study. In a similar fashion, no significant benefit was identified for fetuses less than 28 weeks' gestation; again, total numbers remained small and subsequent neonatal advances may affect future outcomes and recommendations. The question concerning retreatment at 7 days remains unanswered with evidence supporting both sides. New emphasis is also being placed on extrapulmonary effects of steroid therapy including the lowered incidences of necrotizing enterocolitis, bronchopulmonary dysplasia, and patent ductus arteriosus.

Table 12–2.   Evaluation of Antepartum Steroids

I	Liggins and Howie[35,36] (1972, 1977)
II	Block et al.[37] (1976)
III	Taeusch et al.[38] (1979)
IV	Papageorgiou et al.[39] (1979)
V	Morrison et al.[40,41] (1980)
VI	Doran et al.[42] (1980)
VII	Collaborative Group on Antenatal Steroid Therapy[33,34] (1981, 1985)
VIII	Schmidt et al.[43] (1984)

Table 12–3.   Study Inclusion and Exclusion Criteria

I   *Inclusion:* Premature labor; 24–36 weeks gestation. Premature delivery <37 weeks for obstetrical indications.
Exclusion: Corticosteroid therapy contraindicated.

II   *Inclusion:* Premature labor <37 weeks or preterm premature rupture of membranes.

III   *Inclusion:* <33 weeks gestation with premature rupture of membranes or premature labor and cervical examination <5 cm. Patients >33 weeks gestation if L/S ratio <2 or a history of previous infant with respiratory distress syndrome.
Exclusion: Immediate delivery required secondary to vaginal bleeding, chorioamnionitis, patient refusal, obstetrician refusal, severe toxemia, or history of corticosteroid therapy.

IV   *Inclusion:* 25–34 weeks gestation with premature labor or premature rupture of membranes.
Exclusion: Patient had diabetes mellitus, pre-eclampsia, hypertension, Rh sensitization, or evidence of intrauterine growth retardation.

V   *Inclusion:* Premature labor or obstetrical indication for preterm delivery; <34 weeks gestation or documented L/S ratio <2.
Exclusion: corticosteroids contraindicated, history of corticosteroid administration, or delivery was anticipated <24 hours.

VI   *Inclusion:* Premature labor, preterm premature rupture of membranes, planned preterm delivery with an estimated gestational age of 24–34 weeks.
Exclusion: Pre-eclampsia or corticosteroids contraindicated.

VII   *Inclusion:* 26–27 weeks gestation with risk of premature delivery.
Exclusion: Cervical exam >5 cm, delivery anticipated <24 hours or >7 days, evidence of infection, corticosteroids previously administered, or contraindications to steroids, severe Rh disease, follow-up could not be guaranteed; if <34 weeks gestation, could enter study without L/S ratio, otherwise, required; L/S required with history of hyperthyroidism, blood pressures >140/90, suspicion of placental insufficiency, drug addiction, or patient involved in a drug addiction treatment program.

VIII   *Inclusion:* Risk of preterm delivery, 26–32 weeks, estimated fetal weight of 750–1750 g, cervical dilation <5 cm.
Exclusion: Steroids or tocolytics contraindicated.

Studies to be reviewed are listed in Table 12–2 and will subsequently be referred to by number (I-VIII).

The trend of all studies is to concentrate on gestations less than 32 to 34 weeks (Table 12–3). This may reflect a growing expertise in neonatology. There appears to be no significant value for corticosteroid use at 34 weeks or beyond because of the low incidence of RDS beyond this gestational age. Newer studies also reflect a greater emphasis on antepartum assessment of candidates for corticosteroids including greater effort to obtain L/S ratios, phosphatidylglycerol and ultrasound evaluations.

Trends in corticosteroid choice (Table 12–4) appear to favor dexamethasone with betamethasone as a second choice. These drugs appear to have similar placental passage and biologic activity. The preference may be based on the greater availability of dexamethasone as a pure phosphate sold in the United States (betamethasone is most commonly available as a combination of phosphate and acetate salts). The acetate salt is not as well absorbed and may extend the period of steroid exposure for the fetus and mother.

Only two studies (V and VIII) have evaluated hydrocortisone (different dosages and different routes) and widely differing results were reported. The most recent study noted a significant increase in maternal infection in those patients delivered vaginally. Certainly, data are too limited to assess the future of hydrocortisone for antepartum therapy. Methylprednisolone was also evaluated by two groups (II and III). A more certain consensus was reached in regard to its use; no fetal benefit was demonstrated. With regard to other drug exposures, including a wide range of tocolytics, no obvious fetal compromise was demonstrated. It is notable that all patients had strict monitoring for signs of chorioamnionitis (maternal white blood cell count, temperature), and tocolytics were promptly discontinued with any evidence of infection. Several studies (I, II, III, VIII) specifically called for limiting tocolytics to a 48-hour goal; others do not address the length of therapy or specific goals. The role of tocolytics in conjunction with antepartum corticosteroids is not clearly defined. Certainly, with good evidence for a delayed (>24 hours) fetal pulmonary effect from steroids, a strong argument can be made for their use for at least this period of time. The major concern with ruptured membranes would seem to be an increased incidence of maternal febrile morbidity. Thus far, at least with dexamethasone and betamethasone, the majority of studies addressing the problem (I, IV, VI, VII, V, VIII) do not confirm that fear. Interestingly enough, the one study (III) in-

Table 12–4. Drug Regimens

I	Betamethasone 6 mg IM; repeat once at 24 hours.
	Tocolysis to assure 48–72 hour delay (ethanol, salbutamol); antibiotics given for amniorrhexis
II	Betamethasone 12 mg IM; repeat once at 24 hours.
	Methylprednisolone 125 mg IM; repeat once at 24 hours.
	Tocolysis as necessary to achieve 48 hour delay (ethanol).
III	Dexamethasone phosphate 4 mg IM every 8 hours for a maximum of 6 doses.
IV	Betamethasone 12 mg IM; repeat at 24 hours and weekly thereafter to 34 weeks gestation.
	Tocolysis (isoxsuprine) to stop labor.
V	Hydrocortisone 500 mg IV every 12 hours for 4 doses.
	Tocolysis as indicated (ethanol, isoxsuprine, ritodrine).
VI	Betamethasone 6 mg IM; repeat every 12 hours for 4 doses.
	Toxolysis (isoxsuprine, ethanol) as indicated.
VII	Dexamethasone phosphate 5 mg IM; repeat every 12 hours for 4 doses.
	Tocolysis for 48 hours as indicated (ethanol, isoxsuprine).
VIII	Hydrocortisone 250 mg IM; repeat at 24 hours.
	Methylprednisolone 125 mg IM; repeat at 24 hours.
	Betamethasone 12 mg IM; repeat at 24 hours.
	Tocolysis as indicated (isoxsuprine, magnesium sulfate, terbutaline); limited to 48 hours.

volving the use of dexamethasone without tocolytics was the only one to show an increase in maternal infectious morbidity (27 vs 12%; p<.05; two-tailed).

It is unfortunate that such a wide discrepancy exists in defining the disease (Table 12–5) which so much effort is being made to prevent. Very few studies objectively define respiratory distress syndrome in terms of temporal occurrence and actual respiratory status and support requirements (mechanical and F_{IO_2}). As a result, no comparison can be made between studies and only a comparison of trends is possible.

There was variability not only in respiratory distress syndrome definition (Table 12–5), but also in medication type and dosage (Table 12–4), and exclusion criteria for patients (Table 12–3). Also, differences in the gestational age of the fetal population occur (31.4 ± .12 to 35.6 ± 4.4 in studies where information is available; Table 12–6). Nevertheless, the clear trend in every study supports antenatal corticosteroid use. Studies vary in specific recommendations (Table 12–7).

FUTURE ADVANCES IN ANTEPARTUM THERAPY OF RESPIRATORY DISTRESS SYNDROME

Antepartum corticosteroid use will continue. Greater emphasis will be placed on patient selection so that greater efficacy will result. More attention will be focused on treatment of fetuses based on such things as intact membranes, fetal sex, singleton verus multiple gestation, gestational age, route of delivery, and timing and quantity of steroid dosage.

Fibroblast Pneumonocyte Factor (FPF)[44] which has been studied for its role in

Table 12–5.   Respiratory Distress Syndrome Defined

I	Grunting, retraction beginning at <3 hours of age and persisting to >6 hours of age; chest x ray with fine generalized granularity and air bronchograms.
II	Respiratory distress requiring mechanical ventilation or continuous positive airway pressure; radiologic confirmation.
III	Symptoms of respiratory distress persisting >24 hours; clinical and radiologic signs and symptoms.
IV	1. Respiratory rate >60/minute (persisting for >24 hours). 2. Chest retractions (persisting for >24 hours). 3. Grunting (persisting for >24 hours). 4. F_{IO_2} >25% (persisting for >24 hours). 5. P_{CO_2} >50 mm Hg 6. Chest x ray compatible 7. HMD on autopsy 5 of 7 needed for diagnosis
V	Not specified.
VI	1. Tachypnea—respiratory rate >60 for >1 hour 2. Dyspnea: chest retraction, grunting, nasal flaring 3. Poor air exchange; rales 4. Central cyanosis 5. Tachycardia (140 to 160) and cardiac enlargement (slight) 6. Decreased surfactant or L/S ratio in amniotic or tracheal fluid 7. Chest x ray compatible
VII	Retraction, grunting, cyanosis, increased ambient O_2 requirement, hypercarbia; ground glass appearance on chest x-ray with air bronchograms and elevated diaphragms.
VIII	Tachypnea, grunting, retractions with consistent chest x ray

Table 12–6. Patients Evaluated, Exclusions, and Outcome: RDS%

I   Two hundred eighty-seven patients entered (5 excluded)
     Average gestation at delivery 35.6 ± 4.4 weeks

	Betamethasone	Control	p
219 liveborn infants	(122) 9%	(97) 25.8%	<.003
168 liveborn infants in protocol >24h	(93) 4.3%	(75) 24.0%	<.002

II   One hundred sixty-sven patients entered (25 excluded),
      (22 infants excluded—not premature)

	(A) Betamethasone	(B) Methyl Prednisolone	(C) Control	(A vs C) p
128 liveborn infants	(49) 10.2%	(35) 28.6%	(44) 27.3%)	<.05
85 liveborn infants in protocol >24 h	(36) 11.1%	(20) 30%	(29) 20.7%	NS

III   One hundred twenty-two patients entered (115 of 127 infants
       included); average gestation at delivery 32.3 ± 2.4 weeks

	Dexamethasone	Control	p
115 liveborn infants	(50) 14%	(65) 22%	.3*
Infants in protocol >48 h	(30) 7%	(65) 22%	.045*

*One-tailed

IV   One hundred forty patients entered
      (85 of 146 infants excluded)
      Average gestation at delivery 32.2 ± .41 weeks

	Betamethasone	Control	p
61 liveborn infants under protocol >24h	(29) 20.7%	(32) 59.4%	<.005

V   One hundred ninety-six patients entered (70 excluded)

	Hydrocortisone	Control	p
126 liveborn infants	(67) 9%	(59) 24%	.012

VI   One hundred thirty-seven patients entered protocol
      Average gestation at delivery 33.6 ± 4.6 weeks

	Betamethasone	Control	p
140 liveborn infants	(80) 5%	(60) 16.7%	<0.05
95 liveborn infants in protocol >24 h	(53) 1.9%	(42) 9.5%	

VII   Six hundred ninety-six patients registered (35 excluded)
       Average gestation at entry 31.4 ± .12 weeks

	Dexamethasone	Control	p
720 liveborn infants	(361) 12.7%	(359) 18.1%	.04
492 in protocol >24h	(249) 8%	(243) 15.2%	

VIII   One forty-four patients registered (52 excluded)
        1 of 97 liveborn infants excluded. Birth weights <2500 g

	Hydrocortisone	Methyl Prednisolone	Betamethasone	Control
96 liveborn infants	(15) 53%	(17) 35%	(33) 27%	(31) 32%
69 liveborn infants in protocol >24h	(11) 46%	(13) 38%	(26) 15%	(19) 42%
Severe RDS	9%	31%	4%*	26%

*p = .038 (Fisher's Exact Probability Test)

Table 12–7. Conclusions

I	RDS occurs less in premature infants who are treated than in controls. The effect is limited to infants less than 32 weeks' gestation who have been treated for 24 or more hours prior to delivery (population investigated: 24 to 36 weeks gestation).
II	Effectiveness was shown only in those patients with intact membranes in which the L/S ratio was <2.0. The timing between drug dosage and delivery did not appear significant (population studied: <37 weeks' gestation).
III	Those patients receiving a full course of antenatal dexamethasone showed a significant reduction of RDS compared to controls. Increased maternal infection was noted, especially in association with PROM (population studied: <33 weeks' gestation).
IV	A significant reduction in respiratory distress syndrome was found in the betamethasone treated group. Also, a decrease in the severity of RDS was seen and a decrease in neonatal death rate was noted. Prolonged rupture of membranes appeared to be unrelated to respiratory distress syndrome decrease or increase and was not related to infectious morbidity (population studied: 25 to 34 weeks).
V	A significant decrease of RDS was seen in the treatment group. Neonatal survival rates were also improved (population studied: <34 weeks).
VI	The betamethasone-treated group showed a reduction in RDS and neonatal mortality (population studied: 24 to 34 weeks).
VII	The major advantages of antenatal dexamethasone were confined to singleton females. Caucasians showed little effect of therapy. No advantage of treatment was identified in multiple gestations. Infants of dexamethasone-treated mothers had shorter hospitalizations. Primary treatment advantage was seen in the 30-to 34-week category delivered 24 hours to 7 days post-therapy. Patients with PROM received no treatment advantage. No advantage to treatment was seen at <28 weeks' gestation (population studied: 26 to 37 weeks).
VIII	Betamethasone significantly reduced RDS compared to controls if more than 24 hours elapsed to delivery. No increase in neonatal mortality or infection was demonstrated (population studied: 26 to 32 weeks).

the biochemical pathway connecting steroids to increased surfactant release[45,46] may allow a rapid therapeutic intervention in cases of impending delivery. Whereas steroid-mediated effects require 24 hours or more because of protein synthesis requirements,[46,47] FPF appears to have a direct effect which is maximal at 60 minutes.[46] The possible role of percutaneous umbilical blood sampling[48,49] in delivery of this compound will be an additional area of exploration. The evaluation and use of thyroxine[50,51] for its synergistic effect in the development and release of surfactant was originally described more than a decade ago. The most recent update on the Collaborative Groups' work[34] suggests a need for trials evaluating the coincident use of steroids and thyroxine.

The reader is referred to several excellent reviews on RDS and hyaline membrane disease[9,52–54] which discuss further neonatal management.

Future work will concentrate in three major areas:

1. Development of new drug approaches to inhibit labor, which will require earlier recognition of preterm labor. The role of prophylactic measures with high risk groups also demands clarification.

2. Development of both antepartum prophylaxis and postpartum treatments for respiratory distress syndrome must continue. Further, in order to reduce possible risks of different pharmacologic approaches, candidates for therapy must be more clearly defined.

3. Those patients currently excluded from antepartum RDS therapies must

be reconsidered for presently available medications and new options may be developed.

REFERENCES

1. Pritchard, J.A., MacDonald, P.C., Gant, N.F.: Williams Obstetrics, 17th ed., Norwalk, CT, Appleton-Century-Crofts, 1985, p. 749.
2. Eastman, N.J. and Hellman, L.M.: Williams Obstetrics, 12th ed., New York, Appleton-Century-Crofts, 1961, p. 1070.
3. Wood, R.E. and Farrell, P.M.: Edpidemiology of respiratory distress syndrome (RDS). Pediat Res, 8:452, 1974.
4. National Center for Health Statistics: Vital Statistics of the United States, 1980. Volume 1—Natality. Hyattsville, Md, U.S. Department of Health and Human Services, 1984, pp. 1–286.
5. Smith, C.A.: Respiratory physiology and respiratory distress in the newborn infant. Int Anesthesiol Clin, 3:209, 1965.
6. Usher, R., McLean, F. and Maughan, G.B.: Respiratory distress syndrome in infants delivered by cesarean section. Am J Obstet Gynecol, 88:806, 1964.
7. Ballabriga, A., Moragas, A., Gallant-Catala, A., et al.: Respiratory pathology in the immediate postnatal period. Acta Paediatr Scand, 59:497, 1970.
8. Gregory, G.A., Kitterman, J.A., Phibbs, R.H., et al.: Treatment of the idiopathic respiratory distress syndrome with continuous positive airway pressure. N Engl J Med, 284:1333, 1971.
9. Farrell, P.M., and Kotas, R.V.: The prevention of hyaline membrane disease: new concepts and approaches to therapy. Adv Pediatr, 23:213, 1976.
10. Creasy, R.K., Gummer, B.A. and Liggins, G.C.: System for predicting spontaneous preterm birth. Obstet Gynecol, 55:692, 1980.
11. Papiernik, E., Bouyer, J., Yaffe, K., et al.: Women's acceptance of a preterm birth prevention program. Am J Obstet Gynecol, 155:939, 1986.
12, Main, D.M., Richardson, D., Gabbe, S.G., et al.: Prospective evaluation of a risk scoring system for predicting preterm delivery in black inner-city women. Obstet Gynecol, 69:61, 1987.
13. Avery, M.E.: The lungs and its disorders in the newborn infant, 3rd Ed, Philadelphia, W.B. Saunders Co, 1974, p. 191.
14. Fedrick, J. and Butler, N.R.: Hyaline membrane disease. Lancet, 2:768, 1972.
15. Naeye, R.L., Bunt, L.S., Wright, D.L., et al.: Neonatal mortality, the male disadvantage. Pediatr, 48:902, 1971.
16. Gluck, L., Kulovich, M., Borer, R., et al.: Diagnosis of the respiratory distress syndrome by amniocentesis. Am J Obstet Gynecol, 109:440, 1971.
17. Bauer, C.R., Stern, L. and Colle, E.: Prolonged rupture of membranes associated with a decreased incidence of respiratory distress syndrome. Pediatr, 53:7, 1974.
18. Gluck, L. and Kulovich, M.V.: Lecithin/sphingomyelin ratios in amniotic fluid in normal and abnormal pregnancy. Am J Obstet Gyncecol, 115:539, 1973.
19. Glass, L., Rajegowda, B. and Evans, H.: Absence of respiratory distress syndrome in premature infants of heroin addicted mothers. Lancet, 2:685, 1971.
20. Graven, S.N. and Misenheimer, H.R.: Respiratory distress syndrome and the high risk mother. Am J Dis Child, 109:489, 1965.
21. Fleischer, B., Kulovich, M.V., Hallman, M., et al.: Lung profile: sex differences in normal pregnancy. Obstet Gynecol, 66:327, 1985.
22. White, E., Shy, K.K. and Benedetti, T.J.: Chronic fetal stress and the risk of infant respiratory distress syndrome. Obstet Gynecol, 67:57, 1986.
23. Simpson, G.F. and Harbert, G.M., Jr: Use of betamethasone in management of preterm gestation with premature rupture of membranes. Obstet Gynecol, 66:168, 1985.
24. Kero, P., Hirvonen, T. and Välimäki, I.: Prenatal and postnatal isoxsuprine and respiratory distress syndrome. Lancet, 2:198, 1973.
25. Avery, M. and Mead, J.: Surface properties in relation to atelectasis and hyaline membrane disease. Am J Dis Child, 97:517, 1959.
26. Merritt, T.A., Hallman, M., Bloom, B.J., et al.: Prophylactic treatment of very premature infants with human surfactant. N Engl J Med, 315:785, 1986.
27. Hallman, M., Merritt, T.A., Jarvenpaa, A.L., et al.: Exogenous surfactant for treatment of severe respiratory distress syndrome: a randomized prospective clinical trial. J Pediatr, 106:963, 1985.
28. Gitlin, J., Parad, R., Taeusch, H., Jr.: Exogenous surfactant therapy in hyaline membrane disease. Sem Perinatol, 8:272, 1984.
29. Hallman, M., Merritt, A., Schneider, H., et al.: Isolation of human surfactant from amniotic fluid and a pilot study of its efficacy in respiratory distress syndrome. Pediatr, 71:473, 1983.
30. Smyth, J., Metcalfe, I., Duffty, P., et al.: Hyaline membrane disease treated with bovine surfactant. Pediatr, 71:913, 1983.
31. Liggins, G.C.: The foetal role in the initiation of parturition in the ewe, in Wolstenholme, G.E.N.

and O'Connor , M. (eds): Foetal Autonomy. Ciba Foundation Symposium. J.A. Churchill Ltd, London, 1969, p. 142.

32. Liggins, G.C.: Premature delivery of foetal lambs infused with glucocorticoids. J Endocrinal, *45*:515, 1969.

33. Collaborative Group on Antenatal Steroid Therapy. Effect of antenatal dexamethasone administration on the prevention of respiratory distress syndrome. Am J Obstet Gynecol, *141*:276, 1981.

34. Avery, M.E., Aylward, G., Creasy, R., et al.: Update on prenatal steroid for prevention of respiration distress; report on a conference—September 26–28, 1985. Am J Obstet Gynecol, *155*:2, 1986.

35. Liggins, G.C. and Howie, R.N.: A controlled trial of antepartum glucocorticoid treatment for prevention of the respiratory distress syndrome in premature infants. Pediatr, *50*:515, 1972.

36. Liggins, G.C.: Prevention of RDS by maternal betamethasone administration, in Proceedings of the 70th Ross Conference on Pediatric Research, Columbus, Ohio, Ross Laboratories, 1977, pp. 189–198.

37. Block, M.F., Kling, O.R. and Crosby, W.M.: Antenatal glucocorticoid therapy for prevention of respiratory distress syndrome in the premature infant. Obstet Gynecol, *50*:186, 1976.

38. Taeusch, H.W., Frigoletto, F., Kitzmiller, J., et al.: Risk of respiratory distress syndrome after prenatal dexamethasone treatment. Pediatr, *63*:64, 1979.

39. Papageorgiou, A.N., Desgranges, M.E., Masson, M., et al.: The antenatal use of betamethasone in the prevention of respiratory distress syndrome: a controlled double-blind study. Pediat, *63*:73, 1979.

40. Morrison, J.C., Whybrew, W.D., Bucovaz, E.T., et al: Injection of corticosteroids into mother to prevent neonatal respiratory distress syndrome. Am J Obstet Gynecol, *131*:358, 1978.

41. Morrison, J.C., Schneider, J.M., Whybrew, W.D., et al.: Effect of corticosteroids and fetomaternal disorders on the L/S Ratio. Obstet Gynecol, *56*:583, 1980.

42. Doran, T.A., Swyer, P., MacMurray, B., et al.: Results of a double-blind controlled study on the use of betamethasone in the prevention of respiratory distress syndrome. Am J Obstet Gynecol, *136*:313, 1980.

43. Schmidt, P.L., Sims, M.E., Strassner, H.T., et al.: Effect of antepartum glucocorticoid administration upon neonatal respiratory distress syndrome and perinatal infection. Am J Obstet Gynecol, *148*:178, 1984.

44. Smith, B.T.: Fibroblast-pneumonocyte factor, in Stern L. (ed): Neonatal Intensive Care, Vol. 2, New York, Masson Publishing, 1978.

45. Post, M. and Smith, B.T.: Effect of fibroblast-pneumonocyte factor on the synthesis of surfactant phospholipids in type II cells from fetal rat lung. Biochim Biophys Acta, *793*:297, 1984.

46. Post, M. and Smith, B.T.: Fibroblast-pneumonocyte factor purified with the aid of monoclonal antibodies stimulates cholinephosphate cytidylytransferease activity in fetal type II cells. Pediatr Res, *18*:401A, 1984.

47. Floros, J., Post, M. and Smith, B.J.: Glucocorticoids affect the synthesis of pulmonary fibroblast-pneumonocyte factor at a pretranslational level. J Biol Chem, *260*:2265, 1985.

48. Daffos, F., Capella-Pavlovsky, M. and Forestier, F.: Fetal blood sampling during pregnancy with use of a needle guided by ultrasound: a study of 606 consecutive cases. Am J Obstet Gynecol, *153*:655, 1985.

49. Hobbins, J.C., Grannum, P.A., Romero, R., et al.: Percutaneous umbilical blood sampling. Am J Obstet Gynecol, *152*:1, 1985.

50. Redding, R.A., Douglas, W.H.J. and Stein, M.: Thyroid hormone influence upon lung surfactant metabolism. Science, *175*:994, 1972.

51. Redding, R.A., Pereira, C. and Barrett, J.T.: Thyroid function in newborn respiratory distress syndrome. Pediatr Res, *7*:395, 1973.

52. Farrell, P.M. and Avery, M.E.: State of the Art: Hyaline membrane disease. Am Rev Resp Dis, *111*:657, 1975.

53. Hallman, M. and Gluck, L.: Development of the fetal lung. J Perinatal Med, *5*:3, 1977.

54. Stark, A.R. and Frantz, I.D., III: Respiratory distress syndrome. Pediatri Clin North Am, *33*:533, 1986.

Chapter 13

Tocolytic Agents for the Treatment of Preterm Labor

Richard E. Besinger and Jennifer R. Niebyl

Preterm birth and low birth weight are major contributors to perinatal mortality in modern obstetrics. Despite vigorous attempts to avert spontaneous preterm labor with tocolytic agents, it is still unclear whether pharmacologic inhibition of preterm labor has had any signficant impact upon perinatal mortality. Tocolysis appears to have an insignificant effect upon the general low birth weight rate, but may benefit the appropriately selected patient.[1] Even if an ideal inhibitor were available, the maximum reduction of premature delivery would be only 10 to 20%, since many patients are not candidates for labor inhibition.[2,3] Medical and obstetric contraindications to tocolytic therapy preclude the use of these agents in the majority of preterm labor patients. It has been suggested that recent improvements in perinatal mortality attributable to preterm labor are probably due to an overall reduction in the incidence of preterm labor, as well as a advances in neonatal care of the premature infant.[4] Still, the potential benefits to be gained in neonatal morbidity and mortality by delaying delivery are great, particularly between 24 and 28 weeks.[5] Similarly, the use of beta-adrenergic drugs that prolong gestation appear to lower the combined maternal and neonatal medical costs of treating preterm labor prior to 34 weeks of gestation.[6]

Multiple factors are involved in the initiation of human preterm labor. Oxytocin, progesterone withdrawal, elevated estrogen-progesterone ratio, fetal corticosteroids, prostaglandins, catecholamines, increased gap junctions, premature cervical maturation, uterine stretching, and changes in uterine blood flow have all been implicated in the initiation of preterm labor.[7,8] Premature labor may also be associated with identifiable maternal conditions such as abruptio placentae[9] and subclinical amniotic infections.[10–12] Since the triggering event of preterm labor is usually unknown, the therapy is of necessity empiric.

When premature labor is recognized and treated early, there is a greater likelihood of success. Several risk scoring systems based on historic and epidemiologic variables have been proposed to identify those patients at risk for preterm delivery.[13,14] None of these systems have reached the level of discrimination necessary to be recommended for routine clinical use. It appears that precocious cervical ripening can be observed several weeks prior to preterm birth,[15,16] and weekly cervical examinations of high-risk patients may be helpful in predicting the onset of preterm delivery.[17,18] With the advent of sophisticated ambulatory monitoring systems, it may be possible to institute tocolytic therapy in high-risk patients based on pre-labor uterine activity,[19,20] as well as evaluate and manage oral tocolytic therapy in patients being treated for preterm labor.[21] Once uterine activity has been recognized, several investigators have used real-time ultrasound evaluation of fetal breathing to identify those individuals at risk for progressive preterm labor.[22-24] In the absence of fetal breathing, both term and preterm patients with uterine contractions are likely to progress into active labor and deliver. Elevated prostaglandin F metabolite in the maternal serum may also be an indicator of progressive preterm labor.[25]

Whether prophylactic tocolytic agents should be used in patients at high risk for preterm delivery has not been answered. Preliminary studies with low-dose beta-adrenergic agents have failed to demonstrate any significant effect upon prematurity rates in singleton gestations.[26,27] Prophylactic tocolysis in twin gestations may be more effective,[28-30] but further investigation of this important issue is warranted. The use of prophylactic progestational agents in patients at high risk for prematurity is discussed in Chapter 11.

Certain criteria must be fulfilled before a patient is considered a candidate for attempted pharmacologic arrest of preterm labor. The gestational age through which preterm labor should be stopped varies in the literature, from 20 to 36 weeks with estimated fetal weight of 500 to 2500 g. Ritodrine was approved by the FDA for use at 20 weeks and beyond because of the higher risk of anomalous infants at lower gestational ages. At each institution, the survival rates in the neonatal nursery at each specific gestational age should be known and compared with the risk of attempted tocolysis. Ultrasonography is indicated if gestational age is uncertain, particularly if intrauterine growth retardation (IUGR) is suspected. If fetal maturity is still in question, then amniocentesis for fetal lung maturity should be done.[31,32] The presence of a live fetus without life-threatening anomalies should also be assured. Other obstetric contraindications to tocolysis include preeclampsia, reduced uteroplacental blood flow, suspected placental abruption, fetal distress or chorioamnionitis. It is important to realize that initiation of tocolysis may be hazardous, rather than protective, to the fetus in an unfavorable uterine environment.

Before institution of tocolysis, initial baseline clinical data as shown in Table 13–1 should be obtained. If the initial tocolytic agent fails to arrest the uterine

Table 13–1.   Initial Measures Recommended when Tocolysis is Initiated

Bed rest
Admission weight
Baseline vital signs
Vaginal examination to exclude rupture of membranes
Intravenous access line
Continuous fetal monitoring for fetal heart rate and contractions
Aerobic cervical culture
Electrocardiogram
Ultrasonography, if indicated
Laboratory studies:
   Complete blood count
   Electrolytes
   Glucose
   Urinalysis
   Fibrinogen

activity and/or cervical change, then it should be discontinued and alternative therapy considered. When uncomplicated preterm labor appears refractory to initial therapy, a thorough evaluation for silent chorioamnionitis with white cell counts, cervical cultures, and amniotic fluid culture is warranted.[33] Once cervical dilation has progressed to 4 cm, tocolytic therapy should be discontinued since inhibition of labor is rarely successful beyond this point, and this will avoid significant neonatal blood levels of the tocolytic drug at birth. An entirely separate question is whether the benefit of corticosteroids justifies the short-term inhibition of preterm labor to allow time for their maximal effect and this is addressed in Chapter 12.

Premature rupture of membranes makes a significant contribution to the incidence of premature delivery,[34] and most clinicians agree that these patients should be excluded from any long-term attempt to inhibit preterm labor because of the risk of infection. However, several investigators have demonstrated a short-term prolongation of these pregnancies without complications,[35,36] while others have shown no apparent clinical benefit.[37,38]

The clinical evaluation of effectiveness and safety of various tocolytic agents has proven difficult. Few animal models exist to evaluate these medications.[39] A placebo response of approximately 20 to 50% is observed in cases of threatened premature labor, reflecting the inherent difficulties in diagnosing true preterm labor. Universal criteria for the diagnosis of preterm labor have been recommended (Table 13–2) Various parameters for measuring the success rate of tocolytic therapy that have been used include: birth weights, short-term and long-term delay in delivery, and perinatal survival rates. However, the evaluation of success of a tocolytic agent is difficult since cervical dilation and gestational age at the start of treatment differ from patient to patient. For these reasons, only randomized controlled clinical trials should be used to prove the efficacy of any agent used to inhibit preterm labor.

In 1980, the United States Food and Drug Administration approved ritodrine hydrochloride (Yutopar) for inhibition of preterm labor. Among all the tocolytic agents to be discussed in this chapter, this is the only one so approved, and the other agents should be considered experimental. However, the use of approved drugs for non-labeled indications may be entirely appropriate based on medical

Table 13–2.   Criteria for Diagnosis of Preterm Labor[14]

	Gestation 20 to 37 weeks	
	and	
	Documented uterine contractions	
	(4 in 20 minutes or 8 in 60 minutes)	
	and	
Ruptured membranes	or	Intact membranes
		and
		Documented cervical change by a single examiner
		or
		Cervical effacement of >75%
		or
		Cervical dilation of greater than 2 cm

advances extensively reported in the medical literature.[40] The tocolytic agents to be discussed in this chapter with proven clinical utility, as evident in controlled clinical trials, are listed in Table 13–3.

BED REST, HYDRATION, AND SEDATION

In a significant percentage of suspected preterm labor, uterine contractions will subside with bed rest, hydration, and sedation. In a recent study of this phenomenon, 55% of the patients responded to this pretherapy while 45% required tocolytic therapy.[41] However, the lack of randomized, controlled data regarding this issue makes it difficult to differentiate the effects of fluid administration, sedation, and rest.

Medications such as narcotics and barbiturates do not relax the myometrium,[42] but may cause a transitory decrease in uterine activity immediately following administration.[43] Other investigators have shown that meperidine actually has an oxytocic effect,[44,45] and that although the patient may be sedated, she can awaken later in advanced labor. Even more seriously, these drugs can cause CNS depression and respiratory difficulties in the premature infant if given immediately prior to a preterm delivery.

A one-hour observation period prior to initiating tocolytic therapy should be used only if the patient does not meet the criteria for the diagnosis of preterm labor (Table 13–2). Intravenous hydration during this period should not exceed 500 ml as its only purpose is to prevent ketosis, ensure adequate maternal intravascular volume, and improve uteroplacental blood flow (in anticipation of tocolytic therapy). Further hydration may predispose to the development of pulmonary edema,[46] and prolonged observation may ultimately delay the administration of tocolytic agents.

TOCOLYTIC AGENTS

Alcohol

Alcohol was the first clinically useful tocolytic agent used for the prevention of preterm birth.[47] Ethanol inhibits the secretion of both neurohypophyseal hormones, antidiuretic hormone (ADH), and oxytocin.[48] Ethanol may also have a direct effect upon the myometrium. In human labor, oxytocin is released in a series of pulses which increase in frequency as labor progresses. The frequency of oxytocin pulses is reduced during intravenous infusion of alcohol at levels which produce no obvious direct effects upon myometrial contractility.[49] Ethanol inhibits uterine response to endogenous oxytocin elicited by nursing,[50] and uterine contractions induced by prostaglandin PGE_2 infusion.[51] An in vitro study using alcohol levels well above the lethal dosage confirms a possible direct inhibition of myometrial contractility.[52] Therefore, it appears that suppression of uterine activity by ethanol is due to inhibition of oxytocin release and to noncompetitive antagonism at the uterine level.[53]

In the initial clinical study of suppression of preterm labor with alcohol,[47] an inhibitory effect on uterine activity was seen in all cases even when significant postponement of delivery was not achieved. In a later randomized, controlled study, ethanol was shown to be more effective than glucose in water administered as a placebo.[54] Seventeen of 21 patients (80%) in the ethanol group had delivery postponed greater than 72 hours, as opposed to 8 of 21 patients (38%)

Table 13–3. Tocolytic Agents*

Drug	Initial Dose	Maximum Tocolytic Dose	Long-Term Oral Maintenance Dose	Side Effects
Beta Adrenergic Agonists				Maternal and fetal tachycardia
Isoxsuprine	0.10–0.25 mg/min IV	.35 mg/min IV	10–20 mg qid	Hypotension
Ritodrine	0.05–0.10 mg/min IV	.35 mg/min IV	10–20 mg qid	Cardiac arrhythmia
Terbutaline	0.01 mg/min IV	.025 mg/min IV	2.5–5 mg tid	Myocardial ischemia?
Salbutamol	0.01–0.02 mg/min IV	.05 mg/min IV	4 mg qid	Hypokalemia, hyperglycemia, and
				Hyperinsulinemia
				Lactic acidosis
				Fluid retention
				Pulmonary edema?
				Tremor, nervousness, restlessness
				Neonatal hypocalcemia, hypoglycemia, ileus, hypotension, hyperbilirubinemia
Ethanol	9.5% ethanol; 15 mg/kg over 2 hr	1.5 mg/kg over 6–10 hr	—	Restlessness, coma, vomiting and aspiration
				Maternal lactic acidosis and dehydration
				Drug interaction
				Newborn CNS depression
Indomethacin	50 mg p.o.	25 mg p.o. q 4 hr	25 mg p.o. q 4-6 hr	Nausea, gastrointestinal ulceration
				Decreased renal function
				Platelet dysfunction?
				Mask maternal infection?
				Oligohydramnios?
				Closure of fetal ductus arteriosus?
				Neonatal pulmonary hypertension?
Magnesium sulfate	4 g in 10% solution over 10 min	4–6 gm/hr	—	Respiratory depression
				Altered FHR variability?
				Neonatal drowsiness and hypotonia
				Meconium ileus?

*As demonstrated in randomized clinical trials.

who received the placebo. In two other clinical studies of similar design, no significant difference between ethanol and hydration was demonstrated.[55,56] In several other randomized, comparison studies, ethanol was less effective than isoxsuprine,[55] ritodrine,[57] terbutaline,[58] or magnesium sulfate[59] in the inhibition of preterm labor or subsequent prolongation of pregnancy. A comparsion study with salbutamol showed no significant difference in prolongation of pregnancy when compared to ethanol.[60]

Since blood alcohol levels associated with ethanol infusion for the treatment of preterm labor often rise above 100 to 150 mg%, the patient must be monitored closely for the symptoms of inebriation. These serious symptoms include agitation, nausea, vomiting, somnolence and coma, with the danger of aspiration pneumonitis. In the human, ethanol is detoxified by alcohol dehydrogenase in the liver with a half-life approaching 4 hours in the pregnant patient;[61] therefore on average, it will take 10 to 12 hours to eliminate ethanol appreciably from the maternal circulation after discontinuing the intravenous infusion. Newborns metabolize ethanol twice as slowly as the human adult does.[62] Maternal lactic acidosis, dehydration, or maternal liver disease should preclude the use of ethanol for preterm labor inhibition.[63] Ethanol should be used with caution in patients with diabetes mellitus because of the risk of inducing hypoglycemia.

Ethanol readily crosses the placenta, is present in the bloodstream of the newborn infant within 1 minute of maternal administration[61] and equilibrates with maternal levels at 60 minutes.[62] Serum levels in the umbilical artery and vein are lower than or equal to those in the maternal venous blood when drawn simultaneously.[61,62] In sheep preparations, there is no alteration in maternal acid-base status, though a transient metabolic acidosis has been observed.[64,65] These acid-base alterations have not been well described in the human fetus and exposed newborns do not appear to have significant metabolic acidosis at birth.[62]

Adverse effects have been reported in the neonate. While some infants may exhibit CNS depression if born within 12 hours of discontinuing the maternal infusion,[66] this effect is even more pronounced in infants weighing 1000 to 1500 g.[67] Muscular hypotonia has also been described in the exposed neonate.[62] Abnormal bone marrow morphology in the preterm neonate has also been described after ethanol exposure.[68] Despite these observations, there appears to be no significant difference in neonatal mortality between ethanol-exposed newborns and a control group of other premature infants.[66] Long-term evaluation of the growth and mental development of children exposed in utero to ethanol shows no abnormalities when evaluated as a group at age 4 to 7 years; however, alterations in developmental parameters have been suggested in those infants born within 15 hours of terminating the ethanol infusion.[69] To minimize these neonatal effects, it is recommended that an ethanol infusion be discontinued 12 to 15 hours prior to delivery.[66] In contrast, one group of infants between 28 and 32 weeks had a lower incidence and severity of respiratory distress syndrome (RDS) when exposed to ethanol in utero.[70]

In view of its questionable efficacy, significant maternal side effects, and concerns over neonatal toxicity, the use of intravenous ethanol in the modern treatment of preterm labor has been limited.[71]

Beta Adrenergic Agonists

Beta-adrenergic interaction with uterine smooth muscle was one of the earliest recognized inhibitory effects upon uterine contractility. Two types of beta-adrenergic receptors have been described in humans.[72] Beta$_1$ receptors predominate in the heart, small intestine, and adipose tissue, whereas beta$_2$ receptors are more prevalent in the smooth muscle of the uterus, blood vessels, bronchioles and diaphragm. Beta-adrenergic agonists act upon intramembranous beta receptors in these cells, which activate the enzyme adenylate cyclase and cause an increase in the intracellular concentration of cyclic AMP (cAMP).[73] This increased level of cAMP initiates a series of cellular reactions which reduce intracellular calcium levels and decrease the sensitivity of the myosin-actin contractile unit to available calcium.[74] This inhibition of uterine contractility occurs even if oxytocin is given simultaneously.[75] There is no evidence that alpha-adrenergic blockade is of any value in the inhibition of preterm labor. Combined alpha-adrenergic blockade and beta-adrenergic stimulation does not appear to influence the tocolytic effects of ritodrine[76] or isoxsuprine.[77]

The intravenous administration of betamimetic agents can stimulate beta receptors in multiple organ systems and is responsible for the various clinically significant side effects associated with these medications.[78] Maternal cardiovascular side effects are most frequently seen with beta-adrenergic agonists, including hypotension, tachycardia and arrhythmia. Therefore, the use of these agents in patients with intravascular depletion secondary to hemorrhage or dehydration can cause profound effects.

The activation of vascular beta$_2$ adrenergic receptors leads to vasodilation resulting in diastolic hypotension.[79] This results in a reflex compensatory increase in heart rate, stroke volume, cardiac output, and increased systolic blood pressures.[80] Cardiac output during tocolytic therapy with betamimetic agents can be increased 40 to 60% over basal levels.[80,81] The use of M-mode echocardiography during betamimetic therapy demonstrates a marked increase in left ventricular velocity; however, there is no significant incidence of induced cardiac failure and no observed change in cardiac chamber dimensions during therapy.[80,82,83] As well as the predominantly beta$_2$ receptor stimulation, there are probably also some direct inotropic and chronotropic effects.[74] The use of terbutaline with simultaneous beta$_1$ blockade with metroprolol fails to signficantly alter cardiovascular or metabolic effects of betamimetic therapy.[84] Thus, betamimetic tocolytic therapy should not be used in patients with inherent cardiac disease.

Cardiac arrhythmias have been reported with beta-adrenergic therapy. The most common arrhythmia reported is supraventricular tachycardia,[85–88] though atrial fibrillation,[89] atrial premature contractions,[90] and ventricular ectopy[90,91] have also been described. In a recent study 30 patients receiving intravenous ritodrine had continuous electrocardiography. Eighty-four percent of these patients had persistent surpraventricular tachycardia during treatment, 62.5% had atrial premature contractions, and 13% had premature ventricular contractions of greater than 10 per hour.[90] In this study, palpitations or chest pain were not temporally associated with these observed cardiac rhythm abnormalities. Therefore, a careful cardiac history and a screening EKG to rule out underlying cardiac disease should be done prior to the initiation of therapy.[92] Continuous EKG monitoring of the patient receiving intravenous betamimetic therapy may be helpful in identifying the onset of cardiac arrhythmias.

Myocardial ischemia has also been observed with the use of beta-adrenergic agonists. Heart rate and myocardial muscle contractility, both major determinates of myocardial muscle oxygen consumption, are significantly increased by these betamimetic agents.[81] While chest pain is a relatively common symptom during betamimetic therapy, only a few authors have reported EKG changes indicative of myocardial ischemia.[85,93–95] Transient ST segment depression is the most common observation,[85] appears to be dose related[94] and usually resolves with discontinuation of therapy. This ST segment depression has been reversed with sublingual nitroglycerin in some patients suggesting that inadequate coronary blood flow may be responsible.[93] Coronary artery perfusion is partially dependent upon diastolic blood pressures. Diastolic blood pressure during pregnancy is lowered because the placenta acts like an arteriovenous fistula. Beta$_2$ agonists not only lower diastolic pressure further, but also shorten diastolic filling time secondary to tachycardia. All of these factors ultimately decrease coronary artery perfusion and may predispose to myocardial ischemia. Despite these concerning clinical observations, subclinical myocardial damage, as evident by elevated cardiac enzymes or cardiac-specific myoglobin, has not been described in patients receiving betamimetic therapy.[94,96] A closer analysis of these EKG alterations in patients receiving intravenous ritodrine with paired serial EKGs and serum electrolytes suggests that most of these findings can be attributed to electrolyte disturbances and not myocardial ischemia.[97]

As the clinical use of beta-adrenergic agonists has become more widespread, more than 80 cases of pulmonary edema have been reported in the literature.[85,98–117] This life-threatening complication has been reported in up to 5% of patients receiving intravenous betamimetic therapy,[80,85] Although pulmonary edema can occur at any time, it has occurred antepartum in the majority of patients. It has occurred with and without concurrent glucocorticoid therapy for fetal lung maturation. A large percentage of cases of betamimetic-induced pulmonary edema has occurred in twin gestations.[85,99–101,110] Anemia, hypertension, and need for a blood transfusion also appear to be risk factors for the development of pulmonary edema.[111]

The pathophysiology of this serious complication has still not been well defined. Initially, it was attributed to cardiac dysfunction from excessive cardiac stimulation by beta-adrenergic agonists. However, neither non-invasive nor invasive cardiac studies have documented myocardial failure in a previously normal patient.[80,83,84,105]

Non-cardiogenic causes of betamimetic-induced pulmonary edema include increased pulmonary capillary permeability and/or hydrostatic pressures from fluid overload. In the majority of reported cases, compromised patients exhibited a positive fluid balance in excess of 5 liters. An antidiuretic effect of betamimetic agents with sodium and water retention has been described in both animals[118–121] and humans.[122–124] Administration of intravenous saline solutions may increase the risk of pulmonary edema.[107] A significant fall in hematocrit in those patients with subsequent pulmonary edema supports the contention of significant fluid retention.[85,101,103,107] Salt and water retention from steroid administration for fetal lung maturity is probably not signficantly addictive to the effects of beta-adrenergic agonists, since betamethasone and dexamethasone have little mineralocorticoid activity. Although the evidence for altered pulmonary capillary permeability is lacking,[119,120] infection may play a role in the development of pulmonary edema.[110,123] Infection is a leading cause of lung injury in the adult and can result in increased pulmonary capillary permeability with resultant pulmonary edema.

This important observation has recently been reported in 8 out of 12 patients at a single institution with betamimetic-induced pulmonary edema.[123]

Irrespective of the particular mechanism involved in the evolution of pulmonary edema, initial therapy should include discontinuation of the beta-agonist, oxygen administration, upright positioning, and attempted diuresis with furosemide. The presence of significant hypoxia or failure to achieve timely clinical improvement should prompt the initiation of invasive hemodynamic monitoring and preparations to provide ventilator support (with continuous positive airway pressure) based on arterial blood gas monitoring results. It is doubtful that use of cardiac glycosides is helpful in the clinical management of these patients. Avoidance of pulmonary edema is still most important. The current recommendations include limiting intravenous fluid to two liters of 5% dextrose in water or quarter-normal saline solution over each 24-hour period, avoidance of transfusions during intravenous therapy, and choosing alternative tocolytic agents in patients with significant anemia, twin gestation, or hypertension. Careful intake and output monitoring and frequent chest examinations may help identify those individuals developing this life-threatening complication.

Several maternal deaths have been associated with administration of betamimetic therapy.[97,103,117,126,127] While most of these maternal deaths were not directly attributable to the drug, a majority of these patients had a history of cardiac diseases or pulmonary hypertension, pointing out the importance of pretreatment screening for cardiopulmonary disease.

The other major category of beta-adrenergic agonist complications is metabolic including alterations in glucose, insulin, potassium, and lactic acid. Parenteral administration of beta-agonists results in an acute rise in plasma glucose concentration.[126,140] This is probably mediated by direct beta-adrenergic stimulation of the maternal pancreas to secrete glucagon, which in turn results in gluconeogenesis and glycogenolysis.[129,130] Insulin release precedes the onset of induced hyperglycemia due to beta-adrenergic receptor stimulation of the maternal pancreas.[130,131] Thereafter, serum insulin levels parallel the level of hyperglycemia. While these metabolic alterations have been documented with intravenous, subcutaneous or intramuscular administration of these tocolytic agents, the effects of orally administered betamimetic agents upon glucose hemostasis is less clear. The oral form of these betamimetic agents does not appear to cause overt hyperglycemia.[141,142] However, while oral ritodrine is not associated with an abnormal glucose tolerance test,[143,144] it appears that terbutaline may cause such an abnormality.[145,146] This implies that patients placed on chronic oral tocolysis should be screened for gestational diabetes.

The clinical use of betamimetic therapy in insulin-dependent diabetics is controversial.[146,150] Insulin-dependent patients receiving beta-adrenergic agonists have a significantly higher increase in serum glucose, lactate, and free fatty acids when compared to non-diabetic patients receiving these drugs.[151,152] The tendency to develop diabetic ketoacidosis is less dramatic in gestational diabetes and the degree of metabolic alteration seems to parallel the severity of insulin deficiency in the insulin-dependent patient.[151,152] While these metabolic alterations can lead to the development of hyperglycemic ketoacidosis, this potentially hazardous situation for both mother and fetus can be easily controlled with concurrent intravenous insulin administration.[146–148,150] A recent retrospective study of 15 insulin-dependent diabetic patients receiving betamimetic therapy and concurrent insulin therapy revealed no significant difference in perinatal morbidity when compared to a comparable control group.[150] Other authors feel that alternative tocolytic agents should be used in the insulin-dependent diabetic patient in preterm labor.[151] Probably the greatest potential risk in utilizing these agents occurs in the unrecognized diabetic patient. Therefore, it seems prudent to follow serial serum glucose levels and urinary ketones in all patients receiving these tocolytic agents, and institute intravenous insulin therapy in those individuals with evidence of significant hyperglycemia (>200 mg%).

Significant and rapid shifts in serum potassium concentrations have been described in patients receiving parenteral beta-adrenergic agonists.[126,131–133,137–140,153] The maximal drop in serum potassium, generally 0.6 to 1.5 mEq below preinfusion values, occurs at approximately 2 to 3 hours after the initiation of therapy.[126,131,137–139,153] After 10 to 20 hours of continued infusion, the serum potassium concentration normalizes, just as the serum glucose and insulin levels stabilize with continued infusion.[126,131,138,139,149] Parenteral administration of these agents does not significantly increase the urinary excretion of potassium[119,120,154,155] or alter aldosterone-mediated potassium urinary losses.[155,156] Since these shifts in serum potassium parallel the alteration in glucose homeostasis seen with these tocolytic agents, it has been hypothesized that serum potassium is transported intracellularly under the influence of glucose and insulin.[126,131,138,140,153] Although this mechanism of potassium transport clearly exists, direct beta-adrenergic receptor stimulation resulting in translocation of potassium across cellular membranes may also be important.[73,139] Orally-administered betamimetic agents do not appear to significantly alter potassium metabolism.[135,157] Therefore, since total body potassium is apparently not decreased with betamimetic therapy, potassium replacement therapy is rarely necessary. However, intravenous potassium replacement can be considered when serum levels drop below 2.0 mEq/L, a cardiac arrhythmia is present, or if furosemide is administered.

Beta-adrenergic stimulation leads to glycogenolysis and lipolysis. This results in increased lactate production which parallels the previously described alterations in glucose homeostasis and produces a dramatic rise in serum lactate levels.[158–160] In the absence of glucose intolerance, no signficant changes in maternal pH are usually observed.[158,159] However, betamimetic-induced acidosis has been described.[161] While serial determinations of maternal serum pH are not warranted, the use of lactated Ringer's solution during betamimetic therapy should be avoided.

Other maternal effects described with the use of these tocolytic agents include maternal serum transaminase elevations,[162,163] paralytic ileus,[164] cerebral vasospasm in patients with a previous history of migraine syndrome[165] and respiratory arrest due to increased muscle weakness in association with myasthenia gravis.[166]

Placental transfer of these tocolytic agents is rapid[167–175] and induces the typical beta-adrenergic stimulated response in the fetus. Fetal heart rate elevation above pre-infusion levels during maternal betamimetic therapy is common[81,140,175–186] and is presumed secondary to direct beta-receptor stimulation of the fetal myocardium. No significant alteration in fetal electrocardiograms has been observed.[187,188] In vitro fetal heart models have suggested significant cardiac toxicity in the form of myocardial lipid necrosis,[189,190] however, these findings have not been described at the time of neonatal autopsies in infants that were exposed to these medications in utero.[190,191] Recent in utero Doppler investigation of fetal hemodynamics suggest that the increase in fetal heart rate observed augments fetal cardiac output by increasing left ventricular blood flow and also causes a redistribution of fetal blood flow to the upper body.[186] Echocardiographic studies of the exposed fetus have demonstrated significant thickening of the ventricular septum as well.[192] Fetal metabolic alterations associated with betamimetic therapy have not been described, but the weight and histology of the fetal endocrine pancreas appear to be unchanged despite suspected fetal hyperinsulinism.[193]

Alterations in uteroplacental blood flow have been described in both animals[194–199] and humans.[200–204] The results of these investigations are variable with some authors reporting a decrease in uteroplacental blood flow,[194,196,197,199,202,203] other authors reporting an increase in uteroplacental blood flow,[200,201] and others finding no significant change.[195,198,204] These conflicting reports are probably due to differences in the specific beta-adrenergic agent investigated, length of infusion of the medication, concurrent use of sedation or anesthesia, and method of blood flow determination. For the most part, these alterations in uteroplacental blood flow are not associated with a significant alteration in fetal hemodynamics.[194–199,204] Overall, betamimetic agents probably cause a minimal increase in uteroplacental blood flow in the normal human patient; this improvement in placental perfusion is most likely due to vasodilation and increased maternal cardiac output associated with beta-receptor stimulation. The increase in placental perfusion is even more dramatic in those pregnancies with abnormal uteroplacental blood flow as in patients with intrauterine growth retardation and chronic hypertension.[201] Other clinical evidence supporting an increase in uteroplacental blood flow is the abolishment of progressive fetal respiratory acidosis during the second stage of term labor with the administration of intravenous ritodrine.[205] The use of beta-adrenergic agonists during acute fetal distress in those pregnancies with scalp pHs less than 7.25 or prolonged bradycardia result in a signficant improvement in neonatal Apgar scores and umbilical cord pHs.[206–208]

The antepartum adminstration of beta-adrenergic agonists has been associated with a decreased incidence of hyaline membrane disease in the preterm infant.[209,210,213,214] This phenomenon appears to be the result of increased release of surfactant as opposed to increased production prior to birth.[211,212,216,217] The actual clinical utility of the phenomenon has yet to be determined.

Depression of the fetal central nervous system as manifest by Apgar scores has not been reported with any of these tocolytic agents.[140,178,181,183,190,218–224] Likewise, no significant depression of umbilical pHs at the time of delivery has been described with maternal betamimetic therapy.[140,224] Hypoglycemia is common in the preterm infant and beta-adrenergic agonists have been associated with altered glucose homeostasis in the neonate.[140,222,224,225] This phenomenon seems to be related to hyperinsulinism and elevated growth hormone levels induced by beta-stimulation of the fetal pancreas prior to birth.[227,228] While neonatal hypoglycemia following cord clamping has been reported with isoxsuprine,[222] salbutamol,[227] terbutaline[226,227] and fenoterol,[221] it appears to be less significant with ritodrine.[140,224,225] Concurrent alterations in neonatal serum potassium levels have not been described.[224] Therefore, neonates delivered after recent exposure to maternal betamimetic therapy should be monitored for hypoglycemia.

While hypocalcemia in the neonate has been described with maternal isoxsuprine therapy,[222] alterations in neonatal calcium metabolism have not been described with ritodrine therapy.[140,224] Neonatal bilirubin production also appears to be increased with maternal betamimetic therapy,[224,230] but may be a function of other aspects of prematurity.[140] Neonatal thyroid function does not appear to be altered with betamimetic therapy.[228]

While tachycardia is commonly seen in the fetus during intravenous infusion of beta-adrenergic agonists, tachycardia in the neonate at delivery has not been described.[224] However, neonatal supraventricular tachycardia has been described following prolonged maternal administration of ritodrine.[231]

Long-term development evaluation of infants exposed to these betamimetic drugs in utero have been reported. The developmental outcomes assessed after 1 to 9 years in these infants do not significantly differ from preterm controls.[223,232–236] No significant alterations in growth, head circumference, neurologic development, psychomotor or social development have been associated with these specific tocolytic agents.[232–236]

The development of tolerance to the metabolic and cardiovascular effects of beta-adrenergic agonists has been well documented.[126,130,131,138,139,149,237,238] Based on this biologic phenomenon, some investigators have suggested that the ability of these tocolytic agents to arrest premature labor may only be transitory.[239] Chronic administration of betamimetic therapy results in the development of tolerance of smooth muscle relaxation in both animals[240] and humans.[241,242] In vitro studies of human myometrial strips obtained in cesarean delivery in patients receiving chronic betamimetic therapy had signficantly lower cAMP concentrations than control myometrial strips.[241,242] These results suggest that a desensitization of the beta-adrenergic receptor system has occurred with chronic betamimetic therapy and may ultimately limit the efficacy of these tocolytic agents in the prevention of preterm labor.

We will not review the individual betamimetic agents in clinical use today.

ISOXSUPRINE

Isoxsuprine (Vasodilan), which has both beta$_1$ and beta$_2$ activity, was one of the first beta-adrenergic agents used for inhibition of preterm labor. This agent first gained interest in 1961 when it was shown to cause uterine relaxation[177,243,244] and prolong pregnancy[245] in uncontrolled clinical experiences. In two controlled clinical trials, intravenous isoxsuprine followed by oral therapy was found to be significantly more effective than placebo therapy in postponing delivery.[218,246] In one study, delivery was postponed by 1 week in 18 of 25 (72%) of isoxsuprine-treated patients, whereas 6 of 25 (24%) of the placebo-treated pregnancies were postponed by 1 week. In this study, fetal salvage was 84% in the treated group versus 60% in the control group.[246] In the other study, isoxsuprine treatment delayed delivery by a mean of 46 days as compared to 14 days with placebo treatment.[218] The efficacy of isoxsuprine in preventing preterm delivery appeared similar to ethanol in a randomized clinical comparison.[56]

Maternal hypotension and tachycardia are common side effects of intravenous isoxsuprine by virtue of its beta$_1$ adrenergic activity and have subsequently limited the clinical utility of this medication. With the degree of hypotension being dose-dependent, the average decrease in blood pressure is 10 to 20 mm Hg with the standard dosages,[218,244,245] and is seen in 8 to 51% of patients receiving this tocolytic agent.[168,182] Significant maternal tachycardia is also seen in these patients.[168,244,247] Fetal tachycardia is seen in 35 to 55% of pregnancies as well.[168,182,187] While pre-therapy with intravenous hydration and a left lateral decubitus position may prevent some of the hypotensive effects of the drug, these important cardiovascular effects limit the dosage of isoxsuprine and thereby reduce its effectiveness in controlling preterm labor.

Neonatal side effects have also limited the clinical usefulness of isoxsuprine. Several controlled studies of preterm infants whose mothers received isoxsuprine prior to delivery revealed that hypocalcemia, hypoglycemia, hypotension, evidence of ileus, and neonatal death were all more common than in untreated patients.[222,229] Hypocalcemia was seen in 59 to 80% of the treated groups compared to 31 to 61% in the untreated groups; hypoglycemia was seen in 14 to 20% of the isoxsuprine groups compared to 5 to 10% in the control groups. Hypotension was associated with 63% of the isoxsuprine groups and 43 to 45% of the control groups. Prolonged ileus in the neonate was seen in 32 to 40% of infants exposed to isoxsuprine compared to 2.5 to 10% in the untreated group. Neonatal deaths were two to four times more common in the isoxsuprine-treated group.

These dramatic side effects in the neonate are associated with elevated umbilical cord levels of isoxsuprine.[229] Umbilical cord isoxsuprine levels averaged 90% of the maternal serum concentration at the time of delivery. The interval from discontinuing intravenous isoxsuprine to the time when the umbilical drug levels approach a safe range (<10 ng/ml) is greater than 2 hours and it takes over 6 hours before these levels are negligible.[229] Also, clearance of this drug in the neonate is slow with the half-life in the near term neonate of 1.7 hours and as long as 8.0 hours in the 26 to 28 week neonate.[229] Since these complications are related to neonatal drug levels, the drug should be stopped when preterm delivery in less than 2 hours is anticipated.

In view of these clinically significant alterations in maternal and neonatal physiology associated with isoxsuprine administration, newer agents with more specific beta$_2$ beta-adrenergic effects have been developed, including ritodrine, terbutaline, salbutamol, fenoterol and hexaprenaline. Isoxsuprine probably has a limited role in modern tocolytic therapy.

RITODRINE

In 1980, the United States Food and Drug Administration (FDA) approved ritodrine hydrochloride (Yutopar) for the inhibition of preterm labor. This culminated more than 10 years of clinical research with ritodrine in the United States by investigators working at various medical centers and employing different clinical protocols. Ritodrine is a beta-adrenergic agonist with predominant effects on beta 2 receptors and was purported to have similar efficacy and fewer clinical side effects than previously developed tocolytic agents.

The first prospective, double-blind placebo-controlled study of ritodrine from a multicenter trial in Europe was reported in 1971.[178] Patients with or without PROM received an intravenous infusion of ritodrine or placebo followed by oral tablets for a total of 7 days of therapy. Delivery was delayed for at least 7 days in 80% of the ritodrine groups, and in 48% of the placebo controls. Among the

51 patients with intact membranes, the mean interval to subsequent delivery was 28 days in the ritodrine group versus 17 days in the placebo group.[178]

In 1972, a series of prospective, randomized double-blind controlled studies compared ritodrine with either ethanol or placebo in the inhibition of preterm labor at multiple centers throughout the United States.[128,248] A total of 313 singleton patients with intact membranes were studied and constituted the phase III clinical trials for the FDA approval process. Intravenous ritodrine, ethanol, or placebo were initially administered to these patients; for all except the ethanol group, successful parenteral therapy was followed by oral maintenance therapy. Statistically significant prolongation of preterm pregnancies was shown with ritodrine versus alcohol or placebo controls.[248]

Approximately 52% of the ritodrine-treated patients attained 36 weeks of gestation as compared to 38% of the controls and this effect was even more dramatic if enrollment into the study occurred prior to 33 weeks (48 vs 27%). The mean of days gained from initiation of treatment to delivery was 32.6 days for the ritodrine group and 21.3 days for the control group. Similarly, the percentage of pregnancies achieving a birth weight of greater than 2500 g was 58% in the ritodrine group versus 43% in the control group; if treatment was initiated prior to 33 weeks, this difference increased to 53 versus 31%. The neonatal death rate in the ritodrine group was 5% compared to 13% of the controls and the incidence of neonatal RDS was 11 versus 20% respectively. However, the mean gestational age at the time of delivery was only 35.5 weeks for the ritodrine group versus 34.5 weeks for the control group.

Since the controls in these collaborative trials included ethanol as well as placebo, ethanol having already been shown to be more effective than placebo in inhibiting preterm labor,[54] a stronger case for the effectiveness of ritodrine may be provided by these data. However, in this study, those patients who were initially treated with parenteral ritodrine and then randomized to oral ritodrine or placebo therapy were included for analysis in the ritodrine-treated group. Since a proportion of these patients with prolongation of pregnancy were probably not in preterm labor, this may have falsely improved the apparent efficacy of ritodrine. Other criticisms of this study include varying protocols between participating medical centers, as well as too few pregnancies and patients with PROM for a meaningful analysis of these subgroups. Also, no serious maternal complications attributable to ritodrine or the degree of patient intolerance were reported in this study.[128]

Subsequent randomized clinical trials of the efficacy of ritodrine have produced contradictory results. In a study of 29 patients with preterm labor receiving either parenteral ritodrine or placebo with subsequent oral therapy versus placebo, no significant extension of pregnancy (29 vs 27% delivering after 1 week) or increased birth weight (mean birth weight of 1984 vs 1806 g) could be demonstrated.[181] Another comparison of 129 patients with preterm labor from 1980 receiving three different regimens of ritodrine administration and 44 patients receiving placebo and bed rest failed to demonstrate any difference in delay of delivery (57 vs 67% with delivery after 2 weeks), birth weights (56 vs 64% with birth weights greater than 2500 g), or neonatal mortality (8 vs 2% neonatal deaths).[249]

A more recent multicenter European study of 99 patients randomized to receive either intramuscular ritodrine or placebo followed by oral therapy did not show long-term efficacy.[220] The mean gestational age at delivery was 37.2 weeks in the ritodrine group versus 36.3 weeks in the placebo group, whereas the difference in days gained from the initiation of therapy was not statistically significant (34 vs 25 days respectively). The mean birth weight at delivery was also not different at 2845 g in the ritodrine group or 2748 g in the control group. In another study, 106 preterm labor patients were randomized to receive intravenous ritodrine with oral maintenance therapy, or bed rest without tocolytic therapy.[221] There was no statistical difference between the ritodrine versus the bed rest group with regard to mean gestational age at delivery (32.8 vs 32.6 weeks), days gained since initiation of therapy (19.8 vs 15.1 days), or the mean number of days that these neonates required intensive care (14.3 vs 12.4 days). These more recent studies raise serious questions regarding the efficacy of ritodrine in the treatment of preterm labor.

In one comparision study, ritodrine appeared to be more effective than ethanol in preventing prematurity as measured by mean days from initiation of therapy to delivery (46.2 vs 26.6 days respectively), and birth weights greater than 2500 g (72 vs 45%).[57] In other studies comparing the efficacy of terbutaline and ritodrine, it appears that intravenous administration of these drugs has comparable success in arresting preterm labor.[250–252] In these three randomized clinical studies involving a total of 252 patients with intact membranes in preterm labor, there is no statistically significant difference in initial success rates (arrest of preterm labor for greater than 72 hours) with either intravenous ritodrine or terbutaline (26 vs 26%; 67 vs 80%; 69 vs 45%). Several short-term comparison studies between ritodrine and intravenous magnesium sulfate also show no statistical difference in tocolytic success rates.[252–254] In one randomized study of 70 patients with intact membranes with success being defined as arrest of preterm labor for at least 72 hours, a success rate of 88% was achieved with ritodrine and 79% with magnesium sulfate.[254]

Oral maintenance therapy with ritodrine appears to be successful in preventing recurrent preterm labor. In one randomized double-blind study of oral maintenace therapy with ritodrine, 70 patients were initially treated intramuscularly with ritodrine and 59 patients achieved successful tocolysis beyond 24 hours.[219] Fifty-four patients were subsequently randomized to receive either oral ritodrine or placebo therapy. If preterm labor recurred, the sequence of intramuscular injections followed by oral therapy was repeated. The number of days gained after initiation of therapy was similar in both groups (34 days for oral ritodrine vs 36 days for placebo). However, the mean interval between initiation of therapy and the first relapse or delivery was 25.9 days in the ritodrine group compared to 5.8 days in the placebo group. There was a smaller number of relapses requiring repeat intramuscular therapy in the oral ritodrine group (1.1 relapses) than in the placebo group (2.71 relapses). These results suggest that maintenance therapy with an oral betamimetic agent is successful in preventing recurrent preterm labor and allows for the ambulatory management of these patients.

In two randomized, double-blinded studies of 58 and 99 patients respectively with intact membranes, a comparison of oral ritodrine and oral terbutaline as maintenance therapy after successful intravenous tocolysis has been performed.[250,251] Both studies demonstrated a significant difference in the ability of these specific oral betamimetic agents to prolong these pregnancies, despite the fact that initial success rates with the intravenous forms of these drugs were similar (26 vs 26% and 69 vs 80%). In one study, the pregnancy was prolonged for 40 days with intravenous and oral terbutaline, as compared to 22 days with intravenous and oral ritodrine.[250] In the other study, a total of 25.8 days were gained with oral terbutaline compared to 13.1 days with ritodrine therapy.[251] Although these two clinical trials suggest that oral maintenance therapy with terbutaline may be more effective than with ritodrine, a third study of 91 patients randomized to either oral agent after successful intravenous tocolysis[255] showed no significant difference in days gained from initiation of therapy (37.1 days for terbutaline and 38.3 days for ritodrine).

Ritodrine is usually given intravenously at an initial rate of 50 to 100 μg/min and increased every 15 to 20 minutes until uterine contractions have ceased, unacceptable side effects have developed, or the maximum dosage of 350 μg/min has been achieved. Maternal intravenous infusion of ritodrine reaches therapeutic levels quickly with an initial phase half-life of 6 to 9 minutes, followed by a biphasic elimination phase with a half-life of aproximately 2 to 3 hours.[169,221,256] Ritodrine is excreted in free or conjugated forms primarily in the urine.[129] A large range of serum ritodrine concentration at these standard infusion rates is evident (15 to 146 ng/ml), and probably reflects individual variations in the metabolism and excretion rates of this drug.[129,256] There is rapid and appreciable transplacental transfer of intravenous ritodrine,[170–173] with a mean fetal to maternal concentration ratio of 1.17.[171] Once maternal administration of ritodrine has been discontinued, ritodrine levels in the umbilical cord at delivery remain significant for up to 5 hours and are directly related to intravenous dosage schedule and drug discontinuance to delivery interval.[171] Therefore, once tocolysis has failed and delivery is imminent, intravenous ritodrine should be discontinued so as to minimize neonatal levels of the drug.

Ritodrine infusions should be titrated to minimize maternal side effects on an individual basis while ensuring adequate tocolysis. Maternal and fetal side effects from intravenous ritodrine appear to be dose-related, but wide variability exists in serum concentrations and reported side effects between different patients or even during an individual's treatment course.[256] However, these side effects were most commonly observed when the infusion rate and concentration of ritodrine were increasing.[256] Thus, slower increases in infusion rates may allow for continued administration of ritodrine in those individuals experiencing significant side effects. Continuous long-term intravenous betamimetic therapy has been described without significant morbidity,[257] but such long-term intravenous administration of these tocolytic agents requires further investigation.

Some investigators feel that intramuscular ritodrine (5 to 10 mg every 2 to 4 hours) produces superior results, has fewer side effects, and allows use of less intravenous hydration when compared to intravenous ritodrine therapy.[135,219,220,249] Peak serum concentrations of 97 ng/ml ± 5 are achieved within 10 minutes when 10 mg of ritodrine is administered intramuscularly. The subsequent half-life of ritodrine with this route of administration is two hours.[169] However, only one randomized study comparing these two routes of administration suggests any clinical benefit to intramuscular injections.[249] Therefore, without more substantive data, controlled intravenous administration of ritodrine is preferable.

Parenteral administration of ritodrine should be continued for 12 to 24 hours after uterine contractions have ceased and then oral maintenance therapy begun with either 10 mg every 2 hours, or 20 mg every 4 hours of ritodrine. Thereafter, the oral dosage may be maintained at 10 to 20 mg every 4 hours until 36 weeks. Oral administration of 10 mg of ritodrine produces peak serum concentrations of 31 ng/ml $\pm$ 7 in approximately 30 minutes;[169] the reported bioavailability of the oral form is approximately 20 to 30%.[169,258] While metabolic alterations with oral ritodrine appear to be minimal,[135,142,143,151] maternal and fetal cardiovascular responses to oral administration remain significant.[219] There is wide variation in serum ritodrine levels with oral dosage and ritodrine levels are signficantly lower than with intravenous dosages.[258]

Neonatal complications attributable to ritodrine, such as hypoglycemia, hypertension, or hypocalcemia have been minimal.[140,224] However, a fetal death associated with severe ritodrine-induced ketoacidosis has been reported.[259]

The reported clinical experience with betamimetic therapy in twin gestations has been limited. A controlled retrospective comparison study of 23 twins and 23 singletons[185] failed to show any difference in maternal or fetal tachycardia, maternal hypotension, duration of therapy, or delay of delivery. Although patients with multiple gestations appear to be at increased risk for the development of pulmonary edema with these tocolytic agents, the judicious use of ritodrine in these cases is appropriate.

Despite the lack of clinical evidence that ritodrine is more effective than other tocolytic agents, or is associated with a lower incidence of maternal-fetal side effects when compared with other beta-adrenergic agonists, ritodrine remains the only FDA-approved drug for tocolytic therapy in the United States today.

TERBUTALINE

Terbutaline (Brethine/Bricanyl) can also inhibit uterine contractions,[260,261] and has been shown effective in treating premature labor. The first double-blinded placebo-controlled study was reported in 1976, in which 30 patients received intravenous therapy for at least 8 hours, with maintenance subcutaneous and oral therapies being continued until 36 weeks gestation.[175] In 12 of the 15 (80%) terbutaline-treated patients, preterm labor was arrested beyond the treatment period; only 3 of the 15 (20%) placebo-treated patients achieved a gestational age of 36 weeks. The mean birth weight in the placebo-treated group was 2190 g as compared to 3000 g for those patients receiving terbutaline.

A more recent double-blind placebo-controlled study with a similar protocol failed to demonstrate any significant difference in the inhibition of preterm labor in 33 patients.[184] In the 15 patients who received terbutaline and in the 18 patients who received placebo, there was no significant difference in prolongation of pregnancy (30.8 days vs 39.9 days respectively), birth weight (2487 vs 2756 g), or the incidence of RDS (18 vs 5%). Another recent study of short-term intravenous terbutaline or placebo therapy demonstrated no significant efficacy of terbutaline (terbutaline-54% vs placebo-38%) in stopping preterm labor for greater than 48 hours.[262]

In these studies, numbers may have been too small for significance to be achieved. In one comparison study with ethanol,[58] 56 patients with intact membranes received either intravenous terbutaline or ethanol until uterine contractions ceased; then both groups were given oral terbutaline for the next 5 days and observed for recurrent preterm labor. The intravenous terbutaline group had a mean prolongation of pregnancy of 15 days as compared to 10 days in the intravenous ethanol group. Several comparison studies of terbutaline and magnesium sulfate have been reported.[262,263] In one study of 35 patients randomly assigned to receive intravenous therapy with either terbutaline or magnesium sulfate without follow-up maintenance therapy,[262] delay of delivery for greater than 48 hours was not statistically different between the two groups (terbutaline-53% vs magnesium sulfate-37%). In another similar study involving 29 patients, 69% of the terbutaline group had delivery delayed greater than 24 hours as compared to 64% of the magnesium sulfate group.[263]

The ability of maintenance terbutaline therapy to prevent recurrence of preterm labor has been investigated. In one study involving 46 patients who had successful arrest of preterm labor with intravenous ethanol, these patients were then randomized to receive either oral terbutaline or placebo until preterm labor recurred or a gestational age of 38 weeks was obtained.[183] The total days gained until delivery were 42.5 days in the terbutaline group versus 29.4 days in the placebo group. Birth weight (2757 vs 2988 g) and the incidence of RDS (4 vs 23%) were significantly different between the two groups as well. Two clinical studies have sugested that oral terbutaline for maintenance tocolytic therapy is more successful than oral ritodrine.[250,251] However, one study has failed to demonstrate any significant prolongation of pregnancy with terbutaline as compared to oral ritodrine.[255]

Terbutaline is given intravenously at an initial rate of 10 μg/min and increased every 15 to 20 minutes until contractions have ceased, unacceptable side effects develop or a maximum dosage of 25 μg/min has been achieved. Maternal infusion of terbutaline reaches therapeutic levels rapidly with a mean terminal half-life of 3.7 hours.[264] A wide variation in serum plasma concentrations (12.8 to 31.5 ng/ml) with the recommended intravenous dosages has been noted and probably reflects the wide range of urinary excretion of free and conjugated terbutaline by individual patients.[264] In view of these variations, terbutaline infusions should be titrated on an individual basis so as to maximize inhibition of uterine activity and minimize maternal side effects. There is a rapid and appreciable transplacental transfer of terbutaline with maternal-fetal equilibration after 1 hour.[174] Therefore, once preterm delivery seems inevitable, intravenous terbutaline should be discontinued so as to minimize neonatal levels of the drug.

Subcutaneous administration of terbutaline has been advocated as an alternative to intravenous infusion of the drug.[265,266] Terbutaline is absorbed rapidly after subcutaneous administration with an absorptive half-life of 7 minutes.[268] Commonly used treatment regimens are 0.25 mg subcutaneously every 20 to 60 minutes until the contractions have subsided. A recent randomized study involving 77 patients comparing intravenous versus subcutaneous administration of terbutaline revealed similar efficacy and side effects.[266] The ease of administration and avoidance of intravenous hydration make subcutaneous administration of terbutaline a reasonable alternative to intravenous therapy. Effective vaginal administration of terbutaline with apparently fewer side effects has also been described.[269]

Parenteral administration of terbutaline should be continued for 12 to 24 hours after uterine contractions have ceased. Thereafter, oral maintenance therapy with 2.5 to 5.0 mg every 6 to 8 hours is begun. Oral administration of terbutaline results in widely varying peak serum concentrations (1.5 to 8.3 ng/ml) after 1 hour and serum drug levels are significantly lower than seen with intravenous dosages.[264] The schedule for oral maintenance therapy should be individualized on the basis of uterine effects and patient tolerance.

Maternal side effects appear similar with either terbutaline or ritodrine.Most randomized comparison studies have not shown any difference in tachycardia, hypotension, chest pain, arrhythmia, hypokalemia, or jitteriness.[250,252,255] Recent studies also report significant alterations in maternal glucose tolerance with chronic oral terbutaline therapy.[144,145] However, the large cost differential and minimal difference in side effects between these two medications may warrant the substitution of terbutaline for ritodrine.[255]

SALBUTAMOL

Salbutamol has been used extensively outside of the United States for the inhibition of preterm labor.[269–273] Its administration, type of side effects, and effectiveness are similar to other betamimetic agents. In a randomized comparison study with terbutaline, 34 patients received intravenous therapy with follow-up maintenance therapy with either drug.[274] A delay of delivery for greater than 1 week was not statistically different between the two groups (salbutamol-74% vs terbutaline-80%). In another study of 88 patients comparing the efficacy of intravenous salbutamol and ethanol,[275] the mean delay of delivery was similar in both groups (15 vs 20 days).

The initial intravenous dosage of salbutamol is 20 μg/min with a maximum dosage of 50 μg/min. Oral maintenance therapy with 4 mg of salbutamol every 6 to 12 hours is begun once uterine activity has subsided for 12 to 24 hours. Transplacental transfer to the fetus has also been described.[273] The increase in fetal heart rate observed with salbutamol was significantly more common than with terbutaline therapy.[272]

In summary, salbutamol is another effective tocolytic agent without documented superiority to any other betamimetic agent.

OTHER BETA₂ AGONIST AGENTS

Pharmacologic alterations to these beta-adrenergic medications have produced a variety of beta₂ selective tocolytic agents. These agents include fenoterol, hexoprenaline, and orciprenaline. While all of these agents produce significant tocolytic effects,[277–281] controlled clinical trials are currently lacking. Of all of these other beta₂ selective agents, hexaprenaline appears to produce the least effect upon the maternal cardiovascular system.[121,278,281]

Magnesium Sulphate

Physiologists have known for some time that magnesium has the potential to decrease muscle contractility. However, it was not until 1959 that the effect of magnesium therapy upon labor was first described.[282] Subsequently, other investigators reported that the infusion of magnesium sulfate during labor was associated with decreased uterine activity,[43,283,284] although the alteration in uterine activity may be transitory.[285,286] The exact mechanism for the tocolytic action of magnesium sulfate remains unknown. Since magnesium appears to decrease the frequency of depolarization of the smooth muscle cell and uncouples the ATP-linked activation of the actin-myosin unit during in vitro studies, it has been suggested that magnesium competes with calcium for entry into the muscle cell during depolarization.[74,287,288] Serum magnesium concentrations of 4 to 8 mEq/L appear to be necessary for inhibition of uterine activity in humans.[74,284]

Controlled studies evaluating the efficacy of magnesium sulfate in inhibiting preterm labor have been limited. In one study involving 31 patients who received intravenous magnesium sulfate at a rate of 2 g/hr and 9 subsequent patients who received a placebo infusion, delivery was delayed for more than 24 hours in 77% of the magnesium-treated patients and 44% of the placebo-treated patients.[59] In this study, the rate of success was inversely related to the degree of cervical dilation. Another study involving 35 patients randomized to either intravenous magnesium sulfate at 2 g/hr or intravenous hydration failed to show any significant difference in delaying preterm delivery.[262] Intravenous magnesium sulfate delayed delivery for more than 48 hours in only 6 of 16 (38%) patients, as compared to 7 of 19 patients (37%) receiving intravenous hydration.

When intravenous magnesium sulfate and ethanol were compared in their ability to prevent preterm delivery within 24 hours of initiating therapy,[59] magnesium was successful in 24 of 31 (77%) patients as compared to 14 of 31 (45%) patients receiving ethanol. In two studies involving 64 patients, magnesium sulfate and terbutaline were equivalent in their ability to delay preterm delivery for 24 to 48 hours.[262,263] Likewise, short-term tocolytic therapy with magnesium sulfate and ritodrine appear to have similar efficacy in three studies.[252–254] In one study of 63 patients who received either intravenous therapy with magnesium sulfate or ritodrine followed with maintenance terbutaline therapy,[252] the mean days gained until delivery with initial magnesium sulfate were 38 days as compared to 43 days with initial ritodrine therapy. A similar study involving 48 patients who received maintenance ritodrine therapy after the initial randomized therapy,[253] preterm delivery was delayed for greater than 1 week in 21 of 27 (78%) patients of the magnesium sulfate group and 16 of 21 (76%) patients in the ritodrine group.

In a recent study of 70 patients randomized to either intravenous ritodrine or magnesium sulfate followed by oral betamimetic therapy,[254] preterm delivery was delayed for greater than 7 days in 75% of the magnesium sulfate group and 72% of the ritodrine group. These comparison studies suggest that the clinical use of magnesium sulfate as a first-line tocolytic agent is justified.

Magnesium sulfate is given intravenously with an initial 4 g loading dose over 15 to 20 minutes with subsequent continuous infusion rate of 2 to 6 g/hr. An average serum magnesium level of 6.4 mg/dl $\pm$ 1.4 is obtained with an infusion rate of 3 g/hr.[285] Intramuscular magnesium sulfate therapy for preterm labor has not been studied. Magnesium is eliminated almost entirely by renal excretion of the drug.[287] With intravenous infusion of magnesium sulfate, 75% of the administered dose is excreted during a bolus infusion and 90% within 24 hours after treatment.[290] With impaired renal function, it is necessary to check serum magnesium levels frequently in order to prevent magnesium toxicity. All patients receiving magnesium sulfate should be monitored closely for the loss of deep tendon reflexes and respiratory depression. The loss of deep tendon reflexes occurs with serum magnesium levels of 4 to 8 mEq/L and respiratory depression may be seen at 12 to 15 mEq/L.[287] Above this level, cardiac conduction defects and cardiac arrest may occur.

When intravenous magnesium sulfate therapy is maintained in a non-toxic range, maternal side effects remain low. In a recent randomized comparison trial, significant side effects requiring discontinuation of intravenous therapy occurred in only 2% of patients receiving magnesium sulfate as compared to 38% of patients receiving ritodrine and 60% of patients receiving terbutaline.[252] The most common side effects are associated with the loading bolus of magnesium sulfate and include transient hypotension associated with a feeling of heat and flushing.[286,289] There is no maternal tachycardia associated with magnesium sulfate administration[286,291] and cardiac output remains unchanged. A decrease in maternal temperature with magnesium sulfate infusion has been described by several authors,[292,293] but not observed by other investigators.[286] Maternal paralytic ileus secondary to magnesium sulfate infusion has also been described.[294] Pulmonary edema with concurrent magnesium sulfate and steroid administration has been described.[289,295,296] Other large clinical experiences with magnesium sulfate therapy have failed to demonstrate significant maternal morbidity.[297]

Alterations in maternal calcium metabolism have been described with intravenous magnesium sulfate therapy. Serum concentrations of ionized and nonionized calcium fall dramatically with infusion of magnesium sulfate.[290,298,299] This fall in serum calcium is due in part to increased renal excretion of calcium[290,298] and a decrease in serum parathyroid hormone levels.[299,300] The clinical significance of maternal hypocalcemia during magnesium infusion remains unknown.

Maternal magnesium sulfate infusion appears to increase uterine and placental blood flow rates,[291] making it a potential useful tocolytic agent in cases of maternal bleeding or suspected uteroplacental insufficiency. Transplacental transfer of magnesium to the fetus has been confirmed in multiple studies.[301–303] Some investigators have reported a decrease in fetal heart rate variability,[304–305] while others have noted no such fetal heart rate abnormality.[285,306] This appears to be a dose-related phenomenon.

While magnesium levels associated with maternal magnesium sulfate infusion are rarely toxic to the newborn,[283,301–303] significant neonatal hypotonia and drowsiness due to neonatal hypermagnesemia have been described.[302,307–309] Decreased bowel peristalsis mimicking meconium ileus has been reported in two neonates with hypermagnesemia.[310] These cases of hypermagnesemia are usually associated with maternal magnesium infusion of greater than 24 hours, intramuscular injections, or in the premature infant.[302,307,308] In contrast to the adult, the newborn does not excrete a magnesium load satisfactorily[307] and requires up to 48 hours to reach normal serum magnesium levels after maternal infusion.[303] Interestingly, there is no correlation between maternal serum magnesium levels at delivery and concurrent umbilical cord or neonatal levels.[303] Also, maternal magnesium infusion does not appear to cause neonatal hypocalcemia.[303]

The main disadvantage to the clinical use of magnesium sulfate is the lack of an oral preparation for maintenance therapy once the initial uterine contractions have subsided. Some investigators have reported the use of continuous long-term magnesium sulfate infusion to inhibit preterm labor for up to 13 weeks.[311,312] More recently, one group has advocated the use of oral magnesium sulfate for maintenance therapy.[313,314] They report that 1 g of orally-administered magnesium sulfate every 4 hours results in a maternal serum level of 2.16 mEq/L.[313] A recent study involving the use of oral magnesium or oral ritodrine for maintenance tocolytic therapy in 50 patients[314] showed no difference in gestational age at delivery (35.6 vs 34.9 weeks), but did demonstrate a significant difference in maternal side effects (16 vs 40%).

The adjunctive use of magnesium sulfate with ritodrine therapy for the inhibition of preterm labor has been evaluated with conflicting results. The concurrent use of these two agents after a single-agent tocolytic failure has been advocated by some authors.[315,316] In one randomized comparison study, involving 64 patients,[317] 31% of the ritodrine group had delivery delayed greater than 1 week as compared to 59% of the combination therapy group. These authors also reported that while the maternal and fetal side effects were not different between the two groups, the dose requirements of ritodrine and the total duration of therapy were less in the combination group. In a similar blinded study involving 50 patients, adjunctive magnesium sulfate therapy did not alter the metabolic changes associated with ritodrine.[318] However, other investigators have shown no significant difference in efficacy of delaying preterm delivery between these two groups in a study involving 41 patients.[319] The most disturbing aspect of this study was the observation that significant cardiovascular effects were observed in 11 of 24 (46%) patients receiving combination therapy as compared to 1 of 17 (6%) patients receiving ritodrine only. Because of the potential for serious maternal side effects, we do not recommend concurrent use of these drugs.

Sequential therapy with magnesium sulfate in preterm labor patients who fail to respond to therapy with a betamimetic agent has been advocated by several authors.[317,320,321] Based on reports of overall success rates of 40 to 90% with this treatment regimen, it appears that the sequential use of magnesium sulfate may be beneficial in prolonging pregnancy.[252,317,321] While significant progression in cervical dilatation can occur before magnesium sulfate is initiated,[317] it appears that the use of more than one tocolytic agent in a sequential fashion does not decrease the chances for successful therapy.[321] However, since clinical trials where ritodrine failures are randomized to magnesium sulfate or placebo are lacking, the efficacy of sequential magnesium sulfate therapy to treat first-line tocolytic failure remains unproven.

In summary, there is substantial evidence that magnesium sulfate is a reasonable alternative tocolytic agent for the inhibition of preterm labor. While magnesium sulfate has generally been utilized sequentially to prevent preterm delivery after failure of a betamimetic agonist, this tocolytic agent offers the distinct advantages of minimal maternal side effects and no apparent alterations in uteroplacental blood flow. With further investigation and clinical experience, magnesium sulfate may gain widespread use as a primary tocolytic agent.

Prostaglandin Synthetase Inhibitors

Prostaglandin synthetase inhibitors have also been shown to be effective in inhibiting preterm labor. These drugs are easily administered and are well tolerated by the mother.[322–324] However, concern about the effects of prostaglandin synthetase inhibitors upon the fetus has limited their clinical use. Indomethacin (Indocin) is the most widely used prostaglandin synthetase inhibitor in clinical use today.

Prostaglandins are important modulators of uterine contractility. Increased release of prostaglandins has been demonstrated during normal human parturition by a variety of methods.[325–334] More recently, elevated prostaglandin metabolites have been measured in patients with preterm labor.[325] The production of prostaglandins that is associated with uterine contractility appears to be linked with calcium entry across the smooth muscle membrane.[74] All of the currently available prostaglandin synthetase inhibitors act upon the cyclooxygenase enzyme which prevents the cascade of prostaglandins from their precursor, arachidonic acid.[74,336] Indomethacin, naproxen (Naprosyn, Anaprox), and fenoprofen (Nalfon) are more effective inhibitors of prostaglandin synthesis than aspirin.[337] These prostaglandin synthetase inhibitors exhibit marked depressant activity upon uterine contractility in excised uterine muscle strips.[338,339] Administration of either indomethacin[331,340,341] or ritodrine[325,335] during labor in humans results in a significant reduction of plasma prostaglandin levels.

Several studies utilizing prostaglandin synthetase inhibitors have supported the association of prostaglandins and parturition. In pregnant Rhesus monkeys, indomethacin prolongs gestation and prevents the initiation of parturition.[342] In one retrospective study, patients taking high-dose salicylate during pregnancy had a significant increase in the mean length of gestation, the frequency of postdatism and the mean duration of spontaneous labor.[343] In another study, patients taking long-term salicylate during pregnancy had a higher incidence of gestation beyond 42 weeks.[344] In patients undergoing saline-induced mid-trimester abortions, administration of oral indomethacin or aspirin results in prolongation of the injection to abortion interval.[345] In another abortion study involving patients undergoing pregnancy terminations with hyperosmolar urea and oxytocin augmentation, low doses of aspirin prolonged the injection-abortion interval in nulliparous patients.[346] The administration of indomethacin to 16 patients during active term labor resulted in complete cessation of labor in 7 patients and a prolonged active phase in another 7 patients.[347]

Several uncontrolled clinical studies have described the use of indomethacin for the inhibition of preterm labor.[340,348–350] The first clinical use of indomethacin as a tocolytic agent in the treatment of premature labor was reported by Zuckerman in 1974.[348] Fifty women with clinical evidence of preterm labor were initially given 100 mg of indomethacin rectally followed by 25 mg orally every 6 hours; uterine contractions ceased in 40 (80%) of these study patients. Several other early studies described similar results with oral indomethacin in 38 patients who had failed previous tocolytic therapy.[340,349] Another clinical experience involving the use of flufenamic acid, another prostaglandin synthetase inhibitor, in 18 patients resulted in delay of delivery for greater than 48 hours in 15 (83%) patients.[350] The largest clinical experience with indomethacin as a first-line tocolytic agent was reported in 1984 and involved 252 patients with intact membranes in preterm labor.[351] A total of 222 (88%) patients had a prolongation of pregnancy for greater than 1 week. The majority of patients who successfully responded to indomethacin therapy in this study had initial cervical dilation of less than 3 cm.

Controlled clinical studies have clearly demonstrated the efficacy of indomethacin in the inhibition of preterm labor.[341,352] In a prospective, randomized double-blinded study of 30 patients, indomethacin was found to be significantly more effective than placebo in the inhibition of preterm labor during a 24-hour course of therapy.[341] Indomethacin was administered orally, initially as a 50-mg loading dose followed by 25 mg doses every 4 hours for 24 hours, and the patients were observed for recurrent preterm labor. A second 24-hour course of therapy was initiated if recurrent preterm labor occurred. An alternative tocolytic agent was administered if progressive cervical dilation was observed. Treatment failures occurred during therapy in only 1 of 15 (7%) indomethacin-treated patients as compared to 9 of 15 (60%) placebo-treated patients. At 24 hours after therapy, the treatment failure rates were still significantly different (20 vs 67% respectively).

Another controlled, double-blinded study of 36 patients with preterm labor confirms the efficacy of indomethacin as a tocolytic agent.[352] Indomethacin was initially administered as a 100 mg rectal suppository followed by 25 mg orally every 4 hours for 24 hours. Alternative tocolytic therapy was instituted if progressive cervical dilation became evident. Only 1 of 18 (6%) indomethacin-treated patients had delivery within 48 hours as compared to 14 of 18 (78%) of the placebo-treated group. Delay of delivery was also significant with 15 of 18 (83%) indomethacin-treated patients having delivery delayed greater than 7 days as compared to 3 of 18 (17%) patients in the placebo-treated group. Likewise, 78% of the placebo-treated patients delivered an infant less than 2500 g as compared to 17% in the indomethacin group.

Several comparison studies have also been used to demonstrate the efficacy of indomethacin in treating preterm labor.[353,356] In a comparative trial of alcohol, indomethacin and salbutamol involving 62 patients, a combination of ethanol and indomethacin inhibited labor for 48 hours in 70% of the cases as compared to 60% with salbutamol and 32% with ethanol alone.[353] In a double-blinded, randomized trial of ritodrine and a regimen of ritodrine and indomethacin, 22 patients received intravenous/oral ritodrine therapy with 50 mg indomethacin suppositories every 8 hours and the other 22 patients received intravenous/oral ritodrine with placebo suppositories.[354] The mean gain in days from initiation of therapy (41.3 vs 25.9 days), number of pregnancies achieving 37 weeks gestation (15 vs 8) and number of recurrences (7 vs 15) were all signficantly different between the two groups. A similar randomized clinical trial of ritodrine or a combination of ritodrine with indomethacin for 24 hours has been performed with 120 patients.[355] In this study, indomethacin was initially administered as a 100 mg suppository followed by 25 mg orally every 6 hours. The mean number of days gained was significantly different between the two groups (ritodrine group—11.5 days—vs ritodrine/indomethacin group—18.2 days) In a retrospective study matching 16 preterm labor patients treated with indomethacin and 16 patients treated with ritodrine,[356] the initiation of treatment to delivery interval was significantly different between the two groups (indomethacin group—18.0 days vs ritodrine group—4.8 days).

Indomethacin is usually administered initially as a 50-mg oral loading dose, followed with 25 mg every 4 to 6 hours. Indomethacin is rapidly absorbed after oral dosage with peak plasma concentrations occurring in 1 to 2 hours.[357] With women in labor, the peak serum concentrations after oral administration are reached later, but are still reached in 1.5 to 2.0 hours.[323] Comparison with intravenous dosage reveals complete bioavailability with both oral and rectal administration, but the rate of absorption of the drug from rectal suppositories is slower than from oral capsules.[357] The half-life excretion of indomethacin in the non-pregnant adult is approximately 2.2 hours.[323,324] It is readily transferred across the placental unit to the fetus and appears in the fetal blood within 15 minutes.[323,358,359] Fetal concentrations of indomethacin equilibrate with maternal levels within 5 hours.[323] The half-life excretion of indomethacin in the term neonate ranges from 11 to 15 hours[323,324,358] and is prolonged to 19 hours in neonates prior to 32 weeks.[358]

Maternal side effects from indomethacin are minimal. This medication does not alter maternal heart rate or blood pressures.[352,353] The most common maternal complaint associated with oral therapy is nausea and heartburn.[324,351,355] While ingestion of aspirin prior to delivery has been associated with an increased incidence of maternal antepartum and postpartum hemorrhage,[360,361] the effect of indomethacin upon maternal platelet function is reversible[362] and does not subsequently lead to increased maternal perinatal hemorrhage.[324,349,355] However, postpartum hemorrhage was reported in 3 of 16 (19%) term patients who had received a single 100 mg suppository of indomethacin.[347] Chronic maternal ingestion of indomethacin has been associated with altered T-suppressor lymphocyte activity in both the mother and the neonate.[363] Indomethacin should be avoided in patients with a history of peptic ulcer disease or bleeding disorders.

Although prostaglandin regulation of uteroplacental blood flow has been documented,[364,365] indomethacin does not appear to significantly alter this aspect of maternal-fetal physiology. While indomethacin infusion in sheep causes a transient vasoconstriction of systemic and placental blood flow, this phenomenon resolves within 60 minutes.[366] However, the infusion of indomethacin in rhesus monkeys failed to produce any change in maternal-fetal blood flow or fetal oxygenation.[367] In this study, placental blood flow actually increased as uterine contractions were abolished. In one placebo-controlled study with indomethacin in human subjects, the 1 minute Apgar scores (indomethacin group—9.3 vs placebo group—7.8) were significantly greater in the indomethacin group.[352]

The major potential fetal and neonatal complication associated with prostaglandin synthetase inhibitors remains premature closure of the ductus arteriosus and neonatal primary pulmonary hypertension. Indomethacin is used to treat persistent patency of the ductus arteriosus in the preterm neonate.[368-370] However, the clinical response rates in the low birth weight neonate are variable[371-374] and response rates do not appear to correlate well with serum indomethacin concentrations.[375,376] While this literature is contradictory, the preponderance of studies point to a relative resistance to closure of the ductus arteriosus at earlier gestational ages.[324] While in utero closure of the ductus arteriosus has been described in animal studies with indomethacin,[324,377] it has been poorly documented in humans.[378] However, two cases of fetal hydrops associated with maternal indomethacin therapy have been described in the literature.[379,380] A recent uncontrolled report utilizing in utero Doppler flow studies of fetuses suggested some degree of ductus constriction with maternal indomethacin therapy.[381] Utilizing similar techniques, other investigators have been unable to document premature ductal closure in fetuses exposed to indomethacin.[382]

Indomethacin could also theoretically induce a persistent fetal circulation in the neonate by constricting the pulmonary vasculature in the fetus.[324,383] Several anecdotal cases have been reported of persistent fetal circulation in neonates whose mothers had received indomethacin.[379,384-386] However, the majority of clinical experience with this tocolytic agent has failed to substantiate these potential complications. In two large clinical experiences utilizing indomethacin for the inhibition of preterm labor prior to a gestational age of 34 weeks in a total of 464 patients, no cases of premature closure of the ductus arteriosus or persistent fetal circulation were reported.[351,387] Of over 700 patients treated with indomethacin in the clinical studies quoted in this chapter, there are no reported cases of these life-threatening complications. A recent retrospective study of 46 neonates exposed to indomethacin in utero were matched with a group of infants who had received another tocolytic agent and another control group of preterm infants.[388] This study failed to show any significant difference in the incidence of RDS, hypoglycemia, hypocalcemia, patent ductus arteriosus, sepsis or neonatal mortality between the three groups.

Other potential perinatal complications of indomethacin administration include impaired fetal renal function with resultant oligohydramnios, enhanced bleeding in the neonate, and hyperbilirubinemia. Several case reports implicating indomethacin as a cause of oligohydramnios have been described[389–391] and transient oliguria has been described in neonates who are receiving intravenous indomethacin therapy.[392] While aspirin exerts a lasting effect upon hemostasis in the newborn,[344,361] indomethacin produces only transitory effects which resolve as the drug is excreted in the newborn.[358] In one placebo-controlled study, there was no significant evidence of bleeding in the neonate attributable to indomethacin.[341] It has been demonstrated that indomethacin may displace bilirubin from binding sites on albumin,[393] but clinical reports of neonatal hyperbilirubinemia or kernicterus associated with indomethacin therapy are lacking.

In summary, prostaglandin synthetase inhibitors appear to be effective and easily administered tocolytic agents for the treatment of preterm labor. Indomethacin is extremely well tolerated by the mother. Most adverse effects in the fetus and neonate reportedly associated with maternal indomethacin therapy are anecdotal, and may be associated with large doses, long duration of treatment, presence of fetal anomalies, and use after 35 weeks of gestation. Further evaluation of prostaglandin synthetase inhibitors could show that the risk-benefit ratio of these tocolytic agents may justify their routine clinical use.

Diazoxide

Diazoxide, an antihypertensive, non-diuretic thiazide, has received limited clinical use as a tocolytic agent in the treatment of preterm labor. It has been shown to be a potent inhibitor of human myometrial activity[394] and continuous infusion of this medication leads to an arrest of spontaneous labor in baboons.[395] Diazoxide is thought to non-selectively activate adenylate cyclase in smooth muscle cells, thereby decreasing intracellular calcium to cause its apparent relaxant effect.[396] In a study of 16 patients in term labor, a single dose or continuous infusion of diazoxide reduced both the intensity and frequency of uterine contractions.[397] To date, only one study with diazoxide in the treatment of preterm labor has been reported.[398] The use of diazoxide as a tocolytic agent was evaluated in 37 patients. Preterm delivery was delayed for greater than 72 hours in 56% of the patients.

The profound hypotensive effect associated with diazoxide has limited its clinical usefulness as a tocolytic agent. When intravenous diazoxide was used to treat hypertensive disorders of pregnancy in 4 patients, 2 individuals had profound hypotension requiring ephedrine and late decelerations of the FHR were evident in 3 of 4 pregnancies immediately following administration of the drug.[399] Uteroplacental perfusion appears to be profoundly altered when maternal hypotension is present.[400,401] Maternal hypotension and compensatory tachycardia are dose-related, dependent upon individual sensitivity to the drug and may only be transitory with continued infusion.[399] Diazoxide does cross the placenta,[400,402] but appears to cause minimal alterations in fetal hemodynamics[395,400,402] and fetal oxygenation[395] in the absence of maternal hypotension. Moderate maternal and fetal hyperglycemia has also been described with the administration of diazoxide.[400,402] Therefore, the unpredictable nature of this tocolytic agent has hampered its clinical use in the inhibition of preterm labor.

Neonatal effects from maternal diazoxide administration have also been described. While neonatal hypoglycemia secondary to fetal hyperinsulinism might be expected, most infants do not experience alterations in glucose homeostasis.[403] However, several reports of neonatal hyperglycemia have suggested that diazoxide has a direct effect upon the fetal endocrine pancreas.[402,404] No significant long-term abnormalities have been described in children whose mothers received diazoxide.[403]

In summary, diazoxide appears to have a potent tocolytic effect but it produces profound and unpredictable alterations in maternal hemodynamics. These side effects have limited the clinical use of this drug in the treatment of preterm labor.

Calcium Channel Blocking Agents

Calcium channel blocking agents, such as nifedipine (Procardia), nicardipine and verapamil (Calan/Isoptin), are capable of inhibiting uterine contractions. These potential tocolytic agents have been shown to suppress both prostaglandin and oxytocin-induced uterine activity in isolated human and rabbit myometrial preparations,[405–408] These medications can significantly inhibit uterine activity in a dose-related manner in rabbits and ewes[409] and can suppress postpartum uterine activity in humans,[408,412] even after administration of oxytocin, prostaglandin F2 or methergine. In a study of 11 patients undergoing prostaglandin-induced midtrimester abortion,[412] the administration of oral nifedipine reduced the intensity of uterine contractions but had little effect on the frequency of contractions or basal uterine tone.

The clinical experience in the treatment of preterm labor with this group of tocolytic agents has been limited. To date, no controlled, randomized clinical studies have been reported to confirm the efficacy of these tocolytic agents. The first clinical experience with nifedipine was reported from Europe in 1980;[413] 10 patients with suspected preterm labor were administered a 30-mg loading dose with 20 mg doses twice daily for the next 3 days, until uterine contractions subsided. All 10 patients had preterm labor arrested during the study period, with 6 of the 10 (60%) patients requiring only two or less doses. In a similar study of 20 women in preterm labor who received the medication for a total of 3 days,[415] 15 of 20 (80%) patients had delivery delayed for greater than 3 days. In a group of 8 patients with chronic hypertension and preterm labor (mean gestational age at entry—30 weeks) who were placed on continuous therapy with nifedipine,[414] all patients became normotensive and had delivery delayed until after 38 weeks. In another clinical experience from the United States involving 13 patients who had failed other tocolytic therapy,[415] 9 patients (69%) had delivery delayed for greater than 48 hours with oral nifedipine. In a recent case report,[416] the use of nifedipine in addition to oral terbutaline in a patient failing single-agent tocolytic therapy was successful in delaying delivery until 36 weeks.

This diverse group of drugs has the potential to prevent the entry of extra-cellular calcium into smooth muscle cells. These agents apparently block the passage of calcium through the voltage-dependent channels[74,417–419] but may also suppress the release of calcium from the intracellular sarcolemma and increase calcium extrusion from the smooth muscle cell.[419] Smooth muscle relaxation by these medications is non-specific and can result in peripheral vasodilation, as well as slowed atrioventricular conduction in the heart. Verapamil has more cardiac-specific effects than nifedipine and these cardiac side effects have con-traindicated sufficient dosages to suppress uterine activity.[74] The physiologic alterations associated with nifedipine are mainly systemic hypotension and sub-sequent reflex tachycardia,[74,409,410,413,414,420] as well as headache and cutaneous flushing.[413–415,420] In one study utilizing pregnant ewes, the hemodynamic alter-ations observed with nifedipine infusion appeared to be less than those induced by ritodrine.[410]

The major concern restricting the clinical use of calcium channel blocking agents is the effect upon uteroplacental blood flow. While some animal studies report a minimal alteration in placental perfusion with nifedipine infusion,[410,422] other studies suggest a profound decrease in uteroplacental blood flow[421,423] and even fetal demise in the presence of maternal hypertension.[423] Fetal heart rate shows minimal change in response to maternal nifedipine administration.[410,420,423] In vitro study of human placental blood vessels exposed to nifedipine reveals altered auto-regulation of placental blood flow.[424] In the 65 patients who have received nifedipine during pregnancy, no adverse fetal or neonatal side effects have been described.[413–416,420]

Nifedipine is active orally or can be administered parenterally. The usual oral dose is 10 to 20 mg every 4 to 6 hours. Maximum plasma concentrations are achieved in 15 to 90 minutes after oral administration with a plasma half-life of approximately 2 to 3 hours.[74,417] Elimination occurs primarily in the kidneys (70%) and the feces (30%).[417] Sublingual administration results in appreciable serum drug levels within 5 minutes,[417] and may be preferred over oral administration since it allows some control of administration when maternal hypotension be-comes manifest.

Since verapamil has the ability to alter cardiac conduction in the human heart, it has been used to inhibit the cardiovascular side effects of ritodrine during the treatment of preterm labor.[425] In a double-blinded, randomized trial, 83 patients received a combination of intravenous/oral ritodrine and intravenous verapamil, while 99 patients received intravenous/oral ritodrine and an intravenous placebo. There was no apparent difference in prolongation of pregnancy for greater than 1 week (73 vs 62%), but there was a significant difference in maternal cardio-vascular side effects while receiving intravenous ritodrine. With ritodrine in-fusion rates over 200 μg/min, more than 60% of patients treated with ritodrine alone showed intolerance, as compared to no intolerance in the ritodrine/ver-apamil group. No untoward fetal effects from short-term verapamil therapy were reported in this study.

In summary, calcium channel blocking agents represent an apparently pow-erful class of tocolytic drugs. However, the concern over their effect upon the fetus and newborn, as well as their unproven efficacy should limit the clinical use of these agents pending further investigation.

Aminophylline

Aminophylline (Aminophyllin), a methylxanthine, may prove to be an effective tocolytic agent. From investigations of adult asthma, it appears that a combination of terbutaline and aminophylline provides superior bronchodilation when compared to either drug alone.[426] Aminophylline has been shown to decrease uterine activity in the non-pregnant human uterus,[427] as well as suppress induced contractions in myometrial preparations from animals[428,429] and humans. The myometrial relaxation provided with aminophylline appears to be independent of previous terbutaline exposure.[430] It appears that aminophylline inhibits the intracellular enzyme phosphodiesterase, which is responsible for the degradation of cAMP to 5′AMP.[430] Therefore, intracellular levels of cAMP rise and enhance myometrial relaxation, particularly when additional betamimetic receptor stimulation is provided. It has been suggested that aminophylline may complement the tocolytic actions of beta-adrenergic agonists, but this remains unproven.[430]

Several uncontrolled experiences with the clinical use of aminophylline as a primary tocolytic agent in the treatment of preterm labor have been reported.[431,432] In one study, aminophylline delayed delivery for greater than 24 hours in 80% of the preterm labor episodes.[431] In the other non-randomized study, aminophylline appeared to provide similar tocolytic results when compared to salbutamol.[432] In the only randomized comparison study in the literature,[433] 19 patients received intravenous/oral aminophylline and 20 patients received ritodrine. The mean delay of delivery was not signficantly different between the two groups (aminophylline—9.3 weeks and ritodrine—6.8 weeks).

Aminophylline can be administered parenterally or orally. The usual intravenous dose of aminophylline is an initial loading dose of 250 mg over 15 to 20 minutes (5 to 6 mg/kg maximum), followed with a constant infusion of 2 mg/min. Once uterine contractions have subsided, 100 mg of theophylline should be administered orally every 4 to 6 hours. Tachycardia is the only major maternal side effect which is seen in approximately 10% of the cases[431] and fetal tachycardia has also been described.[432] Intravenous aminophylline appears to cause significantly less side effects than intravenous ritodrine.[433]

The preterm fetus receiving aminophylline during pregnancy appears to have accelerated pulmonary maturity after delivery. A retrospective controlled study of preterm infants who were exposed to aminophylline prior to 34 weeks of gestation had only a 10% incidence of RDS, as compared to 29.5% incidence in the non-exposed control group.[434] In several animal models, aminophylline appears to increase phospholipid content and improve lung compliance when administered antenatally.[435–437] It appears that increased de novo production of pulmonary phospholipids is responsible for this phenomenon.[437]

In summary, aminophylline represents a new class of tocolytic agents that may prove effective as a primary therapeutic agent. However, its efficacy as both a tocolytic agent and as preventive therapy for RDS remains unproven at this time.

OTHER CLINICAL USES OF TOCOLYTIC AGENTS

Intrauterine resuscitation with beta-adrenergic agonists for acute intrapartum fetal distress has received considerable attention. A variety of case reports have shown favorable outcomes when these medications were administered for fetal bradycardia or fetal acidosis, particularly when associated with uterine hyper-contractility.[206,207,438–443] Beta-adrenergic agonists cause significant uterine relaxation at term[122,445] and probably cause an increase in uteroplacental blood flow.[201] These medications also abolish the progressive fetal acidosis seen in the second stage of labor[205] and improved fetal pH in cases with prolonged bradycardia.[208,443] Only one prospective, randomized clinical trial involving 50 patients with acute fetal distress has addressed this issue.[446] In this study, both 1 minute Apgar scores and venous cord pHs less than 7.25 were significantly more common in the untreated group. Emergency therapeutic regimens usually consist of ter-butaline 250 μg as a single intravenous bolus or ritodrine 2 mg/min for a total of 3 minutes. These regimens provide high plasma concentrations quickly without serious side effects.[447] A randomized comparison study of ritodrine or fenoterol in treating acute fetal distress showed no significant difference between these two drugs.[448] While this clinical application of betamimetic therapy may be useful, further evaluation is required before it attains widespread use.

Tocolytic therapy may also be useful in the management of placenta previa, particularly when complicated by uterine irritability. Uncontrolled trials with betamimetic agents have reported moderate prolongation of pregnancy.[449,450] Magnesium sulfate may be a better alternative, particularly in the presence of vaginal bleeding, since it produces less alteration in placental blood flow.

Tocolytic therapy appears to be a useful adjunct for external cephalic versions. Several clinical experiences have suggested favorable results when prophylactic tocolysis was used during the procedure,[451–455] but randomized clinical trials are lacking. It remains unclear whether the tocolytic agents' usefulness lies in their ability to prevent contractions during uterine manipulation and/or relaxation of basal uterine tone.

REFERENCES

1. Tejani, N.A., and Verma, U.L.: Effect of tocolysis on incidence of low birth weight. Obstet Gynecol *61*:556, 1983.
2. Zlatnik, F.J.: The applicability of labor inhibition to the problem of prematurity. Am J Obstet Gynecol *113*:704, 1972.
3. Lipshitz, J., and Anderson, G.D.: What is the role of tocolytic drugs in the prevention of premature delivery? Abstract #137 presented at the 6th Annual Meeting of the Society of Perinatal Obstetricians, San Antonio, Texas, Jan-Feb, 1986.
4. Boylan, P., and O'Driscoll, K.: Improvement in perinatal mortality rate attributed to spontaneous preterm labor without use of tocolytic agents. Am J Obstet Gynecol *145*:781, 1983.
5. Goldenberg, R.L., Nelson, K.G., Davis, R.O., et al: Delay in delivery: influence of gestational age and the duration of delay on perinatal outcome. Obstet Gynecol *64*:480, 1984.
6. Korenbrot, C.C., Aalto, L.H., and Laros, R.K. Jr.: The cost effectiveness of stopping preterm labor with beta-adrenergic treatment. N. Engl J Med *310*:691, 1984.
7. Challis, J.R.G., and Mitchell, B.F.: Hormonal control of preterm and term parturition. Sem in Perinatol *5*:192, 1981.
8. Garfield, R.,E.: Control of myometrial function in preterm versus term labor. Clin Obstet Gynecol *27*:572, 1984.
9. Harris, B.A., Gore, H., and Flowers, C.E. Jr: Peripheral placental separation: a possible relationship to premature labor. Obstet Gynecol *66*:774, 1985.
10. Bejar, R., Curbelo, V., Davis, C., et al: Premature labor. II. Bacterial sources of phospholipase. Obstet Gynecol *57*:479, 1981.

11. Handwerker, S.M., Tejani, N.A., Verma, U.L., et al.: Correlation of maternal serum C-reactive protein with outcome of tocolysis. Obstet Gynecol 63:220, 1984.
12. Gravett, M.G., Hummel, D., Eschenbach, DA, et al.: Preterm labor associated with subclinical amniotic fluid infection and with bacterial vaginosis. Obstet Gynecol 67:229, 1986.
13. Creasy, R.K., Gummer, B.A., and Liggins, G.C.: A system for predicting spontaneous preterm birth. Obstet Gynecol 55:692, 1980.
14. Creasy, R.K. and Herron, M.A.: Prevention of preterm birth. Sem in Perinatol 5:295, 1981.
15. Papiernik, E., Bouyer, J., Collin, D., et al.: Precocious cervical ripening and preterm labor. Obstet Gynecol 67:238, 1986.
16. Bouyer, J., Papiernik, E., Dreyfus, J., et al: Maturation signs of the cervix and prediction of preterm birth. Obstet Gynecol 68:209, 1986.
17. Holbrook, R.H., Lirette, M. and Creasy, R.K.: Weekly cervical examination in the patient at high risk for preterm delivery. Abstract #108 presented at the 5th Annual Meeting of the Society of Perinatal Obstetricians in Las Vegas, Nevada, Feb. 1985.
18. Stubbs, T.M., Van Dorsten, P. and Miller, M.D.III: The preterm cervix and preterm labor: relative risks, predictive values, and change over time. Am J Obstet Gynecol 155:829, 1986.
19. Katz, M., Gill, P.J. and Newman, R.B.: Detection of preterm labor by ambulatory monitoring of uterine activity: a preliminary report. Obstet Gynecol 68:773, 1986.
20. Katz, M., Newman, R.B. and Gill, P.J.: Assessment of uterine activity in ambulatory patients at high risk of preterm labor and delivery. Am J Obstet Gynecol 154:44, 1986.
21. Katz, M., Gill, P.J. and Newman, R.B.: Detection of preterm labor by ambulatory monitoring of uterine activity for the management of oral tocolysis. Am J Obstet Gynecol 154:1253, 1986.
22. Castle, B.M. and Turnbull, A.C.: The presence or absence of fetal breathing movements predicts the outcome of preterm labor. Lancet 2:471, 1983.
23. Boylan, P., O'Donovan, P. and Owens, O.J.: Fetal breathing movements and the diagnosis of labor: a prospective analysis of 100 cases. Obstet Gynecol 66:517, 1985.
24. Besinger, R.E., Compton, A.A. and Hayashi, R.H.: The presence or absence of fetal breathing movements as a predictor of outcome in preterm labor. Abstract #169 presented at the 7th Annual Meeting of the Society of Perinatal Obstetricians, Lake Buena Vista, FL, Feb. 1987.
25. Weitz, C.M., Ghodgaonkar, R.B., Dubin, N.H., et al.: Prostaglandin F metabolite concentration as a prognostic factor in preterm labor. Obstet Gynecol 67:496, 1986.
26. Mathews, D.D., Friend, J.B. and Michael, C.A.: A double-blind trial of oral isoxusuprine in the prevention of premature labour. J Obstet Gynaec Brit Cwlth 74:68, 1967.
27. Walters, W.A.W. and Wood, C.: A trial of oral ritodrine for the prevention of premature labour. Br J Obstet Gynaec 84:26, 1977.
28. O'Connor, M.C., Murphy, H. and Dalrymple, I.J.: Double blind trial of ritodrine and placebo in twin pregnancy. Br J Obstet Gynaec 86:706, 1979.
29. Skjaerris, J. and Aberg, A.: Prevention of prematurity in twin pregnancy by orally administered terbutaline. Acta Obstet Gynecol Scand Suppl 108:39, 1982.
30. O'Leary, J.A.: Prophylactic tocolysis of twins. Am J Obstet Gynecol 154:904, 1986.
31. Lipshitz, J., Anderson, G.D., Whybrew, W.D., et al.: Use of fetal lung maturity to improve selection of patients for tocolytic therapy. Abstract #127 presented at the 5th Annual Meeting of the Society of Perinatal Obstetricians, Las Vegas, Nevada, Feb. 1985.
32. Garite, T.J. and Leigh, J: Amniocentesis and management of preterm labor. Abstract #234 presented at the 5th Annual Meeting of the Society of Perinatal Obstetricians, Las Vegas, Nevada, Feb. 1985.
33. Hameed, C., Tejani, N. Verma, U.L., et al.: Silent chorioamnionitis as a cause of preterm labor refractory to tocolytic therapy. Am J Obstet Gynecol 149:726, 1984.
34. Arias, F. and Tomich, P.: Etiology and outcome of low birth weight and preterm infants. Obstet Gynecol 60:277, 1982.
35. Christensen, K.V., Ingemarsson, I., Leideman, T., et al.: Effect of ritodrine on labor after premature rupture of the membranes. Obstet Gynecol 55:187, 1980.
36. Levy, D.L. and Warsof, S.L.: Oral ritodrine and preterm premature rupture of membranes. Obstet Gynecol 66:621, 1985.
37. Garite, T.J., Keegan, K.A., Freeman, R.K., et al. A randomized trial of ritodrine tocolysis vs expectant management in patients with preterm PROM at 25 to 30 weeks. Abstract #4 presented at the 7th Annual Meeting of the Society of Perinatal Obstetricians, Lake Buena Vista, Fl, Feb. 1987.
38. Weiner, C.P., Renk, K. and Klugman, M.: There is no benefit of tocolysis for labor associated with preterm premature rupture of membranes. Abstract #5 presented at the 7th Annual Meeting of the Society of Perinatal Obstetricians, Lake Buena Vista, Fl, Feb. 1987.
39. Hahn, D.W. McGuire, J.L., Vanderhoof, M., et al.: Evaluation of drugs for arrest of premature labor in a new animal model. Am J Obstet Gynecol 148:775, 1984.
40. FDA Drug Bulletin 12:4, 1982.

41. Valenzuela, G., Cline, S. and Hayashi, R.H.: Follow-up of hydration and sedation in the pretherapy of premature labor. Am J Obstet Gynecol *147*:396, 1983.
42. Cibils, L.A. and Zuspan, F.P.: Pharmacology of the uterus. Clin Obstet Gynecol *11*:34, 1968.
43. Petrie, R.H., Wu, R., Miller, F.C., et al.: The effect of drugs on uterine activity. Obstet Gynecol *48*:431, 1976.
44. Sica-Blanco, Y., Rozada, H. and Remedio, M.R.: Effect of meperidine on uterine contractility during pregnancy and prelabor. Am J Obstet Gynecol *97*:1096, 1967.
45. Petrie, R.H., Yeh, Sze-ya, Barron, B.A., et al.: Dose/response effect of meperidine on uterine activity. Abstract #123 presented at the 5th Annual Meeting of the Society of Perinatal Obstetricians, Las Vegas, Nevada, Feb. 1985.
46. Perkins, R.P.: One-hour observation period prior to tocolytic therapy (Letter). Am J Obstet Gynecol *144*:866, 1982.
47. Fuchs, F., Fuchs, A.R., Poblete, V.F., et al.: Effect of alcohol on threatened premature labor. Am J Obstet Gynecol *99*:627, 1967.
48. Fuchs, A.F. and Fuchs, F.: Ethanol for prevention of preterm birth. Semin Perinatol *5*:236, 1981.
49. Gibbens, G.L.D. and Chard, T.: Observations on maternal oxytocin release during human labor and the effect of intravenous alcohol administration. Am J Obstet Gynecol *126*:243 1976.
50. Fuch, A.R. and Wagner, G.: Effect of alcohol on release of oxytocin. Nature *196*:92, 1963.
51. Karim, S. and Sharma, S.: The effects of ethyl alcohol on prostaglandin E_2 and F_2 alpha-induced uterine activity in pregnant women. J Obstet Gynaecol Br Cmwth *78*:251, 1971.
52. Wilson, K.H., Landesman, R., Fuchs, A.R., et al.: The effect of ethyl alcohol on isolated human myometrium. Am J Obstet Gynecol *104*:436, 1969.
53. Mantell, C.D. and Liggins, G.C.: The effect of ethanol on the myometrial response to oxytocin in women at term. Br J Obstet Gynaec *77*:976, 1970.
54. Zlatnik, F.J. and Fuchs, F.: A controlled study of ethanol in threatened premature labor. Am J Obstet Gynecol *112*:610, 1972.
55. Watring, W.G., Benson, W.L., Wiebe, R.A., et al.: Intravenous alcohol—a single blind study in the prevention of premature delivery: a preliminary report. J Repr Med *16*:35, 1976.
56. Castren, O., Siimes, M. and Saarikoski, S.: Treatment of imminent premature labour. Acta Obstet Scand *54*:95, 1975.
57. Lauersen, N.H., Merkatz, I.R., Tejani, N., et al.: Inhibition of premature labor: a multicenter comparison of ritodrine and ethanol. Am J Obstet Gynecol *127*:837, 1977.
58. Caritis, S.N., Carson, D., Greebon, D., et al.: A comparison of terbutaline and ethanol in the treatment of preterm labor. Am J Obstet Gynecol *142*:183, 1982.
59. Steer, C.M. and Petrie, R.H.: A comparison of magnesium sulfate and alcohol for the prevention of premature labor. Am J Obstet Gynecol *129*:1, 1977.
60. Sims, C.D., Chamberlain, G.V.P. and Boyd, I.E.: A comparison of salbutamol and ethanol in the treatment of preterm labour. Br J Obstet Gynaec *85*:761, 1978.
61. Waltman, R. and Iniquez, E.S.: Placental transfer of ethanol and its elimination at term. Obstet Gynecol *40*:180, 1972.
62. Idanpaan-Heikkila, J., Jouppila, P., Akerblom, H.K., et al.: Elimination and metabolic effects of ethanol in mother, fetus, and newborn infant. Am J Obstet Gynecol *112*:387, 1972.
63. Ott, A., Hays, J. and Polin, J.: Severe lactic acidosis associated with intravenous alcohol for premature labor. Obstet Gynecol *48*:362, 1976.
64. Mann, L.I., Bhakthavathsalan, A., Liu, M., et al.: Placental transport of alcohol and its effect on maternal and fetal acid-base balance. Am J Obstet Gynecol *122*:837, 1975.
65. Dilts, P.V.: Effect of ethanol on maternal and fetal acid-base balance. Am J Obstet Gynecol *107*:1018, 1970.
66. Zervoudakis, I.A., Krauss, A. and Fuchs, F.: Infants of mothers treated with ethanol for premature labor. Am J Obstet Gynecol *137*:713, 1980.
67. Wagner, L., Wagner, G. and Guerrero, J.: Effect of alcohol on premature newborn infants. Am J Obstet Gynecol *108*:308, 1970.
68. Lopez, R. and Montoya, M.F.: Abnormal bone marrow morphology in the premature infant associated with maternal alcohol infusion. J Pediatr *79*:1008, 1971.
69. Sisenwein, F.E., Tejani, N.A., Boxer, H.S., et al.: Effects of maternal ethanol infusion during pregnancy on the growth and development of children at four to seven years of age. Am J Obstet Gynecol *147*:52, 1983.
70. Barrada, M.I., Virnig, N.L., Edwards, L.E., et al.: Maternal intravenous ethanol in the prevention of respiratory distress syndrome. Am J Obstet Gynecol *129*:25, 1977.
71. Abel, E.L.: Critical evaluation of the obstetric use of alcohol in preterm labor. Drug & Alcohol Dependence *7*:367, 1981.
72. Lands, A.M., Arnold, A., McAuliff, J.P., et al.: Differentiation of receptor systems by sympathomimetic amines. Nature *214*:597, 1967.

73. Scheid, C.R., Honeyman, T.W. and Fay, F.S.: Mechanism of B-adrenergic relaxation of smooth muscle. Nature *277*:32, 1979.
74. Roberts, J.M.: Current understanding of pharmacologic mechanisms in the prevention of preterm birth. Clin Obstet Gynecol *27*:592, 1984.
75. Krapohl, A.J., Anderson, J.M. and Evans, T.N.: Isoxsuprine suppression of uterine activity. Obstet Gynecol *32*:178, 1968.
76. Siimes, A.S.I. and Creasy, R.K.: Effect of ritodrine on uterine activity, heart rate, and blood pressure in the pregnant sheep: combined use of alpha or beta blockade. Am J Obstet Gynecol *126*:1003, 1976.
77. Jenssen, H.: Inhibition of oxytocin-induced uterine activity in midpregnancy by combined adrenergic alpha blockade and beta stimulation. Acta Obstet Gynec Scand *50*:135, 1971.
78. Benedetti, T.J.: Maternal complications of parenteral beta-sympathomimetic therapy for premature labor. Am J Obstet Gynecol *145*:1, 1983.
79. Schwarz, R. and Retzke, U.: Cardiovascular effects of terbutaline in pregnant women. Acta Obstet Gynecol Scand *62*:419, 1983.
80. Wagner, J.M., Morton, M.J., Johnson, K.A., et al.: Terbutaline and maternal cardiac function. JAMA *246*:2697, 1981.
81. Bieniarz, J., Ivankovich, A. and Scommegna, A.: Cardiac output during ritodrine treatment in premature labor. Am J Obstet Gynecol *118*:910, 1974.
82. Hosenpud, J.D. Morton, M.J. and O'Grady, J.P.: Cardiac stimulation during ritodrine hydrochloride tocolytic therapy. Obstet Gynecol *62*:52, 1983.
83. Finley, J., Katz, M. Rojas-Perez, M., et al.: Cardiovascular consequence of beta-agonist tocolysis: an echocardiographic study. Obstet Gynecol *64*:787, 1984.
84. Ross, M.G., Nicolls, E., Stubblefield, P.G., et al.: Intravenous terbutaline and simultaneous B1-blockade for advanced premature labor. Am J Obstet Gynecol *147*:897, 1983.
85. Katz, M., Robertson, P.A. and Creasy, R.K.: Cardiovascular complications associated with terbutaline treatment for preterm labor. Am J Obstet Gynecol *139*:605, 1981.
86. Fink, B.J. and Weber, T.: Direct current conversion of maternal supraventricular tachycardia developed during the treatment of a pregnant heroin addict with ritodrine. Acta Obstet Gynecol Scan *60*:521, 1981.
87. Kjer, J.J. and Pedersen, K.H.: Persistent supraventricular tachycardia following infusion with ritodrine hydrochloride. Acta Obstet Gynecol Scand *61*:281, 1982.
88. Carpenter, R.J. Jr. and Decuir, P.: Cardiovascular collapse associated with oral terbutaline tocolytic therapy. Am J Obstet Gynecol *148*:821, 1984.
89. Frederiksen, M.C., Toig, R.M. and Depp, R. III: Atrial fibrillation during hexoprenaline therapy for premature labor. Am J Obstet Gynecol *145*:108, 1983.
90. Schneider, E.P., Tejani, N. and Jonas, E.: Continuous ECG monitoring during ritodrine infusion. Presented at the 7th Annual Meeting of the Society of Perinatal Obstetricians, Lake Buena Vista, Fla, Feb. 1987.
91. Chen, W.C. and Lew, L.C.: Ventricular ectopics after salbutamol infusion for preterm labour. Lancet *2*:1383, 1979.
92. Ron-El, R., Caspi, E., Herman, A., et al.: Unexpected cardiac pathology in pregnant women treated with beta-adrenergic agents (ritodrine). Obstet Gynecol *61*:10S, 1983.
93. Tye, K.H., Desser, K.B. and Benchimull, A.: Angina pectoris associated with use of terbutaline for premature labor. JAMA *244*:692, 1980.
94. Yink, Y.K. and Tejani, N.A.: Angina pectoris as a complication of ritodrine hydrochloride therapy in premature labor. Obstet Gynecol *60*:385, 1982.
95. Michalak, D., Klein, V. and Marquette, G.P.: Myocardial ischemia: a complication of ritodrine tocolysis. Am J Obstet Gynecol *146*:861, 1983.
96. Meinen, K.: Radioimmunoassay procedure of serum myoglobin in case of a long-term tocolysis with B-sympathomimetics. Gynecol Obstet Invest *12*:37, 1981.
97. Cohen, G.R., O'Brien, W.F., Knuppel, R.A., et al.: Paired serial electrocardiograms and serum electrolytes in patients receiving IV ritodrine. Presented at the 6th annual meeting of The Society of Perinatal Obstetricians, San Antonio, Texas, January, 1986.
98. Kubli, F.: Preterm Labor, edited by Anderson A., Beard, R., Brundell, M.J., Down, P.M. Proceedings of the Fifth Study Group of the Royal College of Obstetricians and Gynaecologists, 1977, pp.218–220.
99. Elliot, H.R. and Abdulla, U.: Pulmonary oedema associated with ritodrine infusion and betamethasone administration in premature labour. Br Med J *2*:799, 1978.
100. Stubblefield, P.G.: Pulmonary edema occurring after therapy with dexamethasone and terbutaline for premature labor: a case report. Am J Obstet Gynecol *132*:341, 1978.
101. Rogge, M., Young, S. and Goodlin, R.: Pulmonary oedema. Lancet *2*:1026, 1979.
102. Tinga, D.J. and Aarnoudse, J.G.: Postpartum pulmonary oedema associated with preventive therapy for premature labour. Lancet *1*:1026, 1979.

103. Jacobs, M.M., Knight, A.B. and Arias, F.: Maternal pulmonary edema resulting from beta-mimetic and glucocorticoid therapy. Obstet Gynecol 56:56, 1980.
104. Milliez, S., Blot, P.H. and Sureau, C: A case report of maternal death associated with beta-mimetic and betamethasone administration in premature labor. Europ J Obstet Gynecol Repr Biol 2:95, 1980.
105. Niebuhr-Jorgensen, U.: Pulmonary oedema following treatment with ritodrine and beta-methasone in preterm labor. Danish Med Bull 27:99, 1980.
106. Ambramovich, H., Lewin, A., Lissak, A., et al.: Maternal pulmonary edema occurring after therapy with ritodrine for premature contractions. Acta Obstet Gynecol Scand 59:666, 1980.
107. Philipsen, T., Eriksen, P.S. and Lynggard, F.: Pulmonary edema following ritodrine-saline infusion in premature labor. Obstet Gynecol 58:304, 1981.
108. Nagey, D.A. and Crenshaw, M.C.: Pulmonary complications of isoxsuprine therapy in the gravida. Obstet Gynecol 59:38S, 1982.
109. Brodey, P.A. Fisch, A.E. and Huffaker, J.: Acute pulmonary edema resulting from treatment for premature labor. Radiol 140:631, 1981.
110. Benedetti, T.J., Hargrove, J.C. and Rosene, K.A.: Maternal pulmonary edema during premature labor inhibition. Obstet Gynecol 59:33S, 1982.
111. Semchyshyn, S., Zuspan, F.P. and O'Shaughnessy, R.: Pulmonary edema associated with the use of hydrocortisone and a tocolytic agent for the management of premature labor. J Repr Med 28:47, 1983.
112. Alper, M. and Cohen, W.R.: Pulmonary edema associated with ritodrine and dexamethasone treatment of threatened premature labor. A case report. J Repr Med 28:349, 1983.
113. Mabie, W.C., Pernoll, M.L., Witty, J.B., et al.: Pulmonary edema induced by betamimetic drugs. So Med J 76:1354, 1983.
114. Evron, S., Samueloff, A., Mor-Yosef, S., et al.: Pulmonary edema occurring after isoxsuprine and dexamethasone treatment for preterm labor: case report. J Perinat Med 11:272, 1983.
115. Nimrod, C., Rambihar, V., Fallen, E., et al.: Pulmonary edema associated with isoxsuprine therapy. Am J Obstet Gynecol 148:625, 1984.
116. Nimrod, C.A., Beresford, P., Frais, M., et al.: Hemodynamic observations on pulmonary edema associated with a beta-mimetic agent. A report of two cases. J Repr Med 29:341, 1984.
117. MacLennan, F.M., Thomson, M.A.R., Rankin, R., et al.: Fatal pulmonary oedema associated with the use of ritodrine in pregnancy. Case report. Br J Obstet Gynaecol 92:703, 1985.
118. Schrier, R.w., Lieberman, R. and Ufferman, R.C.: Mechanism of antidiuretic effect of beta adrenergic stimulation. J Clin Invest 51:97, 1972.
119. Kleinman, G., Nuwaghid, B., Rudelstorrfer, R., et al.: Circulatory and renal effects of beta-adrenergic-receptor stimulation in pregnant sheep. Am J Obstet Gynecol 149:865, 1984.
120. Hankins, G.D., Hauth, J.C., Keuhl, T., et al.: Ritodrine hydrochloride infusion in pregnant baboons. II. Sodium and water compartment alterations. Am J Obstet Gynecol 147:254, 1983.
121. Hankins, G.D. and Hauth, J.C.: A comparison of the relative toxicities of beta-sympathomimetic tocolytic agents. Am J Perinatol 2:338, 1985.
122. Lammintausta, R. and Erkkola, R.: Effect of long-term salbutamol treatment on renin-aldos-terone system in twin pregnancy. Acta Obstet Gynecol Scand 58:447, 1979.
123. Grospietsch, G., Fenske, M., Girndt, J., et al.: The renin-angiotensin-aldosterone system, antidiuretic hormone levels and water balance under tocolytic therapy with fenoterol and verapamil. Int J Gynaecol Obstet 17:590, 1980.
124. von Oeyen, P., Braden G., Smith, M., et al.: Mechanisms of ritodrine and terbutaline induced hypokalemia and pulmonary edema in the treatment of preterm labor. Abstract #82 presented at the Meeting of the Society of Perinatal Obstetricians, Las Vegas, Nevada, Feb. 1985.
125. Benedetti, T.J. and Johannsen, T.: Infection: A missing link between pulmonary edema and preterm labor inhibition? Abstract #36 presented at the Sixth Annual Meeting of the Society of Perinatal Obstetricians, San Antonio, Texas, 1986.
126. Thomas, D.J.B. and Dove, A.F.: Metabolic effects of salbutamol infusion during premature labour. Br J Obstet Gynaecol 84:497, 1977.
127. Whitehead, M.I., Mander, A.M., Hertogs, K., et al.: Myocardial ischemia after withdrawal of salbutamol for preterm labor. Lancet 2:904, 1980.
128. Barden, T.P., Peter, J.B. and Merkatz, I.R.: Ritodrine hydrochloride: a betamimetic agent for use in preterm labor. I. Pharmacology, clinical history, administration, side effects, and safety. Obstet Gynecol 56:1, 1980.
129. Spellacy, W.N., Cruz, A.C., Buhi, W.C., et al.: The acute effects of ritodrine infusion on maternal metabolism: measurements of levels of glucose, insulin, glucagon, triglycerides, cholesterol, placental lactogen, and chorionic gonadotropin. Am J Obstet Gynecol 131:637, 1978.
130. Lipshitz, J. and Vinik, A.I.: The effects of hexoprenaline, a beta$_2$-sympathomimetic drug, on maternal glucose, insulin, glucagon, and free fatty acid levels. Am J Obstet Gynecol 130:761, 1978.

131. Kirkpatrick, C., Quenon, M. and Desir, D.: Blood anions and electrolytes during ritodrine infusion in preterm labor. Am J Obstet Gynecol 138:523, 1980.
132 Kauppila, A., Tuimala, R., Ylikorkala, O., et al.: Effects of ritodrine and isoxsuprine with and without dexamethasone during late pregnancy. Obstet Gynecol 51:288, 1978.
133. Schreyer, P., Caspi, E., Amidi, S., et al.: Metabolic effects of intravenous ritodrine infusion in pregnancy. Acta Obstet Gynecol Scand 59:197, 1980.
134. Ingemarsson, I., Westgren, M., Lindberg, C., et al.: Single injection of terbutaline in term labor: placental transfer and effects on maternal and fetal carbohydrate metabolism. Am J Obstet Gynecol 139:697, 1981.
135. Schreyer, P., Caspi, E., Snir, E., et al.: Metabolic effects of intramuscular and oral administration of ritodrine in pregnancy. Obstet Gynecol 57:730, 1981.
136. Westgren, M., Carlsson, C., Lindholm, T., et al.: Continuous maternal glucose measurements and fetal glucose and insulin levels after administration of terbutaline in term labor. Acta Obstet Gynecol Suppl 108:63, 1982.
137. Young, D.C., Toofanian, A. and Leveno, K.J.: Potassium and glucose concentrations without treatment during ritodrine tocolysis. Am J Obstet Gynecol 145:105, 1982.
138. Cano, A., Tovar, I., Parrilla, J.J. et al.: Metabolic disturbances during intravenous use of ritodrine: increased insulin levels and hypokalemia. Obstet Gynecol 65:356, 1985.
139. Smythe, A.R. and Sakakini, J.: Maternal metabolic alterations secondary to terbutaline therapy for premature labor. Obstet Gynecol 57:566, 1981.
140. Hancock, P.J., Setzer, E.S. and Beydoun, S.N.: Physiologic and biochemical effects of ritodrine therapy on the mother and perinate. Am J Perinatol 2:1, 1985.
141. Hastwell, G. and Lambert, B.E.: The effect of oral salbutamol on serum potassium and blood sugar. Br J Obstet Gynecol 85:767, 1978.
142. Blouin, D., Murray, M.A.F. and Beard, R.W.: The effect of oral ritodrine on maternal and fetal carbohydrate metabolism. Br J Obstet Gynaecol 83:711, 1976.
143. Main, D.M., Main, E.K., Strong, S.E., et al.: The effect of oral ritodrine therapy on glucose tolerance in pregnancy. Am J Obstet Gynecol 152:1031, 1985.
144. Main, E.K., Main, D.M. and Gabbe, S.G.: Chronic oral terbutaline tocolytic therapy is associated with maternal glucose intolerance. Abstract #19 presented at the Seventh Annual Meeting of the Society of Perinatal Obstetricians, Lake Buena Vista, Fla, 1987.
145. Angel, J.L., O'Brien, W.F., Knuppel, R.A., et al.: Effects of oral terbutaline on glucose tolerance in pregnancy. Abstract #196 presented at the Seventh Annual Meeting of the Society of Perinatal Obstetricians, Lake Buena Vista, Fla, 1987.
146. Thomas, D.J.B., Gill, B., Brown, P., et al.: Salbutamol-induced diabetic ketoacidosis. Br Med J 1:438, 1977.
147. Steel, J.M. Parboosingh, J.: Insulin requirements in pregnant diabetics with premature labour controlled by ritodrine. Br Med J 1:880, 1977.
148. Mordes, D., Kreutner, K., Metzger, W., et al.: Dangers of intravenous ritodrine in diabetic patients. JAMA 248:973, 1982.
149. Hill, W.C., Katz, M., Kitzmiller, J.L., et al.: Tocolysis for the insulin-dependent diabetic woman. Am J Obstet Gynecol 148:1148, 1984.
150. Miodovnik, M., Peros, N., Holroyde, J.C., et al.: Treatment of premature labor in insulin-dependent diabetic women. Obstet Gynecol 65:621, 1985.
151. Lenz, S., Kuhl, C., Wang, P., et al.: The effect of ritodrine on carbohydrate and lipid metabolism in normal and diabetic pregnant women. Acta Endocrinol 92:669, 1979.
152. Wager, J., Fredholm, B., Lunell, N., et al.: Metabolic and circulatory effects of intravenous and oral salbutamol in late pregnancy in diabetic and non-diabetic women. Acta Obstet Gynecol Scand Suppl 108:41, 1982.
153. Cotton, D.B., Strassner, H.T., Lipson, L.G., et al.: The effects of terbutaline on acid base, serum electrolytes, and glucose homeostasis during the management of preterm labor. Am J Obstet Gynecol 141:617, 1981.
154. Smith, S.K. and Thompson, D.: The effect of intravenous salbutamol upon plasma and urinary potassium during premature labor. Br J Obstet Gynaec 84:344, 1977.
155. DiRenzo, G.C. and Anceschi, M.M.: Renin activity, aldosterone levels and urinary sodium and potassium excretion under tocolytic therapy with salbutamol. Europ J Obstet Gynec Repr Biol 13:43, 1981.
156. Bremme, K., Eneroth, P., Hagenfeld, L., et al.: Changes in maternal serum aldosterone, potassium and prolactin levels during beta-receptor agonist treatment in third trimester pregnancies. Horm Metab Res 14:198, 1982.
157. Jovanovic, R.: Serial serum potassium and glucose levels during treatment of premature labor with oral terbutaline. Int J Gyynaecol Obstet 23:399, 1985.
158. Ayromlooi, J., Tobias, M. and Desiderio, D: Effects of isoxsuprine on maternal and fetal acid-base balance and circulation. Obstet Gynecol 57:193, 1981.

159. Richards, S.R., Change, F.E. and Stempel, L.E.: Hyperlactacidemia associated with acute ritodrine infusion. Am J Obstet Gynecol 146:1, 1983.
160. Cano, A., Martinez, P. Parrilla, J.J., et al.: Effects of intravenous ritodrine on lactate and pyruvate levels: role of glycemia and anaerobiosis. Obstet Gynecol 66:207, 1985.
161. Desir, D., VanCoevorden, A., Kirkpatrick, C., et al.: Side effects of drugs: ritodrine-induced acidosis in pregnancy. Br Med J 2:1194, 1978.
162. Suzuki, M., Inagaki, K., Kihira, M., et al.: Maternal liver impairment associated with prolonged high-dose administration of terbutaline for premature labor. Obstet Gynecol 66:14S, 1985.
163. Lotgering, F.K., Lind, J., Huikeshoven, F.J.M., et al.: Elevated serum transaminase levels during ritodrine administration. Am J Obstet Gynecol 155:390, 1986.
164. Nair, G.V., Ghosh, A.K. and Lewis, B.V.: Bowel distension during treatment of premature labour with beta-receptor agonists. Lancet 1:907, 1976.
165. Rosene, K.A.. Featherstone, H.J. and Benedetti, T.J.: Cerebral ischemia associated with parenteral terbutaline use in pregnant migraine patients. Am J Obstet Gynecol 143:405, 1982.
166. Catanzarite, V.A., McHargue, A.M., Sandberg, E.C., et al.: Respiratory arrest during therapy for premature labor in a patient with myasthenia gravis. Obstet Gynecol 64:819, 1984.
167. Meissner, J. and Klostermann, H.: Distribution and diaplacental passage of infused ^{3}H-fenoterol hydrobromide (Partusisten^R) in the gravid rabbit. Int J Clin Pharmacol 13:27, 1976.
168. Brazy, J.E., Little, V., Grimm, J. et al.: Risk:benefit considerations for the use of isoxsuprine in the treatment of premature labor. Obstet Gynecol 58:297, 1981.
169. Gandar, R., deZoeten, L.W. and van der Schoot, J.B.: Serum level of ritodrine in man. Eur J Clin Pharmacol 17:117, 1980.
170. vanLierde, M. and Thomas, K.: Ritodrine concentrations in maternal and fetal serum and amniotic fluid. J Perinat Med 10:119, 1982.
171. Gross, T.L., Kuhnert, B.R. Kuhnert, P.M., et al.: Maternal and fetal plasma concentrations of ritodrine. Obstet Gynecol 65:793, 1985.
172. Borrisud, M., O'Shaughnessy, R., Alexander, M.S., et al.: Metabolism and disposition of ritodrine in a pregnant baboon. Am J Obstet Gynecol 152:1067, 1985.
173. Fujimoto, S., Akahane, M. and Sakai, A.: Concentrations of ritodrine hydrochloride in maternal and fetal serum and amniotic fluid following intravenous administration in late pregnancy. Eur J Obstet Gynecol Reprod Biol 23:145, 1986.
174. Bergman, B., Bokstrom, H., Borgan, O., et al.: Transfer of terbutaline across the human placenta in late pregnancy. Eur J Respir Dis (Suppl 134) 65:81, 1984.
175. Ingemarsson, I.: Effect of terbutaline on premature labor. A double-blind placebo-controlled study. Am J Obstet Gynecol 125:520, 1975.
176. Unbehaun, V.: Effects of sympathomimetic tocolytic agents on the fetus. J Perinat Med 2:17, 1974.
177. Krapohl, A.J., Anderson, J.M. and Evans, T.N.: Isoxsuprine suppression of uterine activity. Obstet Gynecol 32:178, 1968.
178. Wesselius-de Casparis, A., Thiery, M., Sian, A., et al.: Results of double-blind, multicentre study with ritodrine in premature labour. Br Med J 3:144, 1971.
179. Caritis, S.N., Morishima, O., Stark, R.I., et al.: Effects of terbutaline on the pregnant baboon and fetus. Obstet Gynecol 50:56, 1977.
180. Dawson, A.M. and Davies, J.H.: The effect of intravenous and oral salbutamol on fetus and mother in premature labour. Br J Obstet Gynaec 84:348, 1977.
181. Spellacy, W.N., Cruz, A.C., Birk, S.A., et al.: Treatment of premature labor with ritodrine: a randomized controlled study. Obstet Gynecol 54:220, 1979.
182. Schenken, R.S., Hayashi, R.H., Valenzuela, G.V., et al.: Treatment of premature labor with beta sympathomimetics: results with isoxsuprine. Am J Obstet Gynecol 137:773, 1980.
183. Brown, S.M. and Tejani, N.A.: Terbutaline sulfate in the prevention of recurrence of premature labor. Obstet Gynecol 57:22, 1981.
184. Howard, T.E., Jr., Killam, A.P., Penney, L.L., et al.: A double blind randomized study of terbutaline in premature labor. Milit Med 147:305, 1982.
185. Rayburn, W. Piehl, E., Schork, A., et al.: Intravenous ritodrine therapy: a comparison between twin and singleton gestations. Obstet Gynecol 67:243, 1986.
186. Sharif, D.S., Huhta, J.C. Moise, K.J., Jr., et al.: Changes in fetal hemodynamics with preterm labor and terbutaline. Abstract 140 presented at the Seventh Annual Meeting of the Society of Perinatal Obstetricians, Lake Buena Vista, Fl, Feb. 1987.
187. Shenker, L.: Effect of isoxsuprine on fetal heart rate and fetal electrocardiogram. Obstet Gynecol 26:104, 1965.
188. Stawder, R.W., Barden, T.P., Thompson, J.F., et al.: Fetal cardiac effects of maternal isoxsuprine infusion. Am J Obstet Gynecol 89:792, 1964.
189. Weidinger, H., Wiest, W., Schleich, A., et al.: The effects of betamimetic drugs used for tocolysis on the fetal myocardium. J Perinat Med 4:280, 1976.

190. Ingemarsson, I., Arulkumaran, S., Kottegoda, S.R., et al.: Complications of beta-mimetic therapy in preterm labour. Aust NZ J Obstet Gynaecol 25:182, 1985.
191. Karlsson, K.: Beta-receptor agonists in pregnancy. Long term effects in preterm children. Acta Obstet Gynecol Scand Suppl 108:71, 1982.
192. Crawford, C., Bowen, F. and Hall, M.L.: Echocardiographic effects of intrauterine isoxsuprine exposure. Pediatr Res 15:493, 1981.
193. Assche, F.A. and Aerts, L.: The effect of betasympathomimetics on the fetal endocrine pancreas. Europ J Obstet Gynecol Repr Biol 15:395, 1982.
194. Ehrenkranz, R.A. Walker, A.M. Oakes, G.K., et al.: Effect of ritodrine infusion on uterine and umbilical blood flow in pregnant sheep. Am J Obstet Gynecol 126:343, 1976.
195. Ehrenkranz, R.A., Walker, A.M., Oakes, G.K., et al.: Effect of fenoterol (Th1165a) infusion on uterine and umbilical blood flow in pregnant sheep. Am J Obstet Gynecol 128:177, 1977.
196. Ehrenkranz, R.A. Hamilton, L.A. Jr., Brennan, S.C., et al.: Effects of salbutamol and isoxsuprine on uterine and umbilical blood flow in pregnant sheet. Am J Obstet Gynecol 128:287, 1977.
197. Brennan, S.C., McLaughlin, M.K. and Chez, R.A.: Effects of prolonged infusion of beta-adrenergic agonists on uterine and umbilical blood flow in pregnant sheep. Am J Obstet Gynecol 128:709, 1977.
198. Caritis, S.N., Mueller-Heubach, E., Morishima, H.O., et al.: Effect of terbutaline on cardiovascular state and uterine blood flow in pregnant ewes. Obstet Gynecol 50:603, 1977.
199. van de Walle, A.F.G.M. and Martin, C.B., Jr.: Effect of ritodrine on uteroplacental blood flow and cardiac output distribution in unanesthetized pregnant guinea pigs. Am J Obstet Gynecol 154:189, 1986.
200. Lippert, T.H., DeGrandi, P.B. and Fridrich, R.: Actions of the uterine relaxant, fenoterol, on uteroplacental hemodynamics in human subjects. Am J Obstet Gynecol 125:1093, 1976.
201. Brettes, J.P., Renaud, R. and Gandar, R.: A double-blind investigation into the effects of ritodrine on uterine blood flow during the third trimester of pregnancy. Am J Obstet Gynecol 124:164, 1976.
202. Joelsson, S.E.I., Lewander, R., Lundqvist, H., et al.: The effect of beta-receptor-stimulating agents on the utero-placental blood flow. Acta Obstet Gynecol Scand 56:297, 1977.
203. Lunell, N.O., Joelsson, I., Lewander, R., et al.: Utero-placental blood flow and the effect of beta2-adrenoceptor stimulating drugs. Acta Obstet Gynecol Scand Suppl 108:25, 1982.
204. Jouppila, P., Kirkinen, P., Koivula, A., et al.: Ritodrine infusion during late pregnancy: effects on fetal and placental blood flow, prostacyclin, and thromboxane. Am J Obstet Gynecol 151:1028, 1985.
205. Humphrey, M., Chang, A., Gilbert, M., et al.: The effect of intravenous ritodrine on the acid-base status of the fetus during the second stage of labour. Br J Obstet Gynaecol 82:234, 1975.
206. Esteban-Altarriba, J.: The use of beta-adrenergics in fetal distress. Europ J Obstet Gynecol Repr Biol 15:402, 1982.
207. Tejani, N.A., Verma, U.L., Chatterjee, S., et al.: Terbutaline in the management of acute intrapartum fetal acidosis. J Repr Med 28:857, 1983.
208. Ingemarsson, I., Arulkumaran, S. and Ratnam, S.S.: Single injection of terbutaline in term labor. I. Effect on fetal pH in cases with prolonged bradycardia. Am J Obstet Gynecol 153:859, 1985.
209. Kero, P., Hirvonen, T. and Valimaki, I.: Prenatal and postnatal isoxsuprine and respiratory-distress syndrome. Lancet 2:198, 1973.
210. Boog, G. and Gandar, R.: Beta-mimetic drugs and possible prevention of respiratory distress syndrome. Br J Obstet Gynaecol, 82:285, 1975.
211. Enhorning, G., Chamberlain, D., Contreras, C., et al.: Isoxsuprine-induced release of pulmonary surfactant in the rabbit fetus. Am J Obstet Gynecol 129:197, 1977.
212. Gunston, K.D. and Davey, D.A.: Effects of prenatal fenoterol, phenobarbitone, and dexamethasone administration on the total phospholipid content of amniotic fluid. So Afr Med J 54:1141, 1978.
213. Bergman, B. and Hedner, T.: Antepartum administration of terbutaline and the incidence of hyaline membrane disease in preterm infants. Acta Obstet Gynecol Scand 57:217, 1978.
214. Cabero, L., Giralt, E., Navarro, E., et al.: A betamimetic drug and human fetal lung maturation. Europ J Obstet Gynec Repr Biol 9:261, 1979.
215. Dudenhausen, J.W., Kynast, G., Lange-Lindberg, A.M., et al.: Influence of long-term beta-mimetic therapy on the lecithin content of amniotic fluid. Gynecol Obstet Invest 9:205, 1978.
216. Lipshitz, J., Broyles, K., Hessler, J.R., et al.: Effects of hexoprenaline on the lecithin/sphingomyelin ratio and pressure-volume relationships in fetal rabbits. Am J Obstet Gynecol 139:726, 1981.
217. Tzafettas, J.M., Zurnatzi, V. and Papaloucas, A.C.: L/S ratio, biochemical and clinical changes after ritodrine intravenous infusion. Europ J Obstet Gynecol Repr Biol 14:357, 1983.
218. Csapo, A.I. and Herczeg, J.: Arrest of premature labor by isoxsuprine. Am J Obstet Gynecol 129:482, 1977.

219. Creasy, R.K., Golbus, M.S. and Laros, R.K., Jr.: Oral ritodrine maintenance in the treatment of preterm labor. Am J Obstet Gynecol *137*:212, 1980.
220. Larsen, J.F., Eldon, K., Lange, A.P., et al.: Ritodrine in the treatment of preterm labor: second Danish multicenter study. Obstet Gynecol *67*:607, 1986.
221. Leveno, K.J., Guzick, D.S., Hankins, G.D., et al.: Single-centre randomized trial of ritodrine hydrochloride for preterm labour. Lancet *1*:1293, 1986.
222. Brazy, J.E. and Pupkin, M.J.: Effects of maternal isoxsuprine administration on preterm infants. J Pediatr *94*:444, 1979.
223. Brazy, J.E. Eckerman, C.O. and Gross, S.J.: Clinical and laboratory observations. Follow-up of infants of <1500 gm birth weight with antenatal isoxsuprine exposure. J Pediatr *102*:611, 1983.
224. Huisjes, H.J. and Touwen, B.C.L.: Neonatal outcome after treatment with ritodrine: a controlled study. Am J Obstet Gynecol *147*:250, 1983.
225. Essed, G.G.M. Neonatal effects of beta-adrenergic drugs. Europ J Obstet Gynecol Repr Biol *15*:397, 1982.
226. Epstein, M.F., Nicholls, E. and Stubblefield, P.G.: Neonatal hypoglycemia after beta-sympathomimetic tocolytic therapy. J Pediatr *94*:449, 1979.
227. Procianoy, R.S. and Pinheiro, C.E.A. Neonatal hyperinsulinism after short-term maternal beta sympathomimetic therapy. J Pediatr *101*:612, 1982.
228. Desgranges, M.F., Moutquin, J.M. and Peloquin, A.: Effects of maternal oral salbutamol therapy on neonatal endocrine status at birth. Obstet Gynecol *69*:582, 1987.
229. Brazy, J.E. Little, V. and Grimm, J.: Isoxsuprine in the perinatal period. II. Relationships between neonatal symptoms, drug exposure, and drug concentration at the time of birth. J Pediatr *98*:146, 1981.
230. Hopper, A.O., Cohen, R.S. Ostrander, C.R., et al.: Maternal beta-adrenergic tocolysis and neonatal bilirubin production. Am J Dis Child *137*:58, 1983.
231. Hermansen, M.C. and Johnson, G.L.: Neonatal supraventricular tachycardia following prolonged maternal ritodrine administration. Am J Obstet Gynecol *149*:798, 1984.
232. Freysz, H., Willard, D., Lehr, A., et al.: A long term evaluation of infants who received a beta-mimetic drug while in utero. J Perinat Med *5*:94, 1977.
233. Karlsson, K., Krantz, M. and Hamberger, L.: Comparison of various betamimetics on preterm labor, survival and development of the child. J Perinat Med *8*:19, 1980.
234. Svenningsen, N.W.: Follow-up studies on preterm infants after maternal beta-receptor agonist treatment. Acta Obstet Gynecol Scand Suppl *108*:67, 1982.
235. Polowczyk, D., Tejani, N., Lauersen, N., et al.: Evaluation of seven-to- nine-year-old children exposed to ritodrine in utero. Obstet Gynecol *64*:485, 1984.
236. Haddengra, M., Touwen, B.C.L. and Huisjes, J.H.: Long-term follow-up of children prenatally exposed to ritodrine. Br J Obstet Gynaecol *1*:156, 1986.
237. Wager, J., Fredholm, B.B., Lunell, N.O., et al.: Development of tolerance to oral salbutamol in the third trimester of pregnancy: a study of circulatory and metabolic effects. Br J Clin Pharmac *12*:489, 1981.
238. Bredholm, B., Lunell, N.O., Persson, B., et al.: Development of tolerance to the metabolic actions beta2-adrenoceptor stimulating drugs. Acta Obstet Gynecol Scand Suppl *108*:53, 1982.
239. Ryden, G., Andersson, R.G.G. and Berg, G.: Is the relaxing effect of beta-adrenergic agonists on the human myometrium only transitory? Acta Obstet Gynecol Scand Suppl *108*:47, 1982.
240. Benoy, C.J., El-Fellah, M.S., Schneider, R., et al.: Tolerance to sympathomimetic bronchodilators in guinea-pig isolated lungs following chronic administration in vivo. Br J Pharmac *55*:547, 1975.
241. Berg, G., Andersson, R.G.G. and Ryden, G.: Beta-adrenergic receptors in human myometrium during pregnancy: changes in the number of receptors after beta-mimetic treatment. Am J Obstet Gynecol *151*:392, 1985.
242. Berg, G., Andersson, R.G.G. and Ryden, G.: Effects of selective beta-adrenergic agonists on spontaneous contractions, cAMP levels and phosphodiesterase activity in myometrial strips from pregnant women treated with terbutaline. Gynecol Obstet Invest *14*:56, 1982.
243. Bishop, E.H. and Woutersz, T.B.: Isoxsuprine, a myometrial relaxant. Obstet Gynecol *17*:442, 1961.
244. Hendricks, C.H., Cibils, L.A., Pose, S.V., et al.: The pharmacologic control of excessive uterine activity with isoxsuprine. Am J Obstet Gynecol *82*:1064, 961.
245. Bishop, E.H. and Woutersz, T.B.: Arrest of premature labor. JAMA *178*: 812, 1961.
246. Das, R.K.: Isoxsuprine in premature labor. J Obstet Gynecol India *19*:566, 1969.
247. Robertson, P.A. Herron, M., Katz, M., et al.: Maternal morbidity associated with isoxsuprine and terbutaline tocolysis. Europ J Obstet Gynec Repr Biol *11*:371, 1981.
248. Merkatz, I.R., Peter, J.B. and Barden, T.P.: Ritodrine hydrochloride: a betamimetic agent for use in preterm labor. II. Evidence of efficacy. Obstet Gynecol *56*:7, 1980.
249. Larsen, J.F. Hansen, M.K. Hesseldahl, H., et al.: Ritodrine in the treatment of preterm labour.

A clinical trial to compare a standard treatment with three regimens involving the use of ritodrine. Br J Obstet Gynaecol 87:949, 1980.

250. Caritis, S.N., Toig, G., Heddinger, L.A., et al.: A double-blind study comparing ritodrine and terbutaline in the treatment of preterm labor. Am J Obstet Gynecol 150:7, 1984.

251. Kosasa, T.S., Nakayama, R.T., Hale, R.W., et al.: Ritodrine and terbutaline compared for the treatment of preterm labor. Acta Obstet Gynecol Scand 64:421, 1985.

252. Beall, M.H., Edgar, B.W., Paul, R.H., et al.: A comparison of ritodrine, terbutaline, and magnesium sulfate for the suppression of preterm labor. Am J Obstet Gynecol 153:854, 1985.

253. Tchilinguirian, N.G. Najem, R., Sullivan G.B., et al.: The use ritodrine and magenesium sulfate in the arrest of premature labor. Int J Gynaecol Obstet 22:117, 1984.

254. Hollander, D.I., Nagey, D.A. and Pupkin, M.J.: Magnesium sulfate and ritodrine hydrochloride: A randomized comparison. Am J Obstet Gynecol, 156:631, 1987.

255. Kopelman, J.N., Duff, P., Read, J.A., et al.: A randomized trial of oral ritodrine vs oral terbutaline for the prevention of recurrent preterm labor. Abstract #115 presented at the Society of Perinatal Obstetricians Seventh Annual Meeting, Lake Buena Vista, Fl, February, 1987.

256. Caritis, S.N., Lin, L.S., Toig, G., et al.: Pharmacodynamics of ritodrine in pregnant women during preterm labor. Am J Obstet Gynecol 147: 752, 1983.

257. Hill, W.C., Katz, M., Kitzmiller, J.L., et al.: Continuous long-term intravenous beta-sympathomimetic tocolysis. Am J Obstet Gynecol 152:631, 1985.

258. Smit, D.A. Essed, G.G.M. and deHaan, J.: Serum levels of ritodrine during oral maintenance therapy. Gynecol Obstet Invest 18:105, 1984.

259. Schulthuis, M.S., and Aarnoudse, J.G.: Fetal death associated with severe ritodrine induced ketoacdosis. Lancet, 1:1145, 1980.

260. Andersson, K.E., Ingemarsson, I. and Persson, C.G.A.: Effects of terbutaline on human uterine motility at term. Acta Obstet Gynec Scand 54:165, 1975.

261. Andersson, K.E., Bengtsson, L.P., Gustafson, I., et al.: The relaxing effect of terbutaline on the human uterus during term labor. Am J Obstet Gynecol 121:602, 1975.

262. Cotton, D.B., Strassner, H.T., Hill, L.M., et al.: Comparison of magnesium sulfate, terbutaline and a placebo for inhibition of preterm labor. A randomized study. J Repr Med 29:92, 1984.

263. Miller, J.M., Jr., Keane, M.W.D. and Horger, E.O. III: A comparison of magnesium sulfate and terbutaline for the arrest of premature labor. A preliminary report. J Repr Med 27:348, 1982.

264. Lyrenas, S., Grahnen, A., Lindberg, B., et al.: Pharmacokinetics of terbutaline during pregnancy. Eur J Clin Pharmacol 29:619, 1986.

265. Stubblefield, P.G. and Heyl, P.S.: Treatment of premature labor with subcutaneous terbutaline. Obstet Gynecol 59:457, 1982.

266. Moise, K.J. Jr., Dorman, K., Giebel,R., et al.: A randomized study of interavenous versus subcutaneous/oral terbutaline in the treatment of preterm labor. Abstract #276 presented at the Seventh Annual Meeting of the Society of Perinatal Obstetricians, Lake Buena Vista, Fl, February, 1987.

267. Leferink, J.G., Lamont, H., Wagenmaker-Engles, I., et al.: Pharmacokinetics of terbutaline after subcutaneous administration. Int J Clin Pharmacol & Biopharm 17:181, 1979.

268. Kullander, S. and Svanberg, L.: On resorption and the effects of vaginally administered terbutaline in women with premature labor. Acta Obstet Gynecol Scand 64:613, 1985.

269. Liggins, G.C. and Vaughan, G.S.: Intravenous infusion of salbutamol in the management of premature labour. J Obstet Gynaec Br Cmwth 80:29, 1973.

270. McDevitt, D.G., Wallace, R.J., Roberts, A., et al.: The uterine and cardiovascular effects of salbutamol and practolol during labour. Br J Obstet Gynaecol 82:442, 1975.

271. Hastwell, G.B., Halloway, C.P. and Taylor, T.L.O.: A study of 208 patients in premature labour treated with orally administered salbutamol. Med J Aust 1:465, 1978.

272. Gummerus, M.: The management of premature labor with salbutamol. Acta Obstet Gynecol Scand 60:375, 1981.

273. Martin, D.H. and McDevitt, D.G.: Salbutamol in the management of premature labor. J Med Sci 146:224, 1977.

274. Ryden, G.: The effect of salbutamol and terbutaline in the management of premature labour. Acta Obstet Gynecol Scand 56:293, 1977.

275. Sims, C.D., Chamberlain, G.V.P., Boyd, I.E., et al.: A comparison of salbutamol and ethanol in the treatment of preterm labour. Br J Obstet Gynaec 85:761, 1978.

276. Haukkamaa, M., Gumerus, M. and Kleimola, T.: Serum salbutamol concentrations during oral and intravenous treatment in pregnant women. Br J Obstet Gynaec 92:1230, 1985.

277. Lipshitz, J. Baillie, P.: Uterine and cardiovascular effects of beta2-selective sympathomimetic drugs administered as an intravenous infusion. SA Med J 50:1973, 1976.

278. Lipshitz, J., Baillie, P. and Davey, D.A.: A comparison of the uterine beta2-adrenoreceptor selectivity of fenoterol, hexoprenaline, ritodrine and salbutamol. SA Med J 50:1969, 1976.

279. Ayala, L.C. and Karchmer, S.: Comparative study of utero-inhibiting action of two beta-adrenomimetic drugs. Acta Obstet Gynecol Scand 56:287, 1977.

280. Richter, R. and Hinselmann, M.J.: The treatment of threatened premature labor by betamimetic drugs: a comparison of fenoterol and ritodrine. Obstet Gynecol *53*:81, 1979.
281. Lipshitz, J. and Lipshitz, E.M.: Uterine and cardiovascular effects of fenoterol and hexoprenaline in prostaglandin F2a-induced labor in humans. Obstet Gynecol *63*:396, 1984.
282. Hall, D.G., McGaughery, H.S. Jr., Corey, E.L., et al.: The effects of magnesium therapy on the duration of labor. Am J Obstet Gynecol *78*:27, 1959.
283. Hutchinson, H.T., Nichols, M.M., Kuhn, C.R., et al.: Effects of magnesium sulfate on uterine contractility, intrauterine fetus, and infant. Am J Obstet Gynecol *88*:747, 1964.
284. Harbert, G.M., Cornell, G.W. and Thorton, W.N.: Effect of toxemia therapy on uterine dynamics. Am J Obstet Gynecol *105*:94, 1969.
285. Stallworth, J.C., Yeh, S.Y. and Petrie, R.H.: The effect of magnesium sulfate on fetal heart rate variability and uterine activity. Am J Obstet Gynecol *140*:702, 1981.
286. Young, B.K. and Weinstein, H.M.: Effects of magnesium sulfate on toxemic patients in labor. Obstet Gynecol *49*:681, 1977.
287. Petrie, R.H.: Tocolysis using magnesium sulfate. Sem in Perinatol *5*:266, 1981.
288. Guiet-Bara, A., Bara, M. and Durlach, J.: Comparative study of the effects of two tocolytic agents (magnesium sulfate and alcohol) on the ionic transfer through the isolated human amnion. Europ J Obstet Gynecol Repr Biol *20*:297, 1985.
289. Elliott, J.P.: Magnesium sulfate as a tocolytic agent. Am J Obstet Gynecol *147*:277, 1983.
290. Cruikshank, D.P., Pitkins, R.M., Donnelly, E., et al.: Urinary magnesium, calcium, and phosphate excretion during magnesium sulfate infusion. Obstet Gynecol *58*:430, 1981.
291. Thiagarajah, S., Harbert, G.M. and Bourgeois, F.J.: Magnesium sulfate and ritodrine hydrochloride: systemic and uterine hemodynamic effects. Am J Obstet Gynecol *153*:666, 1985.
292. Parsons, M.T., Owens, C.A. and Spellacy, W.N.: Thermic effects of tocolytic agents: decreased temperature with magnesium sulfate. Obstet Gynecol *69*:88, 1987.
293. Rodis, J.F., Vintzileos, A.M., Campbell, W.A., et al.: Maternal hypothermia: An unusual complication of magnesium sulfate therapy. Am J Obstet Gynecol *156*:435, 1987.
294. Hill, W.C., Gill, P.J. and Katz, M.: Maternal paralytic ileus as a complication of magnesium sulfate tocolysis. Am J Perinatol *2*:47, 1985.
295. Elliott, J.P., O'Keefe, D.F., Greenberg, P., et al.: Pulmonary edema associated with magnesium sulfate and betamethasone administration. Am J Obstet Gynecol *134*:717, 1979.
296. Ogburn, P.L. Jr., Julian, T.M., Williams, P.P., et al.: The use of magnesium sulfate for tocolysis in preterm labor complicated by twin gestation and betamimetic-induced pulmonary edema. Acta Obstet Gynecol Scand *65*:793, 1986.
297. Spisso, K.R., Harbert, G.M. Jr. and Thiagarajah, S.: The use of magnesium sulfate as the primary tocolytic agent to prevent premature delivery. Am J Obstet Gynecol *142*:840, 1982.
298. Cholst, I.N., Steinberg, S.F., Tropper, P.J., et al.: The influence of hypermagnesemia on serum calcium and parathyroid hormone levels in human subjects. N Engl J Med *310*:1221, 1984.
299. Penso, C., Abu-Hamad, A., Steel, B.W., et al.: IV magnesium sulfate therapy: interrelationship of magnesium and calcium levels. Abstract #138 presented at the Society of Perinatal Obstetricians Annual Meeting in Las Vegas, Nevada, February, 1985.
300. Olson, R.E.: The hypocalcemia associated with magnesium infusion is mediated through parathyroid hormone. Nutr Rev *42*:315, 1984.
301. Stone, S.R. and Pritchard, J.A.: Effect of maternally administered magnesium sulfate on the neonate. Obstet Gynecol *35*:574, 1970.
302. Savory, J. and Monif, G.R.G.: Serum calcium levels in cord sera of the progeny of mothers treated with magnesium sulfate for toxemia of pregnancy. Am J Obstet Gynecol *110*:556, 1971.
303. McGuinness, G.A. Weinstein, M.M., Cruikshank, D.P., et al.: Effects of magnesium sulfate treatment on perinatal calcium metabolism. II. Neonatal responses. Obstet Gynecol *56*:595, 1980.
304. Lin, C.C. Pielet, B.W., Poon, E., et al.: The effect of magnesium sulfate on fetal heart rate variability in pre-eclamptic patients during labor. Abstract #165 presented at the Sixth Annual Meeting of the Society of Perinatal Obstetricians, San Antonio, Texas, Feb. 1986.
305. Babaknia, A. and Niebyl, J.R.: The effect of magnesium sulfate on fetal heart rate baseline variability. Obstet Gynecol, *51*:2S, 1978.
306. Canez, M.S., Reed, K.L. and Shenker, L.: Effect of maternal magnesium sulfate treatment on fetal heart rate variability. Am J Perinatol *4*:167, 1987.
307. Lipsitz, P.J.: The clinical and biochemical effects of excess magnesium in the newborn. Pediatr *47*:501, 1971.
308. Brady, J.P.F. and Williams, H.C.: Magnesium intoxication in a premature infant. Pediatr *40*:100, 1967.
309. Rasch, D.K., Huber, P.A., Richardson, C.J., et al.: Neurobehavioral effects of neonatal hypermagnesium. J Peds *100*:272, 1982.
310. Koenigsberger, M.R., Rose, J.S. Berdon, W.E., and Santulli, T.V.: Neonatal hypermagnesemia and the meconium-plug syndrome. New Engl J Med *286*:823, 1972.

311. Wilkins, I.A., Goldberg, J.D., Phillips, R.N., et al.: Long-term use of magnesium sulfate as a tocolytic agent. Obstet Gynecol 6738S, 1986.
312. Hill, W.C. and Jurgensen, W.W.: Continuous long-term intravenous magnesium sulfate tocolysis. Abstract #326 presented at the Seventh Annual Meeting of the Society of Perinatal Obstetricians, Lake Buena Vista, Fl, Feb. 1987.
313. Martin, R.W., Gaddy, D.K., Martin, J.N., Jr., et al.: Tocolysis with oral magnesium. Am J Obstet Gynecol 156:433, 1987.
314. Martin, R.W., Martin, J.N., Jr., Gaddy, D.K., et al: The use of ritodrine and magnesium gluconate for ambulatory tocolysis. Abstract #386 presented at the Seventh Annual Meeting of the Society of Perinatal Obstetricians, Lake Buena Vista, Fl, Feb. 1987.
315. Ogburn, P.L., Jr., Hansen, C.A., Williams, P.P., et al.: Magnesium sulfate and beta-mimetic dual-agent tocolysis in preterm labor after single-agent failure. J Repr Med 30:583, 1985.
316. Hatjis, C.G., Nelson, L.H. Meis, P.J., et al.: Addition of magnesium sulfate improves effectiveness of ritodrine in preventing premature delivery. Am J Obstet Gynecol 150:142, 1984.
317. Hatjis, C.G., Swain, M., Nelson, L.H., et al.: Efficacy of combined administration of magnesium sulfate and ritodrine in the treatment of premature labor. Obstet Gynecol 69:317, 1987.
318. Ferguson, J.E. II, Holbrook, H., Jr., Stevenson, D.K., et al.: Adjunctive magnesium sulfate infusion does not alter metabolic changes associated with ritodrine tocolysis. Am J Obstet Gynecol 156:103, 1987.
319. Ferguson, J.E. II, Hensleigh, P.A. and Kredenster, D.: Adjunctive use of magnesium sulfate with ritodrine for preterm labor tocolysis. Am J Obstet Gynecol 148:166, 1984.
320. Valenzuela, G. and Cline, S.: Use of magnesium sulfate in premature labor that fails to respond to beta-mimetic drugs. Am J Obstet Gynecol 143:718, 1982.
321. Karsif, B., Cohen, A.W., Chhibber, G., et al.: Sequential tocolytic therapy for preterm labor. Abstract #134 presented at the Sixth Annual Meeting of the Society of Perinatal Obstetricians, San Antonio, Texas, Feb. 1986.
322. Karim, S.M.M.: On the use of blockers of prostaglandin synthesis in the control of labor. Adv Prostagland & Thrombox Res 4:301, 1978.
323. Niebyl, J.R.: Prostaglandin synthetase inhibitors. Semin Perinatol 5:274, 1981.
324. Repke, J.R. and Neibyl, J.R.: Role of prostaglandin synthetase inhibitors in the treatment of preterm labor. Sem in Repr Endoc 3:3, 259, 1985.
325. Karim, S.M.M. and Devlin, J.: Prostaglandin content of amniotic fluid during pregnancy and labor. J Obstet Gynecol Br Commonw 74:230, 1967.
326. Karim, S.M.M.: Appearance of prostaglandin F2a in human blood during labor. Br Med J 4:618, 1968.
327. Karim, S.M.M. and Hillier, K.: Prostaglandins and spontaneous abortion. J Obstet Gynaecol Br Commonw 77:837, 1970.
328. Keirse, M.J.W.C. and Turnbull, A.C.: Prostaglandins E in amniotic fluid during late pregnancy and labor. J Obstet Gynaecol Br Commonw 80:970, 1973.
329. Lakritz, R., Tulchinsky, D., Ryan, K.J., et al.: Plasma prostaglandin metabolites in human labor. Am J Obstet Gynecol 131:484, 1978.
330. Keirse, M.J.N.C., Mitchell, M.D. and Turnbull, A.C.: Changes in prostaglandin F and 13,14-dihydro-15-keto-prostaglandin F concentrations in amniotic fluid at the onset of and during labour. Br J Obstet Gynaecol 84:743, 1977.
331. Zuckerman, H., Reiss, U., Atad, J., et al.: The effect of indomethacin on plasma levels of prostaglandin F2a in women in labour. Br J Obstet Gynae 84:339, 1977.
332. Dubin, N.H., Johnson, J.W.C., Calhoun, S., et al.: Plasma prostaglandin in pregnant women with term and preterm deliveries. Obstet Gynecol 57:203, 1981.
333. Giannopoulos, G., Jackson, K., Kredentser, J., et al.: Prostaglandin E and F2a receptors in human myometrium during the menstrual cycle and in pregnancy and labor. Am J Obstet Gynecol 153:904, 1985.
334. Nakla, S., Skinner, K., Mitchell, B.F., et al.: Changes in prostaglandin transfer across human fetal membranes obtained during spontaneous labor. Am J Obstet Gynecol 155:1337, 1986.
335. Fuchs, A.R., Husslein, P., Sumulong, L., et al.: Plasma levels of oxytocin and 13,14-dihydro-15-keto prostaglandin F2a in preterm labor and the effect of ethanol and ritodrine. Am J Obstet Gynecol 144:753, 1982.
336. Ramwell, P.W., Foegh, M., Loebr. and Leouey, E.M.K.: Synthesis and metabolism of prostaglandins, prostacyclin and thromboxane: the arachidonic acid cascade. Semin Perinatol 4:3, 1980.
337. Ferreira, S.H., Moncada, S. and Vane, J.R.: Indomethacin and aspirin abolish prostaglandin release from the spleen. Nature WEW Biol 231:237, 1971.
338. Johnson, W.C., Habert, G.M. and Martin, C.B.: Pharmacologic control of uterine contractility. Am J Obstet Gynecol 123:364, 1975.
339. Garrioch, D.B.: The effect of indomethacin on spontaneous activity in the isolated human

myometrium and on the response to oxytocin and prostaglandin. Br J Obstet Gynaecol 85:47, 1978.

340. Wiqvist, N., Lundstrom, V. and Green, K.: Premature labor and indomethacin. Prostaglandins 10:515, 1975.

341. Niebyl, J.R., Blake, D.A., White, R.D., et al.: The inhibition of premature labor with indomethacin. Am J Obstet Gynecol 136:1014, 1980.

342. Novy, M.J., Cook, M.J. and Manaugh, L.: Indomethacin block of normal onset of parturition in primates. Am J Obstet Gynecol 118:412, 1974.

343. Lewis, R.B. and Schulman, J.D.: Influence of acetylsalicylic acid, an inhibitor of prostaglandin synthesis on the duration of human gestation and labour. Lancet 2:1159, 1973.

344. Collins, E. and Turner, G.F.: Salicylates and pregnancy. Lancet 2:1494, 1973.

345. Waltman, R., Tricomi, V. and Palau, A.: Aspirin and indomethacin: effect on installation-abortion time of midtrimester hypertonic saline-induced abortions. Prostaglandins 3:47, 1973.

346. Niebyl, J.R., Blake, D.A., Burnett, L.S. et al.: The influence of aspirin on the course of induced midtrimester abortion. Am J Obstet Gynecol 124:607, 1976.

347. Reiss, U., Atad, J., Rubinstein, I., et al.: The effect of indomethacin in labour at term. Int J Gynaecol Obstet 14:369, 1976.

348. Zuckerman, H., Reiss, U., and Rubinstein, I.: Inhibition of human premature labor by indomethacin. Obstet Gynecol 44:787, 1974.

349. Grella, P. and Zanor, P.: Premature labor and indomethacin. Prostaglandins 16:1007, 1978.

350. Schwartz, A., Brook, I., Iusler, V., et al.: Effect of flufenamic acid on uterine contractions and plasma levels of 15-keto-13,14 dihydroprostaglandin F2a in preterm labor. Gynecol Obstet Invest 9:139, 1978.

351. Zuckerman, H., Shalev, E., Gilad, G., et al.: Further study of the inhibition of premature labor by indomethacin. Part I. J Perinat Med 12:19, 1984.

352. Zuckerman, H., Shalev, E., Gilad, G., et al.: Further study of the inhibition of premature labor by indomethacin. Part II double-blind study. J Perinat Med 12:25, 1984.

353. Spearing, G.: Alcohol, indomethacin, and salbutamol. Obstet Gynecol 53:171, 1979.

354. Gamissans, O., Canas, E., Cararach, V., et al.: A study of indomethacin combined with ritodrine in threatened preterm labor. Europ J Obstet Gynec Reprod Biol 8/3:123, 1978.

355. Katz, Z., Lancet, M., Yemini, M., et al.: Treatment of premature labor contractions with combined ritodrine and indomethacine. Int J Gynaecol Obstet 21:337, 1983.

356. Dillard, T., Witter, F.R. and Dubin, N.H.: Treatment of preterm labor with indomethacin. Abstract #232 presented at the sixth Annual Meeting of the Society of Perinatal Obstetricians, San Antonio, Texas, Feb. 1986.

357. Alvan, G., Orme, M., Bertilsson, L., et al.: Pharmacokinetics of indomethacin. Clin Pharm Ther 18:364, 1975.

358. Bhat, R., Vidyasagar, D., Vadapalli, M.D., et al.: Disposition of indomethacin in preterm infants. J Pediatr 95:313, 1976.

359. Klein, K.L., Scott, W.J., Clark, K.E., et al.: Indomethacin—placental transfer, cytotoxity, and teratology in the rat. Am J Obstet Gynecol 141:448, 1981.

360. Collins, E. and Turner, G.: Maternal effects of regular salicylate ingestion in pregnancy. Lancet 2:335, 1955.

361. Stuart, M.J., Gross, S.J., Elrad, H., et al.: Effects of acetylsalicyclic-acid ingestion on maternal and neonatal hemostasis. N Engl J Med 307:909, 1982.

362. Freidman, ZVI, Whitman, V., Maisels, M.I., et al.: Indomethacin disposition and indomethacin induced platelet dysfunction in premature infants. J Clin Pharmacol 18:272, 1978.

363. Durandy, A., Brami, C., Griscelli, C.: The effects of indomethacin administration during pregnancy on womens' and newborns' T-suppressor lymphocyte activity and on HLA Class II expression by newborns' leukocytes. Am J Repr Immunol & Microbiol 8:94, 1985.

364. Ylikorkala, O., Jouppila, P., Kirkinen, P., et al.: Maternal thromboxane, prostacyclin, and umbilical blood flow in humans. Obstet Gynecol 63:677, 1984.

365. Makila, U.M., Jouppila, P., Kirkinen, P., et al.: Placental thromboxane and prostacyclin in the regulation of placental blood flow. Obstet Gynecol 68:537, 1986.

366. Naden, R.P. Iliya, C.A., Arant, B.S. Jr., et al.: Hemodynamic effects of indomethacin in chronically instrumented pregnant sheep. Am J Obstet Gynecol 151:484, 1985.

367. Novy, M.S.: Effects of indomethacin on labor, fetal oxygenation, and fetal development in rhesus monkeys. Adv Prostaglandin Thromboxane Res 4:285, 1978.

368. Friedman, W.F., Hirschklau, M.J., Printz, M.P., et al.: Pharmacologic closure of patent ductus arteriosus in the premature infant. N Engl J Med 295:526, 1976.

369. Heymann, M.A. Rudolph A.M. and Silverman, N.H.: Closure of the ductus arteriosus in premature infants by inhibition of prostaglandin synthesis. N Engl J Med 295:530, 1976.

370. Merritt, T.A., White, C.L., Jacob, J., et al.: Patent ductus arteriosus treated with ligation or indomethacin: a followup study. J Pediatr 95:588, 1979.

371. Mahony, L., Carnero,V., Brett, C., et al.: Prophylactic indomethacin therapy for patent ductus arteriosus in very-low-birth-weight infants. N Engl J Med 306:506, 1982.

372. McCarthy, J.S., Zies, L.G. and Gelband, H.: Age-dependent closure of the patent ductus arteriosus by indomethacin. Pediatr 62:706, 1978.

373. Ivey, H.H., Kattwinkel, J., Park, T.S., et al.: Failure of indomethacin to close persistent ductus arteriosus in infants weighing under 1000 grams. Br Heart J 41:304, 1979.

374. Cooke, R.W.I. and Pickerine, D.: Poor response to oral indomethacin therapy for persistent ductus arteriosus in very low birth weight infants. Br Heart J 41:30, 1979.

375. Alpert, B.S., Lewins, M.J., Rowland, D.W., et al.: Plasma indomethacin levels in preterm newborn infants with symptomatic patent ductus arteriosus—clinical and echocardiographic assessments of response. J Pediatr 95:578, 1979.

376. Brash, A.R., Hickey, D.E., Graham, T.P. et al.: Pharmacokinetics of indomethacin in the neonate. Relation to plasma indomethacin levels to response of the ductus arteriosus. N Engl J Med 305:67, 1981.

377. Sharpe, G.L., Thalme, B. and Larsson, S.: Studies on closure of the ductus arteriosus. XI. Ductal closure in utero by a prostaglandin synthetase inhibitor. Prostaglandins 8:363, 1974.

378. Van Kets, H., Thiery, M., Derom, R., et al.: Perinatal hazards of chronic antenatal tocolysis with indomethacin. Prostaglandins 18:893, 1979.

379. Goodie, B.M. and Dossetor, J.F.B.: Effect on the fetus of indomethacin given to suppress labour. Lancet 2:1187, 1979.

380. Mogilner, B.M., Ashkenazy, M. Borenstein, R., et al.: Hydrops fetalis caused by maternal indomethacin treatment. Acta Obstet Gynecol Scand 61:183, 1982.

381. Moise, K.J., Jr., Huhta, J.C., Dawod, S., et al.: Indomethacin in the treatment of preterm labor: effects on the human fetal ductus arteriosus. Abstract #14 presented at the seventh annual meeting of the Society of Perinatal Obstetricians, Lake Buena Vista, Fl, Feb. 1987.

382. Kleinman, G., Laird, M., Jennings, J., et al.: Fetal and neonatal effect of indomethacin in the treatment of preterm labor. Abstract #93 presented at the seventh annual meeting of the Society of Perinatal Obstetricians, Lake Buena Vista, Fl, Feb. 1987.

383. Rudolph, A.M.: The effects of nonsteroidal antiinflammatory compounds on fetal circulation and pulmonary function. Obstet Gynecol 58:63S, 1981.

384. Manchester, D., Margolis,H.S., and Sheldon, R.E.: Possible association between maternal indomethacin therapy and primary pulmonary hypertension of the newborn. Am J Obstet Gynecol 126:467, 1976.

385. Csaba, I.F., Sulyok, E. Ertle, T.: Relationship of maternal treatment with indomethacin to persistence of fetal circulation syndrome. J Pediatr 92:484, 1978.

386. Levin, D.L., Fixler, D.E., Morriss, F.C., et al.: Morphologic analysis of the pulmonary vascular bed in infants exposed in utero to prostaglandin synthetase inhibitors. J Pediatr 92:478, 1978.

387. Dudley, D.K.L. and Hardie, M.J.: Fetal and neonatal effects of indomethacin used as a tocolytic agent. Am J Obstet Gynecol 151:181, 1985.

388. Niebyl, J.R. and Witter, F.R.: Neonatal outcome after indomethacin treatment for preterm labor. Am J Obstet Gynecol 155:747, 1986.

389. Cantor, B., Tyler, T., Nelson, R.M., et al.: Oligohydramnios and transient neonatal anuria. A possible association with the maternal use of prostaglandin synthetase inhibitors. J Repr Med 24:220, 1980.

390. Itskovitz, J., Abramovich, H. and Brandes, J.M.: Oligohydramnios, meconium and perinatal death concurrent with indomethacin treatment in human pregnancy. J Repr Med 24:137, 1980.

391. Veersema, D., deJong, P.A. and van Wijck, J.A.M.: Indomethacin and the fetal renal non-function syndrome. Europ J Obstet Gynecol Reprod Biol 16:113, 1983.

392. Cifuentes, R.F., Olley, P.M. Balfe, J.W., et al.: Indomethacin and renal function in premature infants with persistent patent ductus arteriosus. J Pediatr 95:583, 1979.

393. Rasmussen, L.F. and Wennberger, R.P.: Displacement of bilirubin from albumin binding sites by indomethacin. Clin Res 25:2, 1977.

394. Landesman, R. and Wilson, K.H.: The relaxant effect of diazoxide on isolated gravid and nongravid human myometrium. Am J Obstet Gynecol 101:120, 1968.

395. Morishima, H.O., Caritis, S.N., Yeh, M.N., et al.: Prolonged infusion of diazoxide in the management of premature labor in the baboon. Obstet Gynecol 48:203, 1976.

396. Johansson, S., Anderson, R. and Wikberg, J.: Mechanical and metabolic effects of diazoxide on rat uterus. Acta Pharmacol Toxicol 41:328, 1977.

397. Landesman, R., deSouza F., J.A., Coutinho, E.M., et al.: The inhibitory effect of diazoxide in normal term labor. Am J Obstet Gynecol 103:430, 1969.

398. Bert, J. and Adamsons, K.: Clinical use of diazoxide in premature labor. Abstract #202 presented at the 25th Annual Meeting of the Society of Gynecologic Investigation, Atlanta, Georgia, 1978.

399. Neuman, J., Weiss, B., Rabello, Y., et al.: Diazoxide for the acute control of severe hypertension complicating pregnancy: a pilot study. Obstet Gynecol 53:50S, 1979.

400. Nuwayhid, B., Brinkman, C.R. III, Katchen, B., et al: Maternal and fetal hemodynamic effects of diazoxide. Obstet Gynecol 46:197, 1975.
401. Caritis, S., Morishima, H., Stark, R., et al.: The effects of diazoxide on uterine blood flow in pregnant sheep. Obstet Gynecol 456:197, 1975.
402. Boulos, B.M., Davis, L.E., Almond, C.H., et al.: Placental transfer of diazoxide and its hazardous effect on the newborn. J Clin Pharmacol 11:206, 1971.
403. Milner, F.D.G. and Chouksey, S.K.: Effects of fetal exposure to diazoxide in man. Arch Dis Child 47:537, 1972.
404. Milsap, R.L., and Auld, P.A.M.: Neonatal hyperglycemia following maternal diazoxide administration. JAMA 243:144, 1980.
405. Ulmsten, U., Andersson, K.E. and Forman, A.: Relaxing effects of nifedipine on the nonpregnant human uterus in vitro and in vivo. Obstet Gynecol 52:436, 1978.
406. Forman, A., Andersson, K.E., Persson, G.A., et al.: Relaxant effects of nifedipine on isolated, human myometrium. Acta Pharmacol et Toxicol 45:81, 1979.
407. Csapo, A.I., Puri, C.P., Tarro, S., et al.: Deactivation of the uterus during normal and premature labor by the calcium antagonist nicardipine. Am J Obstet Gynecol 142:483, 1982.
408. Forman, A., Gandrup, P., Andersson, K.E., et al.: Effects of nifedipine on spontaneous and methylergometrine-induced activity postpartum. Am J Obstet Gynecol 144:442, 1982.
409. Lirette, M., Holbrook, H. and Katz, M.: Effect of nicardipine HC1 on prematurely induced uterine activity in the pregnant rabbit. Obstet Gynecol 65:31, 1985.
410. Golichowski, A.M., Hathaway, D.R., Fineberg, N., et al.: Tocolytic and hemodynamic effects of nifedipine in the ewe. Am J Obstet Gynecol 151:1134, 1985.
411. Forman, A., Gandrup, P., Andersson, K.E., et al.: Effects of nifedipine on oxytocin-and prostaglandin F2a-induced activity in the postpartum uterus. Am J Obstet Gynecol 144:665, 1982.
412. Andersson, K.E., Ingemarsson, I., Ulmsten, U., et al.: Inhibition of prostaglandin-induced uterine activity by nifedipine. Br J Obstet Gynaecol 86:175, 1979.
413. Ulmsten, U., Andersson, K.E. and Wingerup, L.: Treatment of premature labor with the calcium antagonist nifedipine. Arch Gynecol 229:1, 1980.
414. Ulmsten, U.: Treatment of normotensive and hypertensive patients with preterm labor using oral nifedipine, a calcium antagonist. Arch Gynecol 236:69, 1984.
415. D'Alton, M.E., Jillson, A.E., Hou, S., et al.: Treatment of premature labor with the calcium antagonist nifedipine. Abstract #61 presented at the Society of Perinatal Obstetricians Annual Meeting, Las Vegas, Nevada, Feb. 1985.
416. Kaul, A.F., Osathanondh, R., Safon, L.E., et al.: The management of preterm labor with the calcium channel-blocking agent nifedipine combined with the beta-mimetic terbutaline. Drug Intell Clin Pharmacol 19:369, 1985.
417. Forman, A., Andersson, K.E. and Ulmstein, U.: Inhibition of myometrial activity by calcium antagonists. Sem Perinatol 5:288, 1981.
418. Braunwald, E.: Mechanism of action of calcium-channel-blocking agents. N Engl J Med 307:1618, 1982.
419. Calvin, C., Loutzenhizer, R. and van Breeman, C.: Mechanisms of calcium antagonist-induced vasodilation. Ann Rev Pharmacol Toxicol 23:373, 1983.
420. Walters, B.N.J. and Redman, C.W.G.: Treatment of severe pregnancy-associated hypertension with the calcium antagonist nifedipine. Br J Obstet Gynaecol 91:330, 1984.
421. Lirette, M., Holbrook, R.H. and Katz, M.: Cardiovascular and uterine blood flow changes during nicardipine HCl tocolysis in the rabbit. Obstet Gynecol 69:79, 1987.
422. Veille, J.C., Bissonnett, J.M. and Hohimer, A.R.: The effect of a calcium channel blocker (nifedipine) on uterine blood flow in the pregnant goat. Am J Obstet Gynecol 154:160, 1986.
423. Parisi, V.M., Salinas, J.K. and Stockmar, E.J.: Fetal cardiorespiratory responses to maternal administration of nicardipine in the hypertensive ewe. Abstract #11 presented at the sixth annual meeting of the Society of Perinatal Obstetricians, San Antonio, Texas, Feb. 1986.
424. Maigards, S., Forman, A. and Andersson, K.E.: Effects of nifedipine on human placental arteries. Gynecol Obstet Invest 18:217, 1984.
425. Rodriguez-Escudero, F.J., Aranguren, G., and Benito, J.A.: Verapamil to inhibit the cardiovascular side effects of ritodrine. Int J Gynaecol Obstet 19:333, 1981.
426. Wolfe, J.D., Tashkin, D.P., Calvarese, B., et al.: Bronchodilator effects of terbutaline and aminophylline alone and in combination in asthmatic patients. N Engl J Med 298:363, 1978.
427. Coutinho, E.M. and Lopes, A.C.V.: Inhibition of uterine motility by aminophylline. Am J Obstet Gynecol 110:726, 1971.
428. Jack, P.M.B. and Nathaniel, P.W.: Inhibition of the oxytocic action of prostaglandin F2a on pregnant rabbit uterus by intra-aortic infusion of theophylline in vivo. J Endocr 62:171, 1974.
429. Laifer, S.A., Ghodgaonkar, R.B., Zacur, H.A., et al.: The effect of aminophylline on uterine smooth muscle contractility and prostaglandin production in the pregnant rat uterus in vitro. Am J Obstet Gynecol 155:212, 1986.
430. Berg, G., Andersson, R.G.G. and Ryden, G.: In vitro study of phosphodiesterase-inhibiting

drugs: a complement to beta-sympathomimetic drug therapy in premature labor? Am J Obstet Gynecol 145:802, 1983.
431. Liu, D.T.Y., Measday, B. and Melville, H.A.H.: Premature labour—parameters for comparison employing methylxanthine therapy. Aust NZJ Obstet Gynaec 15:145, 1975.
432. Liu, D.T.Y. and Blackwell, R.J.: The value of a scoring system in predicting outcome of preterm labour and comparing the efficacy of treatment with aminophylline and salbutamol. Br J Obstet Gynaecol 85:418, 1978.
433. Melis, G.B., Fruzzetti, F. and Strigini, F.: Aminophylline treatment of preterm labor. Acta Europ Fertil 15:357, 1984.
434. Hadjigeorgiou, E., Kitsiou, S., Psaroudakis, A., et al.: Antepartum aminophylline treatment for prevention of the respiratory distress syndrome in premature infants. Am J Obstet Gynecol 135:257, 1979.
435. Karotkin, E.H., Kido, M., Cashore, W.J., et al.: Acceleration of fetal lung maturation by aminophyllin in pregnant rabbits. Pediatr Res 10:722, 1976.
436. Barrett, C.T., Sevanian, A., Phelps, D.L., et al.: Effects of cortisol and aminophylline upon survival, pulmonary mechanics, and secreted phosphatidyl choline of prematurely delivered rabbits. Pediatr 12:38, 1978.
437. Sevanian, A., Gilden, C., Kaplan, S.A., et al.: Enhancement of fetal lung surfactant production by aminophylline. Pediatr Res 13:1336, 1979.
438. Lipshitz, J.: Use of beta2-smpathomimetic drug as a temporizing measure in the treatment of acute fetal distress. Am J Obset Gynecol. 129:31, 1977.
439. Arias, F.: Intrauterine resuscitation with terbutaline: a method for the management of acute intrapartum fetal distress. Am J Obstet Gynecol 131:39, 1978.
440. Barrett, J.M.: Fetal resuscitation with terbutaline during eclampsia-induced uterine hypertonus. Am J Obstet Gynecol 150:895, 1981.
441. Hutchon, D.J.R.: Management of severe fetal bradycardia with ritodrine. Br J Obstet Gynaecol 89:671, 1982.
442. Zentner, R.: Ritodrine in the management of a case of acute fetal distress. Aust NZ J Obstet Gynaec 23:250, 1983.
443. Lipshitz, J. and Klose, C.W.: Use of tocolytic drugs to reverse oxytocin-induced uterine hypertonus and fetal distress. Obstet Gynecol 66:16S, 1985.
444. Mendez-Bauer, C., Shekarloo, A., Cook, V. and Freese, U.: Treatment of acute intrapartum fetal distress by B₂-sympathomimetics. Am J Obstet Gynecol, 156:638, 1987.
445. Ingemarsson, I., Arulkumaran, S. and Ratnam, S.S.: Single injection of terbutaline in term labor. II. Effect on uterine activity. Am J Obstet Gynecol 153:865, 1985.
446. Burke M.S., Porreco, R.P., Haverkamp, A.L., et al.: Intrauterine resuscitation with tocolysis. Abstract #321 presented at the 7th annual meeting of the Society of Perinatal Obstetricians, Lake Buena Vista, Fl, Feb 1987.
447. Caritis, S.N., Lin, L.S. and Wong, L.K.: Evaluation of the pharmacodynamics and pharmacokinetics of ritodrine when administered as a loading dose. Am J Obstet Gynecol 152:1026, 1985.
448. Gerris, J., Thiery, M., Bogaert, M., et al.: Randomized trial of two beta-mimetic drugs (ritodrine and fenoterol) in acute intra-partum tocolysis. Eur J Clin Pharmacol 18:443, 1980.
449. Sampson, M.B., Lastres, O., Tomasi, A.M., et al.: Tocolysis with terbutaline sulfate in patients with placenta previa complicated by premature labor. J Repr Med 29:248, 1984.
450. Tomich, P.G.: Prolonged use of tocolytic agents in the expectant management of placenta previa. J Repr Med 30:745, 1985.
451. Wallace, R.L., VanDorsten, J.P., Eglinton, G.S., et al.: External cephalic version with tocolysis. Observations and continuing experience at the Los Angeles County/University of Southern California Medical Center. J Repr Med 29:745, 1984.
452. Brocks, V., Philipsen, T. and Secher, N.J.: A randomized trial of external cephalic version with tocolysis in late pregnancy. Br J Obstet Gynaec 91:653, 1984.
453. Stine, L.E., Phelan, J.P., Wallace, R., et al.: Update on external cephalic version performed at term. Obstet Gynecol 65:642, 1985.
454. Dyson, D.C., Ferguson, J.E. II and Hensleigh, P.: Antepartum external cephalic version under tocolysis. Obstet Gynecol 67:63, 1986.
455. Morrison, J.C., Myatt, R.E., Martin, J.N. Jr., et al.: External cephalic version of the breech presentation under tocolysis. Am J Obstet Gynecol 154:900, 1986.

Chapter 14

*Smoking and Pregnancy**

Gertrud S. Berkowitz

Cigarette smoking is probably the most common addiction among pregnant women in our society. Despite the growing publicity regarding the health hazards of smoking, the overall proportion of adult women who smoke has dropped only slightly over the past two decades and the percentage of heavy female smokers has actually increased.[1] Smoking rates among teenage girls grew substantially up until the late 1970s and have exceeded those of teenage boys.[2,3] Although maternal smoking is detrimental not only to the mother herself, but also to the fetus, only about 20% of pregnant smokers quit during pregnancy.[4] Thus, a greater effort is needed to persuade and help pregnant smokers to alter their behavior.

Current understanding of the effects of maternal smoking on pregnancy and on the developing fetus and child is based on clinical, physiologic, pathologic, experimental, and especially epidemiologic studies, in which an aggregated total of over half a million births have been included.[2,5,6]; The most consistent observation is the reduction in birth weight among infants of smokers, but smoking has also been shown to have other adverse effects on the fetus, the newborn, and the future development of the infant and child. These effects have been found to be proportional to the level of smoking and appear to be prevented or reduced if the mother does not smoke during a subsequent pregnancy.

FETAL GROWTH RETARDATION

Reduced fetal growth is the most frequently reported adverse pregnancy effect associated with maternal smoking. As first reported by Simpson in 1957[7] and since confirmed by more than fifty studies, smokers' babies weigh, on the average, 200 g less at birth than babies of comparable nonsmokers, and the proportion of babies weighing less than 2500 g usually doubles with maternal smoking. It has been estimated that if smoking were eliminated, the number of low birth weight infants would be reduced by 20 to 40%.[8] As shown in Table 14–1, which is based on data from several studies, the reduction in birth weight is dose-related, that is, the more the woman smokes during pregnancy the lower is her baby's birth weight. A recent study has also suggested that the decrease in birth weight may be more pronounced for older smokers than for younger smokers.[9]

The lowered birth weight is primarily due to intrauterine growth retardation since mean gestation is reduced at the most by 1 to 2 days among smokers.[2,5,6]

---

*I am indebted to the late Mary B. Meyer who prepared the chapter on this topic for the first edition. The current version is based in large part on her comprehensive discussion.

Table 14–1. Relationship between Number of Cigarettes Smoked to Birth Weight

		No. Cigarettes			
		0	1–10	11–20	>20
Birth Wt. (g)	(Whites)	3399	3272	3185	3128
Birth Wt. (g)	(Blacks)	3128	2977	2957	2945
% LBW (≤2500 g)	(Whites)	4.8	8.0	9.0	13.4
% LBW (≤2500 g)	(Blacks)	8.3	13.6	17.7	22.7

Abel[6] Hum Biol 52:593, 1980.

Babies of smokers are not only lighter than babies of comparable nonsmokers, they are also shorter.[10–12] Smaller head circumferences and arm circumferences have also been noted.[11,12] Because of the proportional decrease in both weight and length, the ponderal index of smokers' babies is normal. Assessment of skinfold thickness suggests that babies of smokers have a normal layer of subcutaneous fat but a reduction in lean body mass.[11,12] These findings provide further evidence against the argument that the effect of smoking on fetal growth is nutritionally mediated.

The slower fetal growth of smokers' babies has been inferred from measurements made at the time of birth that have shown smoking-related reductions at various gestational ages at delivery. Corroboration is now available from serial ultrasound measurements of biparietal diameters during pregnancy. Figure 14–1 shows growth curves of biparietal diameters (BPD) for fetuses of smokers and nonsmokers based on a study by Persson et al.[13] The BPD increased faster in the nonsmoking group than the smoking group. The difference was significant from 28 weeks onwards and positively correlated with the average number of cigarettes smoked. Others[14] have found a significant decrease in the BPD associated with maternal smoking as early as 21 weeks of gestation.

The generally accepted conclusion is that the association between maternal smoking and reduced fetal growth is a cause-and-effect relationship and not a reflection of different characteristics of smokers and nonsmokers. Evidence in support of this conclusion comes form the consistency of the findings in a wide variety of populations, the relationship between number of cigarettes smoked to the decrement in birth weight, the independence of the association of other factors that affect birth weight (e.g., race, parity, maternal size, maternal weight gain, socioeconomic status, sex of child), the fact that infants of women who stop smoking during pregnancy have birth weights similar to those of infants of nonsmokers, the biologic plausibility of several proposed mechanisms of action, and data from animal studies.[2,5,6,15]

PLACENTAL RATIO

It is well established that the ratio of placental weight to birth weight is higher for smokers than nonsmokers. The definitive study by Wingred et al.[16] used standardized protocols for weighing and examining placentas from 7000 births to members of the Kaiser Foundation Health Plan in California. As shown in Figure 14–2, placental ratios increased with maternal smoking level at each gestational age from 37 through 43 weeks. The increase results from considerable decreases in birth weight accompanied by slight increases in placental weight

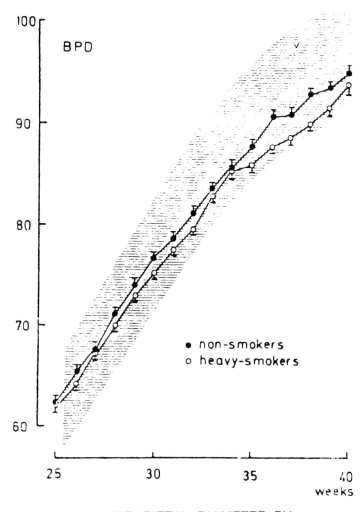

FETAL BIPARIETAL DIAMETER BY
GESTATIONAL AGE, BY MATERNAL SMOKING

Fig. 14–1. Fetal BPD values (means and SEM) of nonsmokers (10 cigarettes/day:lower line) plotted in relation to postmenstrual age against the normal range (shaded area depicts 95% confidence interval).

in heavier smokers. Ratios were higher for black than for white women, and tended to increase as maternal hemoglobin decreased.

PRETERM BIRTH

Although mean gestation is only minimally affected by maternal smoking, there is growing evidence that the risk of a preterm delivery is moderately increased for women who smoke.[8,17–19] In other words, smoking may precipitate a preterm birth in some cases, but it does not cause an overall reduction in the duration of pregnancy. The effect of smoking on preterm births has been found to be independent of other factors that affect pregnancy duration and the risk

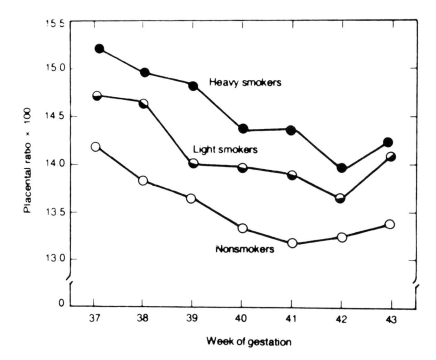

Fig. 14–2. Ratio of placental weight to birth weight by length of gestation and maternal smoking category.

of an early delivery appears to increase with the level of maternal smoking. Of particular concern is the finding from a recent California study that the excess risk is concentrated among the very preterm births[19] (Table 14–2), since it is these infants who have a high risk of mortality. In the latter study, women who smoked one or more packs per day had a 20% increased risk of delivering before 37 weeks of gestation and a 60% increased likelihood of delivering before 33 weeks of gestation. How much of the problem of preterm births can be attributed to maternal smoking depends on the proportion of pregnant women who smoke. In the California study, 4% of preterm births (<37 weeks) and 9% of very preterm births (<33 weeks) were attributable to smoking. Previous studies[2] have generally reported higher attributable risks but in most of these studies the prevalence of smoking was over 40% whereas in the California study the prevalence was 28%.

Table 14–2.   Maternal Smoking and Preterm Birth

Outcome	Adjusted Odds Ratios* Maternal Smoking (Packs per day)			
	None	<1	≥1	AR†
Births <37 wks' gestation	1.0	1.1	1.2	4%
Births <33 wks' gestation	1.0	1.1	1.6	9%

*The adjusted odds ratios give the odds of a preterm delivery for smokers as compared to nonsmokers adjusted for the effect of confounders.
†Percent of preterm births that can be attributed to smoking.
 Adapted from Shiono et al.[19] JAMA 255:82, 1986.

The inverse relationship between the risk of neonatal mortality and gestational age at delivery is well known and is particularly pronounced for the preterm infants. Advances in neonatal care have greatly improved the survival of preterm, low birth weight infants and their potential for normal development. A major part of neonatal intensive care, with its high monetary and emotional costs, is devoted to these small infants. The remarkably improved possibility of keeping them alive does not mitigate the need to seek causes of preterm birth and to prevent it if possible. The extent to which cigarette smoking contributes to the occurrence of preterm birth is undoubtedly one of its more serious consequences.

COMPLICATIONS OF PREGNANCY

Pregnant smokers have a higher incidence of several pregnancy complications, including abruptio placentae, placenta previa, vaginal bleeding during pregnancy, and probably premature rupture of membranes and amnionitis.[2,5,8,20-23] Data from the Ontario Perinatal Mortality Study,[20,24] illustrated in Figure 14-3, show that the risks of abruptio placentae, placenta previa, and premature rupture of membranes are elevated for smokers particularly at early gestational ages. Risks of these complications as well as associated perinatal losses increase with

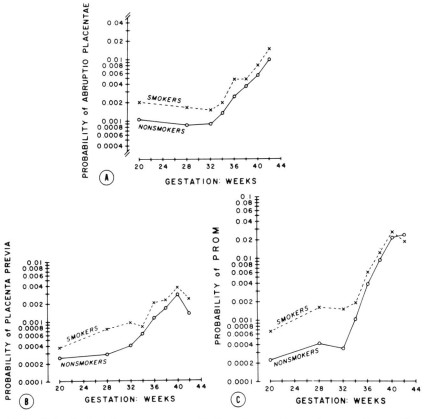

Fig. 14-3. Risk of selected pregnancy complications for smoking and nonsmoking mothers, by period of gestational age at delivery. A. Abruptio placentae: B. Placenta previa; C. Admission diagnosis, rupture of membranes only. (Ontario data.)

the number of cigarettes smoked as shown in Table 14–3. Smoking-level-specific rates of complications, adjusted for the effects of other important factors, have been used to calculate that smoking may be the cause of 10 to 35% in light smokers and 30 to 60% in heavy smokers of the incidence of abruptio placentae, placenta previa, and prolonged rupture of membranes.[24] Although these findings indicate that smoking may precipitate a preterm birth through its effect on placental abnormalities and premature rupture of membranes, the increased risk of a preterm birth could not be completely explained by these pregnancy complications in the California study.[19]

In contrast to the above complications, smokers have consistently been found to have a lower incidence of preeclampsia and toxemia, however defined. This relationship holds true when data are controlled for parity, social class, maternal weight and weight gain, and severity of preeclampsia.[2,21,25] However, if preeclampsia does develop, smokers have a substantially greater risk of perinatal mortality than nonsmokers.[21,25,26] It has been suggested that the negative association may be due to the hypotensive effect of thiocyanate which is derived from the cyanide in cigarette smoke and has been regularly found in the blood of smokers.[27] Reduced fetal growth rate and a lower gain in blood volume have also been hypothesized as contributing factors.[28]

PERINATAL MORTALITY

Although the risk of perinatal mortality is generally higher for smokers than nonsmokers, the relationship between maternal smoking and perinatal loss is less consistent than that between smoking and birth weight. Several reasons can be given for this discrepancy. First is the observation that other important variables that affect perinatal mortality might influence the results if they were unequally distributed in comparison groups of smokers and nonsmokers. For example, perinatal mortality rates in the United States are higher for black than for white babies, but until recently black women smoked less than white women. Selection of births on the basis of smoking alone would include more nonsmokers who were black and at high risk and more smokers who were white and at a lower risk, thereby minimizing the apparent effects of maternal smoking on perinatal loss. Large studies which have controlled for the effect of other relevant factors have demonstrated an independent effect of maternal smoking on perinatal mortality.[5,8] Second is the finding that cigarette smoking increases the risk of perinatal death most for women who are already at high risk. In general, young, healthy, low-parity women have little increase in perinatal loss, espe-

Table 14–3. Pregnancy Complications: Incidence and Associated Perinatal Mortality by Maternal Smoking Level (Ontario data.)

	Rates/1000 Total Births					
	Incidence			Perinatal Deaths		
	Packs/Day			Packs/Day		
	0	<1	1+	0	<1	1+
Placenta Previa	6	8	12	0.9	1.1	2.2
Abruptio Placentae	16	20	28	4.6	7.0	9.0
Bleeding During Pregnancy	116	142	180	5.4	10.8	16.5
ROM >48 hours	16	24	36	1.9	3.9	7.5

cially if they are light smokers, whereas women with other perinatal risk factors are at high risk, especially if they are heavy smokers.[8,29,30] Other factors may also play a role. For example, the occasional observation that young primaparous, light smokers who are healthy and well-off may have slightly lower perinatal mortality rates than comparable nonsmokers may reflect the reduced incidence of preeclampsia in these women. Data from several large studies are given in Table 14–4 to illustrate the variation in perinatal mortality rate according to some of these factors.

Perhaps an even more important reason why the impact of smoking on perinatal mortality appears to be less than what might be expected is the predominance of intrauterine growth retardation rather than prematurity among infants of smokers. Although survival data have traditionally focused on birth weight, the importance of joint assessment of gestational age and birth weight is increasingly being recognized. Specifically, Goldenberg et al.[31] have shown that for infants within the same low birth weight groups those with intrauterine growth retardation had one half to one sixth of the neonatal mortality rate of infants who evidence no growth retardation. The influence of growth retardation may also explain the so-called paradoxical finding that the perinatal mortality rate among low birth weight babies of smokers tends to be lower than among low birth weight babies of nonsmokers. In addition, as Goldstein[32] has demonstrated, the lower mortality is to be expected since the low birth weight babies of smokers have a higher average birth weight than those of nonsmokers.

Cause of Death

To gain insight into the mechanisms by which maternal smoking may cause a fetal or a neonatal death, data from the Ontario study were used to analyze relationships between excess deaths of smokers' babies and specific causes of death.[24] Smoking-associated fetal deaths were most frequently coded in the category of "unknown cause" and also in the categories of "anoxia" and "maternal cause." Excess neonatal deaths of smoking women were due to "prematurity alone" and the related category of "respiratory difficulty."[20] These findings are corroborated by other studies in which perinatal deaths have been reported by maternal smoking habit and by cause.[5] The tentative conclusion is that fetuses and neonates whose deaths were related to maternal smoking had little or no recognizable pathologic condition, but had died in utero from anoxia or maternal causes, or had suffered the consequences of preterm delivery.

Complications of Pregnancy and Perinatal Mortality

If the cause of death of smokers' babies is not found in the baby, it is logical to expect an increase in pregnancy complications that carry high risks of perinatal loss. Analysis of excess smoking-related deaths in the Ontario data revealed highly significant associations of fetal deaths with bleeding after 20 weeks of pregnancy and with abruptio placentae. Neonatal deaths of smokers' infants, on the other hand, were significantly associated with a history of bleeding before 20 weeks and with premature and prolonged rupture of membranes.[24] Similar associations between maternal smoking and these complications have also been reported in other studies.[5,21]

Because perinatal deaths occur most frequently before term, the probability of perinatal death for all fetuses in utero has been calculated from the Ontario

Table 14–4. Examples of Perinatal Mortality by Maternal Smoking Status Related to Other Subgroup Characteristics[2,5]

Study Population	Number of Births		Category		Perinatal or Neonatal Deaths/1000 Births		Relative Risk[1]
	Nonsmoker	Smoker			Nonsmoker	Smoker	
Butler: British Perinatal Mortality Survey, England All Births	11,145	4,660	Social Class				
				1–2 (high)	25.8	26.3	1.02
				3–5	33.5	46.6	1.39
Comstock: Washington Co. Maryland, White	7,646	4,641	Fathers' Education				
				9+ years	14.4[2]	16.1[2]	1.12
				≤8 years	17.6[2]	38.0[2]	2.16
Rantakallio: N. Finland White	8,898	2,346			23.2	23.4	1.01
Yerushalmy: California Middle to Upper Middle Class			Race				
	6,067	3,726		White	11.0[2]	11.3[2]	1.03
	2,219	1,071		Black	17.1[2]	21.5[2]	1.26
Niswander & Gordon: Collaborative Perinatal Study. 12 U.S. Centers			Race & Cigs/day				
	8,521	11,369		White	31.4		
				1–10		31.5	1.00
				11+		38.2	1.22
	9,862	8,160		Black	38.5		
				1–10		41.5	1.08
				11+		57.4	1.49
Ontario Perinatal Mortality Study. All single births in 10 teaching hospitals 1960–61			Packs/day				
	8,833	6,307	Parity	0			
				None	21.5		
				<1		22.8	1.06
				1+		26.9	1.25
	15,341	11,697		1–3			
				None	22.4		
				<1		26.2	1.17
				1+		29.5	1.32
	4,111	3,822		4+			
				None	30.6		
				<1		44.3	1.45
				1+		51.8	1.69

[1] Ratio of smoker rate:nonsmoker rate
[2] Neonatal only.

data for smokers and nonsmokers at each period of gestational age from 20 weeks on as shown in Figure 14–4.[24] Probabilities of perinatal loss were significantly higher for smoking women at 20 to 32 weeks of gestation. As was shown in Figure 14–3, there is also an increased probability that smoking women will experience early placental complications and premature rupture of membranes. These findings suggest that maternal smoking increases the risk of perinatal mortality at least partly because it increases the incidence of these complications, which in turn may cause anoxic fetal death or early delivery. These complications occur in a minority of births, but are an important cause of perinatal mortality. Discouragement of smoking during pregnancy should reduce the risk of complications and of perinatal mortality, especially if women at high risk for other reasons can be identified.

SPONTANEOUS ABORTION

Several case-control and prospective studies[33–36] have indicated that maternal smoking increases the risk of spontaneous abortions. However, the effect has

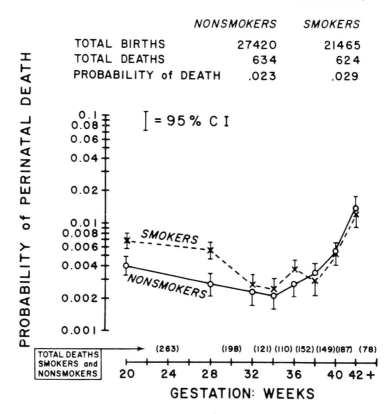

Fig. 14–4. Probability of perinatal death for smoking and nonsmoking mothers, by period of gestational age. Bars show 95% confidence intervals.

generally been small, particularly in studies that have controlled for confounding factors.[35,37] There is some evidence, albeit not entirely consistent, that the risk of abortion among smokers is concentrated among chromosomally normal conceptions.[34,35] In the light of the latter observations and the methodological problems of studying early pregnancy losses, further clarification is needed of the role of maternal smoking in spontaneous abortion.

CONGENITAL MALFORMATION

There are reports of increased frequencies of anencephaly,[38] congenital heart defects,[39] and orofacial clefts[21,39] but a decreased frequency of Down's syndrome[40] among infants of smokers as compared to controls. The lack of consistency among studies and the absence of an effect in other investigations[6,37] argue against a teratogenic effect of tobacco smoke.

OTHER EFFECTS

Smoking-related behavioral effects during the pregnancy and neonatal periods have been reported. These include alterations in fetal vital signs and possible neonatal functional deficits. Other miscellaneous findings include a protective effect against neonatal respiratory distress syndrome and decreased breast feeding among smoking mothers.

Fetal Behavior

The most consistent acute effect of cigarette smoking on the fetal behavioral state is a reduction in the number of fetal movements[41,42] or an increase in the number of epochs without fetal movement.[43] The changes in fetal heart rate and fetal breathing appear to be more complex. While it has traditionally been believed that maternal smoking results in fetal tachycardia,[5] Goodman et al.[42] found no significant increase in the fetal heart rate during or after maternal smoking but did observe significant reductions in beat-to-beat variability and in the number of accelerations.

The findings with respect to fetal breathing movements are also at variance. Early findings that maternal smoking was associated with a decrease in fetal breathing movements[44] have not been confirmed by more current data,[41-43] although some alteration in fetal breathing movements has been noted.[43] These conflicting results have been attributed to improved monitoring methods.[43]

Neonatal Functioning

With some exceptions,[45] maternal smoking has generally not been found to have any effect on Apgar scores.[33,46] A few investigators have reported that maternal smoking adversely affects other neonatal behavioral characteristics, such as visual alertness and auditory response.[47,48] Saxton's study of newborn infants of smoking and nonsmoking mothers, using the Brazelton Neonatal Behavioral Assessment Scale, showed deficiencies of smokers' infants on tests with important auditory components. The author concluded that some effect on the normal hearing mechanism had occurred in infants of smokers, and suggested that this might be due to the hypoxic effect of carbon monoxide on the cochlear organ.[47] It is obvious that other antepartum and intrapartum factors can influence early neonatal behavior. However, the latter study controlled for a number of potential confounders including obstetric anesthesia.

Neonatal Respiratory Distress Syndrome

While cigarette smoking generally exerts an adverse effect on fetal growth and neonatal well-being, recent studies [49,50] have found a beneficial effect of maternal smoking on the development of neonatal respiratory distress syndrome (RDS). However, the risk of nenonatal death attributable to RDS was not diminished for infants of smokers.[50] The reduction in risk of RDS with maternal smoking remained after adjustment for demographic factors, pregnancy complications, gestational age, and method of delivery.[50] This finding is consistent with the theory that conditions of chronic intrauterine stress may accelerate lung maturity.[51]

Breast Feeding

Women who smoke are much less likely to nurse their babies than non-smokers, as shown in Table 14–5. Although a common personality type may be responsible for this association, there is also some evidence that maternal smoking may have a direct effect on lactation. Andersen et al.[52] observed normal suckling induced increments in serum prolactin levels among breast-feeding smokers but lower basal prolactin levels among heavy cigarette smokers as compared to nonsmokers. The smokers also weaned their babies significantly earlier than the nonsmokers, a finding which Andersen et al. suggested may be related to the basal prolactin levels. Studies in animals also show inhibition of milk production by nicotine.[53] New studies are needed to find out whether women who want to nurse their babies would be more successful if they did not smoke. Possible effects of nicotine transmitted to the infant through breast milk also need to be evaluated.[5]

LONG-TERM EFFECTS OF MATERNAL SMOKING

An increasing number of studies is finding that maternal smoking may affect morbidity, mortality, growth and development beyond the perinatal period. Evaluating these findings, however, is hampered by the difficulty of separating out the independent effect of in utero exposure from postnatal passive exposure and other characteristics of the home environment of smoking parents.

Postneonatal Morbidity and Mortality

Studies of infant and child morbidity and mortality by the mother's smoking habits both before and after birth have shown adverse effects of maternal smoking at least up to the age of 5. Hospitalization rates for pneumonia and bronchitis

Table 14–5. Type of Infant Feeding at Discharge (%) by Amount Smoked by Mother During Pregnancy

Feed Type	Amount Smoked by Mother (packs/day)		
	0	<1	1+
Bottle	47.9	55.1	61.4
Breast	51.6	44.0	37.4
Gavage	0.5	0.8	1.1
Total no. fed	14,610	10,882	4,927

Source: Ontario Perinatal Mortality Study English-speaking Canadian women (unpublished data).

were found to be higher for infants of mothers who smoked during the pregnancy as compared to infants of nonsmokers in studies in Israel[54] and Finland[55] especially below the age of 1. In the Finnish study, postneonatal mortality, from 28 days to 5 years, was significantly higher for smokers' children, with rates of 11.1 per 1000, compared with 3.9 per 1000 for children of nonsmokers. In addition, smokers' children were more often hospitalized, stayed in the hospital longer, and had more visits to doctors and greater use of specialized services. A subsequent follow-up study of the Finnish children up to the age of 14 revealed that the children of smokers continued to be more prone to respiratory diseases after the age of 5, but that the difference between them and the controls diminished over time.[56] Since paternal smoking was found to be as important as maternal smoking in this analysis, it does not settle the issue of the relative contribution of prenatal and postnatal exposure.

Several studies have reported a positive association between maternal smoking and sudden infant death syndrome (SIDS).[2,5,57] In a case-control study by Bergman and Wiesner,[57] the mothers of SIDS victims did not differ from matched controls in their use of such substances as caffeine-containing beverages but did differ significantly in their smoking habits, both during and after pregnancy as shown in Table 14–6. Again, however, it is not clear whether the association reflects in utero exposure to cigarette smoke or passive exposure postnatally, or both.

Because of the higher incidence of cancer in smokers than nonsmokers, there is concern that the offspring of smokers may be more prone to malignancies. While most studies have found no signficant association between maternal smoking and cancer in the offspring,[58-60] transplacental and/or early childhood exposure to cigarette smoke has recently been related to an excess risk of adulthood leukemia/lymphoma[61] and childhood cancer, particularly Hodgkin's lymphoma, acute lymphoblastic leukemia and Wilms' tumor.[62] Further research is needed to confirm or refute these disturbing findings.

Growth and Development

Several long-term studies now give evidence that children of smoking mothers have slight but measurable deficiencies in physical growth, intellectual development, and behavior. According to the National Child Development Study,[63] which has followed up more than 12,000 British children at ages 7 and 11, children whose mothers smoked 10 or more cigarettes a day during pregnancy were on average 1.0 cm shorter and between 3 to 5 months retarded in reading, mathematics and general ability, as compared with the offspring of nonsmokers. These effects were evident after allowing for associated social and biologic factors but were relatively small compared to those attributable to social class or number

Table 14–6.   Parental Smoking and SIDS

Smoking Habits	% Smoking		
	SIDS	Controls	p
Mothers: During pregnancy	61	42	<.05
Mothers: After pregnancy	59	37	<.02
Fathers	53	43	NS

Bergman and Wiesner[57] Pediatrics 58:665, 1976

of siblings. Similar findings of impaired cognitive functioning have been shown in the Finnish follow-up study,[56] a Canadian longitudinal study,[64] as well as by data from the Collaborative Perinatal Project comparing the intellectual performance of siblings whose mothers had smoked during one but not in the other of the two pregnancies.[65] Although the children whose mothers had smoked during pregnancy scored only 2 to 5% lower on spelling and reading tests in the latter investigation, the built-in control for genetic factors and many environmental influences strengthen the possibility that these deficits were caused by smoking. In contrast, a study of inner city, lower class women failed to detect any significant association between maternal smoking and intellectual ability of offspring at 4 or 7 years of age,[66] but this may be due to the small sample size.

In addition to intellectual impairments, smokers' children have been found to exhibit short attention spans and hyperactive behavior more frequently than children of nonsmokers.[65,67] Since the behavioral abnormalities in children of smokers were associated with raised neonatal hemoglobin levels and low birth weights, fetal hypoxemia has been suggested as a possible factor in the development of these behavioral abnormalities.[65]

MECHANISMS

Cigarette smoke contains approximately 2000 different compounds. It seems likely that some observed effects of maternal smoking may be physiologic responses to the action of certain of these compounds, especially those that interfere with the fetal oxygen supply. The extent to which these responses either succeed or cause harm may depend on the level of smoking, the nature of the adaptation, and the reserve capacity of the system.

Carbon Monoxide

Carbon monoxide in cigarette smoke may cause chronic tissue hypoxia both by decreasing the oxygen transport capacity of blood and by reducing the pressure at which oxygen is released to the fetal tissue. Carbon monoxide, which has a higher affinity for hemoglobin than oxygen, combines with hemoglobin to form carboxyhemoglobin and thereby reduces the oxygen-carrying capacity of blood. Carboxyhemoglobin levels in pregnant nonsmokers reportedly vary from 0.4 to 4.4%, while concentrations in chronic smokers range from 2 to 14%.[68] At equilibrium, fetal carboxyhemoglobin levels are 10 to 15% higher than maternal levels.[69] The hypoxic effects of maternal smoking are also magnified in the fetus because the oxygen-carrying capacity of both blood supplies is decreased and because the driving pressure of oxygen is reduced twice, once as it crosses the placenta and again as it enters the fetal tissues. Since carboxyhemoglobin concentrations of 4 to 5% are associated with alterations in mental ability and other performance functions in adults,[69] the tissue hypoxia may not only be responsible for the reduced birth weight but also the reported retardation of mental abilities in infants of smokers.

Nicotine

Pharmacologic and physiologic effects of nicotine, based on studies in humans and experimental animals, are highly complex and include short term increases in maternal catecholamine levels, pulse rates, and blood pressure, decreases in uteroplacental blood flood, and alterations in fetal heart rate. The effect of nicotine on sympathetic and parasympathetic ganglia, skeletal muscles, and the central nervous system is similar to that of acetylcholine, first stimulating then depressing. Nicotine also produces cardiovascular changes by release of epinephrine from the adrenal medulla. Thus, it can produce widely differing effects depending upon the dosage, the time since smoking, and the site of action, making interpretation or prediction of these effects extremely difficult.[2,5]

A major hypothesis linking nicotine with adverse fetal effect is that nicotine stimulates the release of catecholamines which in turn produce uteroplacental vasoconstriction and, as a result, decreased nutrient and/or oxygen flow to the fetus.[6,21,70] Quigley et al.[71] noted that in moderate to heavy smokers, after 34 weeks' gestation, smoking two cigarettes in 10 minutes was associated with a 60% increase in maternal plasma norepinephrine and epinephrine and a 20% increase in serum cortisol concentrations. Lehtovirta and Forss[72] assessed the acute effects of smoking on placental intervillous blood flow using the 133 xenon method and found that intervillous flow decreased 22% immediately after smoking. Philipp et al.[73] have similarly shown that smokers have a higher rate of poor placental perfusion patterns than nonsmokers.

Maternal nicotine administration has been shown to reduce uterine blood flow in sheep[74] and in rhesus monkeys.[75] There is also evidence in rhesus monkeys that nicotine infusion results in marked cardiovascular disturbances in both mother and fetus and acidosis and hypoxia in the fetus.[15,75] Since nicotine rapidly crosses the placenta,[76] nicotine may have a direct detrimental effect on the fetus. The available animal data, however, suggest that the nicotine-induced decrease in uterine blood flow is a major factor responsible for fetal hypoxemia and metabolic acidosis.[75]

Other Components

Cyanide is another constituent of tobacco smoke that may interfere with tissue growth. Cyanide and thiocyanate levels have been found to be increased in the blood and urine of smokers' infants as compared to controls.[77] Vitamin B_{12} and sulfur-containing amino acids are necessary in the detoxification of cyanide. The depletion of these important nutrients may affect the growth and development of the fetuses of smokers.

Cadmium, also a component of tobacco smoke, appears to concentrate in the placentas of smokers. Since placental cadmium concentrations have been reported to exceed those of both maternal and fetal blood, it has been suggested that the placenta may act as a barrier to this metal.[78] Van der Velde et al.[79] have speculated that the increased cadmium concentrations may play a role in the structural changes that have been observed in the placentas of smokers (see below).

Placental Changes

Placentas of women who smoke have an increased incidence of degenerative changes, with calcification and patchy subchorionic fibrin appearing earlier in smokers' than in nonsmokers' placentas.[80] This is consistent with other reports that smoking causes "premature aging." Microscopic assessment of placentas of smokers and nonsmokers has also revealed a smaller diameter of the villous capillaries, a decrease in vasculosyncytial membranes and a thickening of villous basement membranes in smokers' placentas.[79,81] However, the extent to which these structural changes in the placenta interfere with normal fetal growth is not known.

Certain placental changes, such as the increased placental ratios, are believed to represent adaptive mechanisms to the reduced oxygen supply in pregnant smokers. The increased placental ratio should improve oxygen delivery, while a smaller fetus should have a reduced oxygen demand. However, other placental changes that may occur in response to hypoxia have limits beyond which they may fail or may become part of pathologic processes. For example, Christianson's findings that smokers had a significant reduction of the distance from the edge of rupture of membranes to the placental margin and an increased placental diameter-thickness ratio[80] is consistent with the finding of an increased probability of placenta previa among smokers. It is of interest that the placental ratio, the ratio of placental diameter to thickness, and the incidence of placenta previa all increase significantly with increasing altitude. Although placental hypertrophy appears to be more marked in the case of high altitude than with smoking, the physiologic effects of altitude on pregnancy appear to be similar in many respects to the effects of smoking.

Currently, the most widely accepted explanation for the detrimental effects of smoking on the fetus and newborn is that smoking causes intrauterine hypoxia through increased carboxyhemoglobin levels and/or reduced uteroplacental blood flow. It is likely that the increased placental ratios as well as the reported higher neonatal hemoglobin levels in infants of smokers[65] represent physiologic responses to the hypoxic state. However, Bureau et al.[82] have concluded that the hematologic compensatory mechanisms are trivial and that the fetus does not have the biologic capacity to accommodate to maternal smoking.

SUMMARY AND RECOMMENDATIONS

The most consistent result of maternal smoking is a reduction in fetal growth rate. Smoking during pregnancy is also associated with an increased risk of preterm deliveries, stillbirths and nenonatal deaths, and possibly spontaneous abortions. Many of the perinatal deaths and preterm births seem to be mediated through a smoking-related increase in the incidence of complications related to the placenta and, probably, the fetal membranes. In addition, maternal smoking may increase the incidence of morbidity and mortality in infancy and childhood and may result in slight but measurable deficits in long-term physical growth, intellectual performance and behavioral development.

Since maternal smoking represents one of the few known preventable causes of perinatal morbidity and mortality, it should be strongly discouraged. Recommendations for obstetricians to motivate their patients to stop smoking include the giving of information about known risks, special efforts to be applied to pregnancies with other risk factors, measurement of exhaled CO or of carboxyhemoglobin as part of the routine prenatal examinations, prohibition of smoking in all areas of the prenatal care clinic, and financial incentives for not smoking or for cessation efforts. A recent randomized trial of smoking cessation methods also suggests that health education methods tailored to pregnant women are more effective in changing smoking behavior than standard smoking cessation techniques.[83]

Suggested Steps To Help Reduce Smoking Among Pregnant Women.*

1. At the first prenatal visit, cigarette smoke should be included in the list of drugs known to have adverse effects on the fetus, and to be avoided. It might be mentioned that cigarette smoke contains over 1000 "drugs," and is of special concern during pregnancy.

2. Physicians should consider direct measurement of their patients' smoking by obtaining a carboxyhemoglobin or expired carbon monoxide level during the first prenatal visit. The patient should be shown the results and told that levels of carboxyhemoglobin in the fetal blood will be increased similarly to her own, and that the risk posed to the fetus by high levels can be lowered only if she stops smoking. Repeat testing at each prenatal visit will serve to monitor cessation efforts, will help to motivate the patient, and will reinforce the physicians' advice.

3. Extra effort should be made with smoking women likely to be at particularly high risk of detrimental effects. These include: any women with previous history of perinatal loss, bleeding, or placental complications; women of older age or high parity; and especially women with anemia, bleeding, placental complications, or premature rupture of membranes during the current pregnancy.

4. Health facilities and physicians' offices should not permit smoking in any areas where staff and patients come in contact. Prominent "No Smoking" signs should be displayed in all patient areas, and abstinence enforced.

5. Physicians should obtain a list of reputable local smoking cessation clinics and provide this information to pregnant patients who smoke, with the suggestion that peer groups may help the patients to stop smoking.

6. Blue Cross, commercial insurers, and Medicaid should consider inclusion of coverage for approved smoking cessation activities in all subscriber contracts, especially for pregnant women. Insurers should be encouraged to charge lower premiums to individuals and families who will sign a certified affidavit that they are nonsmokers.

REFERENCES

1. U.S. Department of Health and Human Services. Health, United States, 1984. DHHS Publication No. 85-1232, pp.86–89.
2. U.S. Department of Health, Education and Welfare. The Health Consequences of Smoking for Women: A report of the Surgeon General, 1980. DHEW Publication No. 79-50069.
3. Johnston, L.D., O'Malley, P.M., and Bachman, J.G.: Use of Licit and Illicit Drugs by America's High School Students 1975–1984. National Institute on Drug Abuse, Washington, D.C., DHHS Publication No. (ADM) 85-1394, 1985. p.48.
4. Prager, K., Malin, H., Spiegler, D., et al.: Smoking and drinking behavior before and during pregnancy of married mothers of live-born infants and stillborn infants. Public Health Reports, *99*:117, 1984.
5. U.S. Department of Health, Education and Welfare. Smoking and Health: A Report of the Surgeon General, 1979. DHEW Publication No. 79-50066.
6. Abel, E.L.: Smoking during pregnancy: A review of effects on growth and development of offspring. Hum Biol, *52*:593, 1980.
7. Simpson, W.J.: A preliminary report on cigarette smoking and the incidence of prematurity. Am J Obstet Gynecol, *73*:808, 1957.
8. Meyer, M.B., Jonas, B.S., and Tonascia, J.A.: Perinatal events associated with maternal smoking during pregnancy. Am J Epidemiol, *103*:464, 1976.
9. Cnattingius, S., Axelsson, O., Eklund, G., et al.: Smoking, maternal age, and fetal growth. Obstet Gynecol, *66*:449, 1985.

*Based on recommendations by the Massachusetts Department of Health.[84]

10. Miller, H.C., Hassanein, K., and Hensleigh, P.A.: Fetal growth retardation in relation to maternal smoking and weight gain in pregnancy. Am J Obstet Gynecol, *125*:55, 1976.
11. D'Souza, S.W., Black, P., and Richards B.: Smoking in pregnancy: Associations with skinfold thickness, maternal weight gain, and fetal size at birth. Br Med J, *282*:1661, 1981.
12. Harrison, G.G., Branson, R.S., and Vaucher, Y.E.: Association of maternal smoking with body composition of the newborn. Am J Clin Nutr, *38*:757, 1983.
13. Persson, P.H., Grennert, L., Gennser, G., et al.: A study of smoking and pregnancy with special reference to fetal growth. Acta Obstet Gynecol Scand Suppl, *78*:33, 1978.
14. Murphy, J.F., Drumm, J.E., Mulcahy, R., et al.: The effect of maternal cigarette smoking on fetal birth weight and on growth of the fetal biparietal diameter. Br J Obstet Gynaecol, *87*:462, 1980.
15. Suzuki, K., Horiguchi, T., Comas-Urrutia, A.C., et al.: Pharmacologic effects of nicotine upon the fetus and mother in the rhesus monkey. Am J Obstet Gynecol, *111*:1092, 1971.
16. Wingred, J., Christianson, R., Lovitt, W.V, et al.: Placental ratio in white and black women: Relation to smoking and anemia. Am J Obstet Gynecol, *124*:671, 1976.
17. Fedrick, J., and Anderson, A.B.M.: Factors associated with spontaneous preterm birth. Br J Obstet Gynaecol, *83*:342, 1976.
18. Berkowitz, G.S., Holford, T.R.,, and Berkowitz, R.L.: Effects of cigarette smoking, alcohol, coffee and tea consumption on preterm delivery. Early Human Dev, *7*:239, 1982.
19. Shiono, P.H., Klebanoff, M.A., and Rhoads, G.G.: Smoking and drinking during pregnancy: Their effects on preterm birth. JAMA, *255*:82, 1986.
20. Meyer, M.B., and Tonascia, J.A.: Maternal smoking, pregnancy complications, and perinatal mortality. Am J Obstet Gynecol, *8*:494, 1977.
21. Andrews, J., and McGarry, J.M.: A community study of smoking in pregnancy. J Obstet Gynecol Br Commonw, *79*:1057, 1972.
22. Naeye, R.L.: Abruptio placentae and placenta previa: Frequency, perinatal mortality, and cigarette smoking. Obstet Gynecol, *55*:701, 1980.
23. Naeye, R.L.: Effects of maternal cigarette smoking on the fetus and placenta. Br J Obstet Gynaecol, *85*:732, 1978.
24. Meyer, M.B.: Smoking and pregnancy, in Drug Use in Pregnancy. Niebyl, J.R., (ed), Philadelphia: Lea & Febiger, 1982, pp.133–153.
25. Butler, N.R., and Alberman, E.D. (eds): Perinatal Problems. The Second Report of the 1958 British Perinatal Mortality Survey. London: E. and S. Livingstone, Ltd., 1969, pp.36–84.
26. Russell, C.S., Taylor, R., and Law, C.E.: Smoking in pregnancy, maternal blood pressure, pregnancy outcome, baby weight and growth, and other related factors. A prospective study. Br J Prev Soc Med, *22*:119, 1968.
27. Andrews, J.: Thiocyanate and smoking in pregnancy. Br J Obstet Gynaecol, *80*:810, 1973.
28. Pirani, B.B.K., and MacGillivray, I.: Smoking during pregnancy: Its effect on maternal metabolism and fetoplacental function. Obstet Gynecol, *52*:257, 1978.
29. Meyer, M.B., Tonascia, J.A., and Buck, C.: The interrelationship of maternal smoking and increased perinatal mortality with other risk factors. Further analysis of the Ontario perinatal mortality study, 1960–61. Am J Epidemiol, *100*:443, 1974.
30. Crosby, W.M., Metcoff, J., Costiloe, J.P., et al.: Fetal malnutrition: An appraisal of correlated factors. Am J Obstet Gynecol, *128*:22, 1977.
31. Goldenberg, R.L., Nelson, K.G., Koski, J.F., et al.: Low birth weight, intrauterine growth retardation, and preterm delivery. Am J Obstet Gynecol, *152*:980, 1985.
32. Goldstein, H.: Smoking in pregnancy: Some notes on the statistical controversy. Br J Prev Soc Med, *31*:13, 1977.
33. Kullander, S., and Kaellen, B.: A prospective study of smoking and pregnancy. Acta Obstet Gynecol Scand, *50*:83, 1971.
34. Alberman, E., Creasy, M., Elliott, M., et al.: Maternal factors associated with fetal chromosomal anomalies in spontaneous abortions. Br J Obstet Gynaecol, *83*:621, 1976.
35. Kline, J., Stein, Z., Susser, M. et al.: Environmental influences on early reproductive loss in a current New York City study, in Human Embryonic and Fetal Death. Porter, I.H., Hook, E.B. (eds), New York: Academic Press, 1980.
36. Harlap, S., and Shiono, P.: Alcohol, smoking and incidence of spontaneous abortions in the first and second trimester. Lancet, *2*:173, 1980.
37. Hemminki, K., Mutanen, P., and Saloniemi, I.: Smoking and the occurrence of congenital malformations and spontaneous abortions: Multivariate analysis. Am J Obstet Gynecol, *145*:61, 1983.
38. Naeye, R.L.: Relationship of cigarette smoking to congenital anomalies and perinatal death. Am J Pathol, *90*:289, 1978.
39. Fedrick, J., Alberman, E., and Goldstein, H.: Possible teratogenic effect of cigarette smoking. Nature, *231*:529, 1971.

40. Hook, E.B., and Cross, P.K.: Cigarette smoking and Down syndrome. Am J Hum Genet, *37*:1216, 1985.
41. Thaler, I., Goodman, J.D.S., and Dawes, G.S.: Effects of maternal cigarette smoking on fetal breathing and fetal movements. Am J Obstet Gynecol, *138*:282, 1980.
42. Goodman, J.D.S., Visser, F.G.A., and Dawes, G.S.: Effects of maternal cigarette smoking on fetal trunk movements, fetal breathing movements and the fetal heart rate. Br J Obstet Gynaecol, *91*:657, 1984.
43. Eriksen, P.S., Gennser, G., Lofgren, O., et al.: Acute effects of maternal smoking on fetal breathing and movements. Obstet Gynecol, *61*:367, 1983.
44. Manning, F.A., and Feyerabend, C.I.: Cigarette smoking and fetal breathing movements. Br J Obstet Gynaecol, *83*:262, 1976.
45. Garn, S.M., Johnston, M., Ridella, S.A., et al.: Effect of maternal cigarette smoking on Apgar scores. Am J Dis Child, *135*:503, 1981.
46. Hingson, R., Gould, J.B, Morelock, S., et al.: Maternal cigarette smoking, psychoactive substance use, and infant Apgar scores. Am J Obstet Gynecol, *144*:959, 1982.
47. Saxton, D.W.: The behavior of infants whose mothers smoke in pregnancy. Early Hum Dev, *2*:363, 1978.
48. Picone, T.A., Allen, L.H., Olsen, P.N., et al.: Pregnancy outcome in North American women. II. Effects of diet, cigarette smoking, stress, and weight gain on placentas, and on neonatal physical and behavioral characteristics. Am J Clin Nutr, *36*:1214, 1982.
49. Curet, L.B., Rao, A.V., Zachman, R.D., et al.: Maternal smoking and respiratory distress syndrome. Am J Obstet Gynecol, *147*:446, 1983.
50. White, E., Sky, K.K., Daling, J.R., et al.: Maternal smoking and infant respiratory distress syndrome. Obstet Gynecol, *67*:365, 1986.
51. Gluck, L., and Kulovich, M.V.: Lecithin/sphingomyelin ratios in amniotic fluid in normal and abnormal pregnancy. Am J Obstet Gynecol, *115*:539, 1973.
52. Andersen, A.N., Lund-Andersen, C., Larsen, J.F., et al.: Suppressed prolactin but normal neurophysin levels in cigarette smoking breast-feeding women. Clin Endocrinol, *17*:363, 1982.
53. Blake, C.A., and Sawyer, C.H.: Nicotine blocks the suckling-induced rise in circulating prolactin in lactating rats. Science, *177*:619, 1972.
54. Harlap, S., and Davies, A.M.: Infant admissions to hospital and maternal smoking. Lancet, *1*:527, 1974.
55. Rantakallio, P.: The effect of maternal smoking on birth weight and the subsequent health of the child. Early Hum Dev, *2*:371, 1978.
56. Rantakallio, P.: A follow-up study up to the age of 14 of children whose mothers smoked during pregnancy. Acta Paediatr Scand, *72*:747, 1983.
57. Bergman, A.B., and Wiesner, L.A.: Relationship of passive cigarette-smoking to sudden infant death syndrome. Pediatrics, *58*:665, 1976.
58. Neutel, C.I., and Buck, C.: Effect of smoking during pregnancy on the risk of cancer in children. J Natl Cancer Inst, *47*:59, 1971.
59. Manning, M.D., and Carroll, B.E.: Some epidemiologic aspects of leukemia in children. J Natl Cancer Inst, *19*:1087, 1957.
60. Van Stensel-Moll, H., Valkenburg, H.A., Vandenbroucke, J.P., et al.: Are maternal fertility problems related to childhood leukaemia? Int J Epidemiol, *14*:555, 1985.
61. Sandler, D.P., Everson, R.B., Wilcox, A.J., et al.: Cancer risk in adulthood from early life exposure to parents' smoking. Am J Publ Health, *75*:487, 1985.
62. Stjernfeldt, M., Berglund, K., Lindsten, J., et al.: Maternal smoking during pregnancy and risk of childhood cancer. Lancet, *1*:1350, 1986.
63. Butler, N.R., and Goldstein, H.: Smoking in pregnancy and subsequent child development. Br Med J, *4*:573, 1973.
64. Dunn, H.G., McBurney, A.K., Ingram, S., et al.: Maternal cigarette smoking during pregnancy and the child's subsequent development. II. Neurological and intellectual maturation to the age of 6½ years. Can J Pub Health, *68*:43, 1977.
65. Naeye, R.L., and Peters, E.C.: Mental development of children whose mothers smoked during pregnancy. Obstet Gynecol, *64*:601, 1984.
66. Hardy, J.B., and Mellits, E.D.: Does maternal smoking during pregnancy have a long-term effect on the child? Lancet, *2*:1332, 1972.
67. Denson, R., Nanson, J.L., and McWatters, M.A.: Hyperkinesis and maternal smoking. Can Psychiatr Assoc J, *20*:183, 1975.
68. Heron, H.J.: The effects of smoking during pregnancy: A review with a preview, NZ Med J, *61*:545, 1962.
69. Longo, L.D.: The biological effects of carbon monoxide on the pregnant woman, fetus, and newborn infant. Am J Obstet Gynecol, *129*:69, 1977.
70. Longo, L.: Some health consequences of maternal smoking: Issues without answers. Birth Defects, *18*:13, 1982.

71. Quigley, M.E., Sheehan, K.L., Wilkes, M.M., et al.: Effects of maternal smoking on circulating catecholamine levels and fetal heart rates. Am J Obstet Gynecol, *133*:685, 1979.
72. Lehtovirta, P., and Forss, M.: The acute effect of smoking on intervillous blood flow of the placenta. Br J Obstet Gynaecol, *85*:729, 1978.
73. Philipp, K., Patersky, N., and Endler, M.: Effects of smoking on uteroplacental blood flow. Gynecol Obstet Invest, *17*:179, 1984.
74. Resnik, R., Brink, G.W., and Wilkes, M.M.: Catecholamine-mediated reduction in uterine blood flow after nicotine infusion in the pregnant ewe. J Clin Invest, *63*:1113, 1979.
75. Suzuki, K., Minel, L.J., and Johnson, E.E.: Effect of nicotine upon uterine blood flow in the pregnant rhesus monkey. Am J Obstet Gynecol, *136*:1009, 1980.
76. Suzuki, K., Horiguchi, T., Comas-Urrutia, A.C., et al.: Placental transfer and distribution of nicotine in the pregnant rhesus monkey. Am J Obstet Gynecol, *119*:253, 1974.
77. Pettigrew, A.R., Logan R.W., and Willocks, J.: Smoking in pregnancy—Effects on birth weight and on cyanide and thiocyanate levels in mother and baby. Br J Obstet Gynaecol, *84*:31, 1977.
78. Roels, H., Hubermont, G., Buchet, J.P., et al.: Placental transfer of lead, mercury, cadmium and carbon monoxide in women: III. Factors influencing the accumulation of heavy metals in the placenta and the relationship between metal concentration in the placenta and in maternal and cord blood. Environ Res, *16*:236, 1978.
79. Van der Velde, W.J., Copius Peereboom-Stegeman, J.H.J., Treffers, P.E., et al.: Structural changes in the placenta of smoking mothers: A quantitative study. Placenta, *4*:231, 1983.
80. Christianson, R.E.: Gross differences observed in the placentas of smokers and nonsmokers. Am J Epidemiol, *110*:178, 1979.
81. Asmussen, I.: Ultrastructure of the villi and fetal capillaries in placentas from smoking and non-smoking mothers. Br J Obstet Gynaecol, *87*:239, 1980.
82. Bureau, M.A., Shapcott, D., Berthiaume, Y., et al.: Maternal cigarette smoking and fetal oxygen transport: A study of P50, 2-3-diphosphosphoglycerate, total hemoglobin, hematocrit, and type F hemoglobin in fetal blood. Pediatrics, *72*:22, 1983.
83. Windsor, R.A., Cutter, G., Morris, J., et al.: The effectiveness of smoking cessation methods for smokers in public health maternity clinics: A randomized trial. Am J Public Health, *75*:1389, 1985.
84. Fielding, J.E.: Smoking and pregnancy. N Engl J Med, *298*:337, 1976.

Chapter 15

*Alcohol Use in Pregnancy**

Ernest L. Abel and Robert J. Sokol

Alcohol is now recognized as the leading known teratogen in the western world. Although the total impact of exposure to alcohol during pregancy has yet to be fully determined, it is known that the incidence of fetal alcohol syndrome (FAS), one of the major consequences of drinking during pregnancy, is about 2.2/1000 live births in the United States and 1.9/1000 live births worldwide.[1] The number of children born with alcohol-related birth defects is unknown, but undoubtedly far exceeds this number. This chapter will summarize some of the relevant information concerning FAS alcohol-related birth defects, identification of at-risk pregnancies and the potential for prevention of abnormal pregnancy outcomes related to prenatal exposure to alcohol.

HISTORIC BACKGROUND

One of the earliest scientific studies documenting alcohol's adverse effects on pregnancy outcome was reported in 1899 by an English physician, Dr. William Sullivan.[2] Sullivan was a physician in a Liverpool jail for women where he conducted a case-control study of 120 alcoholic women prisoners and their non-drinking female relatives. Sullivan found that infant mortality and stillbirth rates for the alcoholic's children were 2.5 times higher than rates among their non-drinking relatives. He also found that women who entered prison early in their pregnancy had a more favorable pregnancy outcome than alcoholic women who entered later in pregnancy. Presumably, this was because the women who entered earlier had less opportunity to drink during pregnancy. Although this was a rather dramatic finding, little attention was paid to the effects of drinking during pregnancy until 1973 when Jones and Smith described a pattern of malformations in children born to alcoholic women.[3,4] These publications focused international interest on a set of birth defects whose causal agent, alcohol, was widely used throughout the world and was previously unsuspected of having any damaging effects on the unborn child.

CRITERIA FOR FETAL ALCOHOL SYNDROME

Alcohol is now recognized as a teratogen capable of producing a wide spectrum of defects ranging from spontaneous abortion at one extreme to subtle behavioral effects in the absence of physical anomalies at the other. FAS refers to a pattern of such defects occurring in children born to alcoholic women.

In 1980, the Fetal Alcohol Study Group of the Research Society on Alcoholism proposed strict criteria for diagnosis of FAS.[5] These criteria stated that at least

*Supported in part by grants NIAAA #AA05631, DA06334-1 and NIAAA DAO6571.

one characteristic from each of the following three categories had to be present for a valid diagnosis of the syndrome:
1. Growth retardation before and/or after birth;
2. Facial anomalies including small palpebral fissures, indistinct or absent philtrum, epicanthic folds, flattened nasal bridge, short length of nose, thin upper lip, low set, unparallel ears, and retarded mid-facial development;
3. Central nervous system dysfunction including microcephaly, varying degrees of mental retardation or other evidence of abnormal neurobehavioral development, such as attention deficit disorder with hyperactivity.

None of these features is individually pathognomonic for fetal alcohol exposure, making diagnosis difficult. Instead, these individual anomalies are nonspecific and may be seen even in the absence of maternal drinking. However, when the pattern of abnormalities is present, a reasonable diagnosis of FAS may be made. Confirmatory clinical evidence for this diagnosis would include a history of heavy maternal drinking during pregnancy.

Alcohol-related birth defects are even less specific than FAS. In addition to individual features of the syndrome, such defects include cardiac abnormalities, including atrial and ventricular septal defects, and genitourinary abnormalities such as hydronephrosis and hypospadias. Clinical recognition of such abnormalities is often not difficult, but attributing their presence in the neonate to prenatal exposure to alcohol is considerably less certain.

PREVALENCE

Most of the identified cases of FAS in the United States come from study areas where a majority of the mothers were black or Indian, and their socioeconomic status was low. In such areas, the rate has varied from 0.4 to 19.5 per 1000 live births.[6–10] The overall rate from these sites is 2.6/1000 live births. In contrast to these estimates, the estimated incidence from study sites where women were mainly white and of middle socioeconomic status (e.g. Denver, Loma Linda, and Seattle) has ranged from 0 to 1.3/1000.[11–14] The overall rate from these sites is 0.6/1000.

The highest frequency of FAS (19.5/1000) has been noted among women of the Apache and the Ute tribes of the American Southwest.[10] These Indian tribes seem to be at especially high risk for FAS. It is unclear if this is related to a high frequency of abusive drinking among women of these tribes and/or to some type of so far undefined genetic susceptibility.

The overall rate in North America is 2.2/1000,[6–15] compared to a slightly lower rate of 1.8/1000 in Europe and other countries.[16–24] Reasons for these differences between North America and other countries may be (1) difficulty in ascertainment of FAS because the facial features are not easily recognized; (2) a true difference in the frequency of FAS in these different areas; and/or (3) a higher survivability of children in North America so that when studies are done of children after birth, more are available for inclusion compared to studies in other countries where less advanced neonatal medical support is available.

The overall worldwide rate of FAS is 1.9/1000. In 1984, 3,697,000 children were born in the United States. Using this rate of 1.9 cases/1000 births, this would put the number of children born with FAS in 1984 in the United States at 7,024.

About 60% of American women drink to some extent and about 3 to 4% drink at abusive levels.[25] The estimated incidence of pregnancies resulting in FAS offspring among women identified as problem drinkers or alcohol abusers is considerably higher than among the general population, and ranges from 24/1000 to 259/1000.[7,8,12,26–31] The overall incidence of FAS pregnancies among these women is 59/1000.

Although the causes of the large majority of birth defects still remain to be determined, based on the prevalence of alcohol abuse in pregnant women and the relative risks now identified for alcohol, we have estimated that about 5% of all congenital anomalies may be due to prenatal alcohol exposure.[32] This implies that a significant proportion of previously unaccounted for anomalies may be related to prenatal alcohol exposure and such exposure may in fact be a major contributor to abnormal fetal development.

ECONOMIC IMPACT

There is no evidence that drinking at abusive levels by women has decreased[33] and no evidence that the incidence of FAS has decreased since its original recognition in 1973. The high prevalence of FAS is noteworthy not only because of its impact on the individual and society, but also because of its economic impact. We have recently estimated the annual cost of treatment for individuals with FAS in the USA at $321,000,000 per year.[1] Based on annual costs for 24-hour residential care, the annual economic impact of FAS is greater than that for Down Syndrome.[1] Mental retardation related to prenatal alcohol exposure may, in fact, account for as much as 11% of the annual cost for all mentally retarded institutionalized residents in the United States.

SPECIFIC ADVERSE OUTCOMES OF DRINKING DURING PREGNANCY

Spontaneous Abortion

The risk for spontaneous abortion is increased approximately two-fold by maternal drinking during pregnancy,[34,35] although this increase is possibly due to 3 to 5% of the heaviest drinking women.[6,36] Pregnant monkeys also tend to abort early in pregnancy following alcohol exposure.[37] Rodents likewise have increased rates of resorption (the analog of spontaneous abortion) following maternal alcohol exposure.[38] Our recent study[39] showed that there may be synergism between alcohol and other drugs (e.g. marijuana), so that at doses of either drug that individually do not significantly increase the spontaneous abortion rate, when combined, this rate is increased above what might be expected from the additive effects of these drugs. This has not yet been confirmed in the human.

Stillbirth

Studies of stillbirth rate after prenatal alcohol exposure are equivocal. In an early study from Cleveland, Ohio,[26] we did not observe any significant increase in the stillbirth rate. In France, an early study reported an increase in the stillbirth rate following drinking during pregnancy, but this was not corroborated in the second study.[40–41] Recently, we studied pregnancy losses from a sample of over 8,000 pregnancies, and have been able to identify a signfican relationship between heavy embryonic alcohol exposure later in pregnancy and stillbirth.[7] It was hypothesized that damage to the embryo may have been insufficient to lead to spontaneous abortion, but severe enough to produce later stillbirth.

Physical Anomalies

FAS is usually diagnosed on the basis of morphologic anomalies and growth deficiency. To the experienced dysmorphologist, the facial features described above are easily recognized. These craniofacial anomalies can be reproduced in animal studies.[42] In fact, nearly all the congenital anomalies associated with FAS have now been duplicated in various animal models.[43] As noted above, other physical anomalies include heart and kidney defects, urogenital anomalies, and limb and joint disorders.

Lowered Birth Weight

Decreased birth weight is the most reliable effect of prenatal alcohol exposure in both humans and animals. We reviewed more than 300 reported cases of FAS and found the average birth weight of such children to be about 2000 g[44] compared to a median birth weight for all infants in the United States of about 3300 g.[45] The high incidence of children with birth weights below 2500 g is of concern since low birth weight is a marker for significant increases in risk for infant mortality and morbidity. Children with low birth weights often require intensive care immediately after birth and repeated hospitalization for continued failure to thrive. We recently estimated the annual cost associated with FAS-related intrauterine growth retardation in the United States at approximately $118,000,000.[1]

CNS Dysfunction

FAS is now the leading known cause of mental retardation in the western world. It exceeds the incidence of Down Syndrome and cerebral palsy.[1] In general, the extent of mental retardation is positively related to severity of dysmorphogenesis.[33,46]

Although other anomalies can be treated surgically, the anomalies associated with brain damage, such as mental retardation, are untreatable and irreversible. The average IQ scores for patients with FAS is about 65.[33]

Children prenatally exposed to alcohol may also be physically unremarkable, but still have behavioral disorders. For example, Majewski[46] found that two-thirds of the 95 alcohol-exposed children he encountered were "hyperactive." In the United States, Shaywitz[47] found that of 82 children brought to their attention because of learning problems, 15 were hyperactive and had physical features compatible with FAS or had mothers who were known to be alcoholic during pregnancy. Significant difficulties with perceptual problems, e.g. eye-hand coordination and visual form perception, have also been noted.[48]

Speech and language problems seem especially common among children with FAS.[30,33,47–50] Iosub et al.[49] reported that 3 of 63 children with FAS whom they encountered had hearing impairments. More recently, Church et al.[51] reported that 90% of the 12 FAS children they examined had hearing losses requiring hearing aids. Serous otitis media was also a common occurrence among these children, and myringotomy was required to treat the problem. Larsson et al.[30]

reported an incidence of 40 to 46% of speech disorders in children born to alcohol abusers, compared to a 15% incidence in children born to social drinkers.

Abnormal Neuronal Development

Microcephaly is a common feature associated with FAS and is probably a result of an overall decrease in brain growth. Autopsy studies of children born to alcoholic women have shown gross neural pathologic conditions including abnormal growth patterns and migration of neural cells and absence of corpus callosum.[52,53] Studies in animals have shown that subtle changes may occur in brain structure which are compatible with life and which presumably underlie many of the behavioral anomalies observed in connection with prenatal alcohol exposure.

The hippocampus appears to be a particularly vulnerable area for such anomalies. Studies in animals, for example, have shown that mossy fibers which carry neural impulses from the dentate gyrus of the hippocampus terminate in areas of the hippocampus in which they do not normally end.[54] Other studies have shown decreases in specific cells in the hippocampus,[55] and dendrite structure may also be abnormal in this area.[56]

Brain electrical activity is also abnormally affected in children with FAS. Havlicek et al.[57] and Chernick et al.[58] have observed abnormally high amplitude EEGs during various sleep states in these children.

SOCIAL DRINKING

Reports of the effects of social drinking during pregnancy are considerably more difficult to evaluate than reports of heavy prenatal exposure. As noted above, although spontaneous abortion rates have been reported to be increased among social drinkers,[6,34,35] we question whether the women in these studies were, in fact, social drinkers. Difficulties associated with evaluating reports concerning the effects of social drinking include the many different ways drinking histories are taken. What is documented in such studies is reported drinking, not actual drinking. Self reports may underestimate actual drinking considerably. Recommendations regarding risk identification and clinical instrumentation are included in a later section of this chapter.

NEED FOR FURTHER RESEARCH

More studies need to be focused on the effects of moderate and low doses of alcohol. More information is also needed concerning alcohol abuse and dependence among young women, especially information about the development of abusive drinking. Better descriptions of drinking before or during pregnancy would enable researchers to estimate the risks of moderate drinking with respect to outcome.

There is no longer any doubt that alcohol is a teratogen. It would seem that eliminating this teratogen would be a relatively simple matter, but alcohol abuse has been an intractable problem. To be effective, prevention will require improved methods of identification and treatment of pregnant women with alcohol problems.[59,60] Considerably more needs to be determined regarding the mechanisms for alcohol's teratogenicity and maternal risk factors for teratogenicity.[7] Thresholds for various alcohol-related effects need to be determined. Studies in animals will undoubtedly be of value for determining both mechanisms and thresholds; however, ultimately determination of thresholds for specific adverse outcomes will have to come from clinical studies.

There have been considerable efforts by federal, state, and local agencies to alert the public concerning the dangers of drinking during pregnancy. The National Institute on Alcohol Abuse and Alcoholism published "Alcohol and Your Unborn Baby,"[61] and the Surgeon General's Advisory Committee on Alcohol and Pregnancy produced a report.[62] These messages appear to have had little impact on the drinking behavior of abusive drinkers or on the frequency of FAS. For example, Little et al.[63] found that three-quarters of the people they interviewed thought that abstinence during pregnancy was not necessary and that an average of about 3 drinks per day was a safe level of drinking. Such findings suggest that public education and prevention programs have not had their intended impact. An alternative is involvement of professional education and intervention originating in the physician's office.[60] This represents an opportunity to focus on early identification and counseling.

CLINICAL RISK IDENTIFICATION

Just as the physician does with respect to other habits, e.g. smoking and marijuana use, one should obtain an alcohol history for all reproductive age women as part of the routine Ob/Gyn history. From both the medical and medicolegal perspectives, it is a good idea to document this history in the medical record.

Both alcohol abuse and alcohol dependence are marked by psychologic denial of alcohol problems by the patient. Identifying women whose drinking is placing their fetuses at risk is difficult. If the clinician merely asks the patient how much she drinks, denial will be triggered leading to under-identification of risks and underestimation of fetal alcohol exposure. Rather than focusing on volume and frequency of intake, the clinician should look for evidence of *tolerance*. From the late teenage years to the early 30s, the large majority of women seldom drink more than twice a week. When these young women do drink, they seldom consume over 3 drinks. Moreover, most women begin to feel "high" after drinking 2 to 3 drinks. The type of alcoholic beverage is not critical from the perspective of exposure of the fetus—a glass of wine, a can of beer, and a mixed drink have the same amount of absolute alcohol in them, viz., ½ oz. Wine drinking does not rule out the development of a drinking problem.

From the clinical perspective, if a woman drinks more frequently than twice a week or typically drinks more than 2 to 3 drinks per occasion, and/or in particular, if she does not feel "high" after 2 to 3 drinks, she may be developing an alcohol problem. In such circumstances, her drinking behavior deserves further investigation.

ADVICE TO PATIENTS

A large majority of women seen in clinical practice will not be problem drinkers. Based on our current state of knowledge, patients can be offered the following advice:

1. If a patient is seen prior to pregnancy, a physician can suggest that limiting her drinking or completely quitting is reasonable when pregnancy is planned. The concept here is similar to that for women with diabetes

mellitus for whom attaining euglycemia prior to conception may decrease the risk of birth defects.

2. Regardless of when a patient is seen during pregnancy, it is reasonable to inform her that limited drinking or abstinence can help her have a healthier baby. Minimally, she should limit her drinking, and certainly she should not get "drunk." If the patient has had an occasional drink before pregnancy was diagnosed, it is unlikely that this will constitute a significant risk to the fetus and it should not be a major concern to the patient. On the other hand, if the patient is a problem drinker, different advice is warranted.

3. Women with chronic alcohol problems who continue to drink heavily during pregnancy may have a high enough rate of abnormal pregnancy outcome to warrant consideration of therapeutic abortion. However, even among heavy-drinking women, only a limited proportion will have infants with full FAS. There is also good evidence that abusive drinkers who are able to stop prior to the third trimester can have normal-appearing infants even if they drank heavily early in pregnancy. Therapeutic abortion is clearly not warranted in every case. Nonetheless, considering the psychosocial disruption often surrounding the lives of alcohol abusers, the option for abortion may be considered.

During pregnancy, women are motivated to improve their health practices. It is often therapeutic just to ask the patient about her alcohol use. Many gravidas, including those who drink heavily, become abstinent during pregnancy. If the physician indicates a concern about drinking, this tendency can be maximized. Clinical experience indicates that many pregnant women who abuse alcohol report that it is easier to decrease or stop drinking during pregnancy than to decrease or stop cigarette smoking.

MANAGEMENT GUIDELINES

With regard to antenatal management, it is crucial that the clinician maintain contact with the problem drinker. At each antenatal visit, the patient should be asked how well she is controlling her drinking. The clinician must maintain a non-judgmental supportive attitude and provide repeated and continued encouragement to maintain abstinence, or at least, to minimize drinking episodes. If, despite such an approach, the patient continues to drink heavily, consultation with an alcohol rehabilitation unit or referral to Alcoholics Anonymous can be helpful. Clinical experience indicates that it is difficult to motivate these patients to see professionals other than the primary physician so that the major responsibility for antenatal care and for attaining abstinence remains with the obstetrician/gynecologist.

We have found that alcohol-abusing women tended to have antepartum admissions related to the development of pneumonia and pancreatitis.[26] There is an increased risk for intrauterine growth retardation and possibly abruptio placentae, as well as premature rupture of the membranes. These pregnancies should thus be considered at increased maternal/fetal risk. A protocol of increased frequency of antenatal visits as well as antepartum fetal monitoring is warranted.

The neonate may show signs of early neonatal depression. If the mother has taken high doses of alcohol just prior to the onset of labor, she may have a high circulating blood alcohol level (which can be measured in cord blood) and may well have a tendency toward acidosis. Determining cord blood pH and base excess may be warranted. In the nursery, these infants may show signs of jitteriness, but severe withdrawal symptomatology is usually not observed.

For women with major alcohol problems, the impact of a new infant should be carefully assessed. Even among women who are able to attain abstinence or near abstinence during pregnancy, heavy drinking may resume postpartum. The impact of a disrupted lifestyle on the ability of the mother to care for her infant should definitely be considered. Clinical experience indicates that infants of alcoholic mothers often require placement outside the home. Adding to the problem of care of the neonate is the impact of prenatal alcohol exposure on infant behavior. Sleep state regulation may be disrupted, and attention deficit syndrome with hyperactivity may also develop. Dealing with a difficult infant or child may lead to life stress for the alcohol-abusing woman. Such stress could further impact adversely on the development of the child.

RECOMMENDATIONS

Although a wide range of specific alcohol-related outcomes has been identified, considerably more research is needed to identify possible susceptibility factors, relationship to morbidity, and longevity and transgenerational effects. Thresholds for specific alcohol-related defects need to be defined, so that the frequently asked question about safe levels of drinking, the answer to which is currently unknown, can be addressed.

Public education efforts have been successful in alerting most Americans to the dangers of drinking during pregnancy. However, awareness of such dangers does not seem to have been translated into changes in behavior. Alternatively, more emphasis on professional education including improvement in methods for detection of abusive drinking and treatment methods are needed. Education based on a firm scientific foundation will undoubtedly result in a better understanding of alcohol's impact on the embryo/fetus and how this impact may be reduced.

Based on what is currently known about alcohol as a teratogen, clinicians should attempt to obtain an alcohol history from all reproductive age women. Focusing on tolerance to the effects of alcohol is a clinically useful technique. Pregnant alcohol-abusing women and their fetuses deserve intense antepartum/intrapartum and neonatal monitoring and care. The impact of maternal problem drinking on development of the infant may require long term medical follow-up.

Alcohol appears to affect all developing systems, but the most serious consequence of drinking during pregnancy is brain damage as reflected in mental retardation. FAS will undoubtedly continue to be a major societal problem with major economic implications.

REFERENCES

1. Abel, E.L. and Sokol, R.J.: Incidence of fetal alcohol syndrome and economic impact of FAS-related anomalies. Drug and Alcohol Dependence, in press.
2. Sullivan, W.C.: A note on the influence of maternal inebriety on the offspring. J Ment Sci 45:489, 1899.

3. Jones, K.L., and Smith, D.W.: Recognition of the fetal alcohol syndrome in early infancy. Lancet 2:999, 1973.
4. Jones, K.L., Smith, D.W., Streissguth, A.P. et al.: Patterns of malformation in offspring of chronic alcoholic women. Lancet 1:1267, 1973.
5. Rosett, H.L.: A clinical perspective of the fetal alcohol syndrome. Alcoholism: Clin Exp Res 4:119, 1980.
6. Sokol, R.J.: Alcohol and spontaneous abortion. Lancet 2: 1079, 1980.
7. Sokol, R.J., Ager, J., Martier, S., et al.: Significant determinants of susceptibility to alcohol teratogenicity. NY Acad Sci: 1986, in press.
8. Ouellette, E.M., Rosett, H.L., Rosman, N.P., et al.: Adverse effects on offspring of maternal alcohol abuse during pregnancy. N Engl J Med 297:528, 1977.
9. Hingson, R., Alpert, J.J., Day, N., et al.: Effects of maternal drinking and marijuana use on fetal growth and development. Pediatr 70:539, 1982.
10. May, P.A., Hymbaugh, K.J., Aase, J.M. et al.: Epidemiology of fetal alcohol syndrome among American Indians of the Southwest. Soc Biol 30:374, 1983.
11. Kuzma, J.W., and Sokol, R.J.: Maternal drinking behavior and decreased intrauterine growth, Alcoholism: Clin Exp Res 6:396, 1982.
12. Hanson, J.W., Streissguth, A.P., and Smith, D.W.: The effects of moderate alcohol consumption during pregnancy on fetal growth and morphogenesis. J Pediatr 92:457, 1978.
13. Little, R.E.: Moderate alcohol use during pregnancy and decreased infant birth weight. Am J Pub Health 67:1154, 1977.
14. Tennes, K., and Blackard, C.: Maternal alcohol consumption, birth weight, and minor physical anomalies. Am J Obstet Gynecol 138:774, 1980.
15. Fried, P.A.: Alcohol and the newborn infant. In: Toxicology and the Newborn, eds S. Kacew and M.J. Reasor. Elsevier Science Publishers B.V. 1984, pp. 87–100.
16. Gibson, G.T., Baghurst, P.A. and Colley, D.P.: Maternal alcohol, tobacco, and cannabis consumption and the outcome of pregnancy. Aust N Zeal J Obstet Gynecol 23:15, 1983.
17. Yla-Outinen, A. and Tuimala, R.:The effect of moderate alcohol consumption during pregnancy on the birth weight and early outcome of the infant. Upsala J. Med Sci (suppl) 37:64, 1983.
18. Dehaene, P.H., Samaille-Villette, C.H., Samaille, P.P. et al.: Le syndrome d'alcoolisme foetal dans le nord de la France. (The fetal alcohol syndrome in the north of France.) Rev Alcool 23:145, 1977.
19. Dehaene, P., Crepin, G., Delahousse, G., et al.: Aspects epidemiologiques du syndrome d'alcoolisme foetal. Nouv Press Med 10:2639, 1981.
20. Olegard, R., Sabel, K.G., Aronsson, M., et al.: Effects on the child of alcohol abuse during pregnancy. Acta Paediat Scand Suppl 275:112, 1979.
21. Larsson, G., Ottenblad, C., Hagenfeldt, L., et al.: Evaluation of serum gamma-glutamyl transferase as a screening method for excessive alcohol consumption during pregnancy. Am J Obstet Gynecol 177:654, 1983.
22. Halperin, D.S., Assimacopoulos, A., Lacourt, G., et al.: Gamma-glutamyl transferase serique maternelle et depistage prenatal du syndrome de l'alcoolism foetal. Helv Paediat Acta 40:183, 1985.
23. Fricker, H.S., Burgi, W., Kaufmann, H., et al.: Schwangerschaftsverlauf in einem reprasentativen Schweizer Kolletiv (Aarauer Schwangerschafts-und Neurgeborenenstudie. II Genussmitdtel in der Schwangerschaft. Schweiz Med Wschr 115:381, 1985.
24. Wright, J.T., Barrison, I.G., Lewis, I.G. et al.: Alcohol consumption, pregnancy, and low birth weight. Lancet 1:663, 1983.
25. Noble, E.P. (ed): Alcohol and Health, Third Special Report to the U.S. Congress. U.S. Government Printing Office, Washington, D.C., 1978.
26. Sokol, R.J., Miller, S.I., and Reed, G.: Alcohol abuse during pregnancy: an epidemiologic study. Alcoholism: Clin Exp Res 4:135, 1980.
27. Seidenberg, J., and Majewski, F.: Zur Haufigkeit der alkoholembryopathie in den verschiedenen Phasen der mutterlichen alkoholkrankheit. (On the frequency of alcohol embryopathy in the different phases of maternal alcoholism.) Suchtgefahren 24:63, 1978.
28. Halliday, H.L., MacReid, M,., and McClure, G.: Results of heavy drinking in pregnancy. Br J Obstet Gynaecol 89:892, 1982.
29. Vitez, M., Koranyi, G., Gonczy, E., et al.: A semiquantitative score system for epidemiologic studies of fetal alcohol syndrome. Am J Epidemiol 119:301, 1984.
30. Larsson, G., Bolin, A.B. and Tunell, R.: Prospective study of children exposed to variable amounts of alcohol in utero. Arch Dis Child 60:316, 1985.
31. Aronson, M.: Children of Alcoholic Mothers. Goteborg, Sweden, University of Goteborg, 1984, p. 8.
32. Sokol, R.J.: Alcohol and abnormal outcomes of pregnancy. Can Med Assoc J 125:143, 1981.
33. Streissguth, A.P., Herman, C.S. and Smith, D.W.: Intelligence, behavior and dysmorphogenesis in the fetal alcohol syndrome: a report on 20 clinical cases. J Pediatr 92:363, 1978.

34. Harlap, S. and Shiono, P.H.: Alcohol, smoking, and incidence of spontaneous abortions in the first and second trimester. Lancet 2:173, 1980.
35. Kline, J., Shrout, P., Stein, Z., et al.: Drinking during pregnancy and spontaneous abortion. Lancet 2:176, 1980.
36. Sokol, R.J.: Alcohol and spontaneous abortion (letter to the editor). Lancet 2:1079, 1980.
37. Altshuler, H.L. and Shippenberg, T.S.: A subhuman primate model for fetal alcohol syndrome research. Neurobehav Toxicol & Teratol 3:121, 1981.
38. Randall, C.L., Taylor, W.J., and Walker, D.W.: Ethanol-induced malformations in mice. Alcoholism: Clin Exp Res 1:219, 1977.
39. Abel, E.L.: Fetal Alcohol Exposure and Effects. Westport, Conn., Greenwood Press, 1985.
40. Kaminski, M., Ruimeau-Rouquette, C., and Schwartz, D.: Alcohol consumption in pregnant women and the outcome of pregnancy. Alcoholism: Clin Exp Res 2:155, 1978.
41. Kaminski, M., Franc, M., Lebouvier, M., et al: Moderate alcohol use and pregnancy outcome. Neurobehav Toxicol Teratol 3:173, 1981.
42. Sulik, K.K., Johnston, M.C., and Webb, M.A.: Fetal alcohol syndrome: embryogenesis on a mouse model. Science 214:936, 1981.
43. Abel, E.L.: Fetal Alcohol Syndrome and Fetal Alcohol Effects, New York, Plenum Press, 1984.
44. Abel, E.L.: Marihuana, Tobacco, Alcohol and Reproduction. Boca Raton, FL, CRC Press, 1983.
45. US Department of Health and Human Services: Monthly vital statistics report: annual summary for the Untied States, 1979. Hyattsville, MD, National Center for Health Statistics, 1980.
46. Majewski, F.: Uber schadigende einflusse des alkohols aux die nachkommenen. Nervenarzt 49:410, 1978.
47. Shaywitz, S.E. Cohen, D.J., and Shaywitz, B.A.: Behavior and learning difficulties in children of normal intelligence born to alcoholic mothers. J Pediatr 96:978, 1980.
48. Aronson, M., Kyllerman, M., Sabel, K.G., et al.: Children of alcoholic mothers. Development, perceptual and behavioral characteristics as compared to matched controls. Acta Paediat Scand 74:27, 1985.
49. Iosub, S., Fuchs, M., Bingol, N., et al.: Fetal alcohol syndrome revisited. Paediatrie 68:475, 1981.
50. Sparks, S.N.: Speech and language in fetal alcohol syndrome. ASHA 26:27, 1984.
51. Church, M.W. and Gerkin, K.P.: Hearing disorders in children with fetal alcohol syndrome: findings from case reports. Submitted for publication.
52. Clarren, S.K., and Smith, D.W.: The fetal alcohol syndrome. N Engl J Med 298:1063, 1978.
53. Peiffer, J., Majewski, F. Fischbach, H., et al: Alcohol embryo-and fetopathy: neuropathology of three children and three fetuses. J Neurol Sci (Amsterdam) 41:125, 1979.
54. West, J.R., Hodges, C.A., and Black, A.C., Jr. Prenatal exposure to ethanol alters the organization of hippocampal mossy fibers in rats. Science 211:957, 1981.
55. Barnes, D.E., and Walker, D.W.: Prenatal ethanol exposure permanently reduces the number of pyramidal neurons in rat hippocampus. Dev Brain Res 1:3, 1981.
56. Abel, E.L., Jacobson, S. and Sherwin, B.T.: In utero alcohol exposure: functional and structural brain damage. Neurobehav Toxicol Teratol 5:363, 1983.
57. Havlicek, V., Childiaeva, R., and Chernick, V.: EEG frequency spectrum characteristics of sleep rates in infants of alcoholic mothers. Neuropaediatrie 8:360, 1977.
58. Chernick, V., Childiaeva, R., and Isoffe, S.: Effects of maternal alcohol intake and smoking on neonatal electroencephalogram and anthropometric measurements. Am J Obstet Gynecol 146:41, 1983.
59. Rosett, H.L., Weiner, L. and Edelin, K.C.: Strategies for prevention of fetal alcohol effects. Obstet Gynecol 57:1, 1981.
60. Sokol, R.J., Miller, S.I., and Martier, S.: Preventing fetal alcohol effects: a practical guide for ob/gyn physicians and nurses. NIAAA National Clearinghouse for Alcohol Information. Rockville, Md., 1981.
61. National Institute on Alcohol Abuse and Alcoholism. *Alcohol and Your Unborn Baby.* Dept. Health and Human Services, 1982.
62. Surgeon General's Advisory Committee on Alcohol and Pregnancy Report. FDA Drug Bulletin 11:9, 1981.
63. Little, R.E., Grathwohl, H.L., Streissguth, A.P., et al.: Public awareness and knowledge about the risks of drinking during pregnancy in Multnomah County, Oregon. Am J Pub Health 71:312, 1981.

Chapter 16

Narcotic Addiction in Pregnancy

Loretta P. Finnegan and Ronald J. Wapner

The epidemic of psychotropic drug use continues to escalate. In addition to adolescents experimenting with drugs and individuals with chronic heroin dependence, large numbers of emotionally distraught individuals use psychotropic medications which are procured through licit as well as illicit sources. A general complacency exists with regard to licit psychotropic medications. Moderate utilization of these agents is rarely feared and is often believed to be safe and beneficial. However, large numbers of psychotropic drug users are women of childbearing age. The extent of drug use during pregnancy is often underestimated, as are the effects of maternal drug use on the fetus and neonate. This awareness is related in part to a common tendency to minimize the existence of problems that one finds socially unattractive. Nevertheless, the prevalence and sequelae of both licit and illicit psychotropic drug use during pregnancy indicate that the phenomenon represents a significant problem which must be recognized and addressed by health care delivery systems providing optimal medical care.

Menstrual abnormalities are found in 60 to 90% of women dependent upon heroin. Amenorrhea is most frequently reported.[1-4] Polydrug abuse may also accentuate menstrual irregularities.[5] Other frequent contributory factors in menstrual problems of the narcotic addict are malnutrition, hepatitis, pelvic infection, and other physical illnesses, as well as the stress of the unstable social, economic, and emotional environment in which the women is involved.

Women taking legally prescribed narcotics for underlying medical conditions and those enrolled in methadone maintenance programs usually do not have difficulty with their menstrual cycle.[1] Similarly, discontinuation of illicit heroin with subsequent abstinence is associated with a return to menstrual regularity in 57 to 88% of women.[6,7] Many reports of a high incidence of amenorrhea in women on methadone maintenance have been based on histories obtained from women during the first 3 to 6 months of methadone maintenance treatment. In most patients receiving chronic methadone maintenance treatment for heroin addiction, menses become normal during the first 6 months of treatment. Eighty to 93% of women on chronic high-dose methadone maintenance treatment have reported a return of normal menstrual cycles during the first 6 to 12 months of treatment,[3,8] but in a few patients, up to 2 years were required for menses to return to normal.[1,3,6-9] During methadone maintenance treatment, contraception therefore is necessary to avoid unwanted pregnancies. When pregnancy is desired, it is usually possible in those patients whose menstrual cycles have returned to normal.

Fertility is difficult to assess in any population and especially in heroin addicts. Proper prospective studies cannot be carried out because of difficulties in identification and maintenance of this population. A comparison of the reported high frequency of sexual activity with the number of known pregnancies and births in this population has led to the impression that fertility is diminished. In one retrospective study, 61% of active heroin users were considered infertile. Despite the fact that all 100 former female heroin addicts interviewed had frequent sexual exposure without contraceptives while using heroin, only 39 became pregnant during this period.[9,10] This may be compared to an estimated prevalence of infertility of 13% in non-addicted women.

It must be emphasized, however, that although anovulatory cycles are frequent, pregnancy may indeed occur. The need for family planning and dissemination of birth control information is therefore apparent. Once a narcotic addict becomes pregnant, the course of the pregnancy may not be smooth. Increased risk exists for abortion, birth of premature infants, intrauterine fetal distress, and narcotic withdrawal in the neonatal period. It therefore becomes quite important to diagnose pregnancy in the narcotic addict as early as possible, so that adequate medical and psychologic care can be instituted.

DIAGNOSIS OF PREGNANCY

The three most common indicators of pregnancy are (1) a history of amenorrhea; (2) a positive pregnancy test; and (3) palpation of the gravid uterus.

Unfortunately, in the addict, none of these indicators are reliable. Amenorrhea as discussed above is common. In addition, the early signs or symptoms of pregnancy, such as fatigue, headaches, nausea and vomiting, hot sweats, or pelvic cramps may be interpreted as withdrawal symptoms by both physician and patient. Not infrequently, the onset of these symptoms compels the drug addict to seek more drugs which not only are ineffective in alleviating her symptoms, but also expose the fetus to increased risk secondary to changing serum levels of narcotics and other drugs.

Many of the older pregnancy tests using latex agglutination such as Pregnosis or Pregnosticon gave a false-positive reaction in 5% of women addicts secondary to the direct effects of the heroin. False-positive pregnancy tests were also obtained from methadone-maintained patients. In one series of over 500 pregnancy tests in women maintained on methadone, 24% of the results were false-positive when the Gravindex slide test was used, and 5% false-positive when the Pregnosticon slide test was used.[11] However, there was less than 0.2% incidence of false-positive results when the 2-hour Pregnosticon or UCG tube tests were used. It is postulated that the false-positive tests are due to an in vitro effect of methadone metabolites which apparently interfere with the inhibition of latex particle agglutination in the slide tests.[6] With the current use of bioassays or radioimmunoassays, specific for beta HCG, there are no false-positive results and therefore, these tests are recommended.

For several reasons, it may be extremely difficult on bimanual pelvic examination to palpate an early intrauterine pregnancy in these patients. The generally poor physician-addict interrelationship tends to make these women quite uncooperative while undergoing a pelvic examination. Pelvic infections, which are common in this population, may lead to patient discomfort or distorting masses. Constipation with fecal impaction, a problem for opiate addicts, may also distort the examination.

The single most reliable aid for diagnosis of pregnancy and fetal age is ultrasonography, a non-invasive technique that has a high safety factor for both the mother and fetus.[12] Normal early intrauterine pregnancy may be readily diagnosed with this method at 5 to 6 weeks after the last normal menstrual period or 3 weeks post-conception. Furthermore, since it has been shown that early onset symmetrical intrauterine growth retardation is seen in drug dependent women, ultrasound evaluations are essential in this population for early dating.[13]

Some patients may consider pregnancy termination for social reasons, and after appropriate counselling these wishes should be accommodated. However, mandatory abortion in a heroin-dependent woman or a methadone-maintained patient should never be advocated. These patients need all the assurance and support that can be provided to overcome their problems; to urge abortion against the patient's wishes is certainly not part of that support.

DIAGNOSIS OF NARCOTIC ADDICTION

The diagnosis of heroin dependency based on history and physical examination in the pregnant woman is similar to that in a non-pregnant heroin addict. The presence of pupillary constriction, dermatologic signs of intravenous injection such as "track marks," thrombotic veins, subcutaneous abscesses or nodules, and localized edema over superficial veins are all suggestive of addiction. Lymphadenopathy and hepatomegaly may be quite pronounced in parenteral drug users. The possibility of illicit injections must be considered when lymphadenopathy is unilateral. Bizarre behavior or a labile affect may also be apparent. A history of drug associated disease such as hepatitis, bacterial endocarditis or cellulitis adds suspicion. Certain other features may provide additional evidence such as poor attendance at prenatal care. Frequently, the first suspicion will develop when the patient consistently fails to have prenatal laboratory work preformed because of a lack of available veins.

Features associated with previous pregnancies that should be noted are a past history of low birth weight infants or poor to absent prenatal care. An increase in fetal activity in the present pregnancy may be observed when unstable serum levels of narcotics occur secondary to irregular or changing heroin doses.

It should be emphasized that the administration of narcotic antagonists to diagnose heroin dependency in pregnancy is contraindicated. The inducing of even mild withdrawal may result in severe adverse fetal effects. The most definitive method of diagnosing heroin or polydrug abuse is by analysis of urine specimens, and the observation of early signs and symptoms of abstinence.

The application of toxicology studies to the management of pregnant methadone-maintained women is extremely beneficial because at least 98% of women on methadone maintenance will use an additional drug at least once. These drugs may include diazepam, heroin, amphetamines, or cocaine. Typically, women who use one type of depressant are likely to be using another. Many of the women attempt to induce a particular effect with anti-anxiety or anti-depressant agents and possibly to augment the effects of their methadone. It is important, therefore, to know the specific agents that the mother is using, in addition to her methadone, not only in an attempt to monitor the mother's physical and psychologic well being, but also in the treatment of the infant who may undergo abstinence.[14]

Thin Layer Chromatography (TLC) is a practical, economical, and sensitive method for detection of drugs in urine specimens. Drugs detectable with TLC and acid hydrolysis include: heroin, morphine, amphetamines, barbiturates, codeine, cocaine, glutethimide (Doriden), methadone, methaqualone (Quaalude), phenothiazines, and quinine.

It should be emphasized that urine screening is not completely accurate since intermittent injections and dilute urine can result in negative results. False-positive TLCs, although rare, may occur when spots of identical coloring and motility caused by different drugs are seen on the chromatograph. Legally prescribed cough medications may yield a positive TLC for morphine since a portion of the codeine is transformed into morphine in the body.

The Enzyme Monitored Immunoassay technique (EMIT) is another sensitive and relatively easy technique for identifying drugs of abuse. Drugs detectable with the EMIT include: opiates, amphetamines, barbiturates, methadone, benzodiazepines, propoxyphene (related chemically to methadone but tested for separately), cocaine, and anticonvulsants.

If the patient has a bacterial urinary tract infection, a false-positive reaction with EMIT may occur with each test, giving the impression that polydrug use is present. When there is an actual or potential urinary tract infection, the presence of lysoenzyme should be determined to rule out the possibility of a false-positive reaction. Finally, the expertise of the testing laboratory may determine the reliability of the results. Even the best labs have a high incidence of none-reproducible results.

ANTEPARTUM MEDICAL MANAGEMENT

A complete and comprehensive medical and drug history, especially with respect to polydrug abuse, is of prime importance in the management of the narcotic dependent woman. Over the past several years, most methadone clinics have experienced a marked increase in the number of cocaine-using individuals. In our program in Philadelphia, the incidence of cocaine use in methadone-maintained women has increased from 7 to 58% over the last 3 years. It is important to detect the use of this drug because various prenatal complications such as abruptio placentae, precipitous labor, fetal distress, and an increased need for an emergency cesarean section are seen more frequently in cocaine users. Fetal losses are greater and infant size and gestational age are diminished, as well as an increase in infant morbidity.[15]

In general, all pregnant patients who are substance abusers, regardless of the particular agent abused, are considered to be in a higher than normal risk category because of the complications of illicit drug use. Chronic parenteral drug abuse during pregnancy has a variety of concomitant obstetric and medical complications due to the method of drug administration, potential withdrawal from reduced availability of drugs, and lack of prenatal care for identification and treatment of problems. Infections account for a high percentage of related medical complications (Table 16–1) and they may have profoundly harmful effects on the pregnant addict and her unborn child—particularly if they remain untreated throughout gestation. Especially frequent are: types A, B, and non-

Table 16–1.   Medical Complications Encountered in Pregnant Addicts

Anemia	Tetanus
Bacteremia	Tuberculosis
Cardiac disease, especially endocarditis	Urinary tract infection:
Cellulitis	Cystitis
Poor dental hygiene	Urethritis
Edema	Pyelonephritis
Hepatitis—acute and chronic	Venereal disease:
Phlebitis	Condyloma acuminatum
Pneumonia	Gonorrhea
Septicemia	Herpes
	Syphilis

A, non-B hepatitis, bacterial endocarditis (often with a variety of unusual organisms), septicemia, cellulitis, and venereal disease.[7,9,16–23]

An additional concern with regard to infection in pregnant drug-dependent women is the ongoing epidemic of acquired immune deficiency syndrome (AIDS). Seventy-five percent of infants and children who acquire this disease are born to women who have risk factors for acquiring AIDS. Because of sharing needles and sexual practices, the drug-dependent woman is at extremely high risk for the development of AIDS. Therefore, in the antepartum medical management of these women, it is appropriate to take a clear history with regard to needle sharing and sexual practices. Moreover, these women should be asked if they would be willing to have an ELISA test done. This is helpful not only in managing them during pregnancy, but also for the management of the newborn child. Furthermore, if the women is HIV positive, she should be advised about the various methodologies available to her concerning the prevention of birth of future children. Also, from a public health standpoint, she needs to be advised as to how she should prevent others from acquiring the disease. Women who are HIV positive should be advised that breastfeeding their infants is contraindicated.[24]

Active clinically apparent hepatitis occurs in some addicts while many others have infection or liver damage but are without clinical symptoms. Several studies have shown that over 60% of heroin addicts in methadone maintenance or drug-free treatment have persistent abnormalities of liver function tests due to chronic liver disease. This is most frequently a post-viral hepatitis disorder such as chronic persistent hepatitis, chronic active hepatitis, or cirrhosis. Occasionally, these abnormalities may be attributable to alcoholic liver disease or a mixture of the types mentioned above.[17,19,20,25,26] Liver function tests, therefore, need to be checked routinely. The use of contaminated needles during active heroin addiction is probably the most common cause of the high incidence of viral hepatitis. Since over 12% of heroin addicts and former heroin addicts are chronic carriers of the hepatitis B antigen,[26] a heptatitis-associated antigen (HAA) should be included in the initial evaluation and, if positive, an e-antigen should be ordered. If the mother is found to be a carrier of this antigen (and especially if she is e-antigen-positive), a cord blood HAA should be obtained at delivery and treatment of the neonate with hepatitis B immunoglobulin and vaccine should be initiated.[27]

A high incidence of biologic false-positive serologies for syphilis occurs in both active and former heroin addicts.[7,16,18] Similarly, persistent elevations of the immmunoglobulins IgM and IgG are commonly observed in this group.[7,21] Therefore, Treponema-specific tests, such as the fluorescent Treponema antibody (FTA) or the Microhemoglutination Inhibition Treponema Pallidum (MHA-TP) should be used to confirm the diagnosis of syphilis. On the other hand, care must be used in ascribing a positive result to drug abuse since this population is also at a high risk for reinfection with syphilis. In general, if one is not able to be assured that the test result is a biologic false-positive, then treatment is indicated to protect the fetus.

Obstetrical complications associated with heroin addiction are those usually seen in any woman lacking prenatal care. A frequent result is the birth of a low weight infant who has an array of problems due to prematurity, and whose withdrawal symptoms are therefore difficult to manage. In some cases, death of the pregnant woman and/or her fetus may occur from these untreated complications.

Methadone maintenance, in and of itself, is not sufficient to reduce perinatal complications but must be offered in conjunction with prenatal care reinforced by psychosocial counseling. With this combination of services, complications can be identified and treated, thereby reducing maternal and infant morbidity and mortality.[7,28]

Following the initial history, comprehensive physical (Table 16-2) and laboratory diagnostic evaluations (Table 16-3), a therapeutic plan must be formulated to manage the pregnant woman through the remainder of her pregnancy as well as during labor, delivery, and the postpartum period. The formulation of this plan is dependent upon both the duration of the pregnancy and the character of the narcotic dependency present when the patient is first seen.

PRENATAL TREATMENT

In addition to the regular care that any pregnant woman receives, an addicted woman needs special close attention with emphasis on assessment of nutritional status and detection of occult venereal disease. Shortly after the patient's first

Table 16–2. Area of Special Concern in the Physical Examination of Pregnant, Narcotic Dependent Women

Dermatologic:	Presence of infections, abscesses, thrombosed veins, herpes infections, pyodermas, icterus.
Dental:	Status of dental hygiene. Existence of pyorrhea or abscessed cavities.
Otolaryngeal:	Rhinitis, excoriation of nasal septum.
Respiratory:	Presence of asthma, rales, signs of interstitial pulmonary disease.
Cardiovascular:	Presence of increased pulmonary artery pressure or murmurs indicative of endocarditis or pre-existing valvular disease.
Gastrointestinal:	Hepatomegaly, scars from injuries, incisional or umbilical hernias.
Genitourinary:	Presence of infections such as: condyloma acuminatum, trichomonas vaginitis, herpes vaginitis, gonorrheal urethritis, salpingitis, tubal abscesses. a) Uterus: Size, configuration, fetal position, fetal heart rate, fetal activity. b) Breast: Evidence of trauma, "lumps or bumps," nipples, used breast vein for injection.
Musculoskeletal:	Pitting edema, distortion of muscular landmarks due to subcutaneous abscesses or brawny edema.

Table 16–3. Initial Routine Laboratory Tests

Complete blood count with indices	Serology (VDRL & FTA)
Urine:	Cervical-rectal culture for N. gonorrhea
Urinalysis—routine and microscopic	Cervical culture
Urine colony count and culture and	Hepatitis associated antigen (HAA)
sensitivity	HIV[1]
Urine for drug screen	Cervical Pap smear
Chest roentgenogram or T.B. skin test	Blood type; Rh and indirect Coombs
Electrocardiogram	Alpha-feto-protein if between 16 and 18
SMA-6	weeks' gestation[1]
SMA-12	Ultrasound scan:
Sickle prep[1]	1. For confirmation of pregnancy
Rubella titer	after 6 weeks' gestation
	2. For biparietal diameter between 20
	and 30 weeks' gestation[1]

[1]Where appropriate—not necessarily routine procedures

visit, an initial hospitalization of 3 to 4 days is of benefit to both patient and medical staff in assessing the drug dependent state and physical status. After discharge, prenatal clinic visits should be every 2 weeks until the patient has been stabilized. Urinalysis for drugs should be performed at every visit. Not only should weight, blood pressure, and a uterine fundus examination be performed, but time should be allowed to communicate with the patient. This will enable (1) the medical team to determine the patient's ability to conform to the regulations of the methadone clinic; (2) the patient to elaborate her feelings and problems; and most importantly, (3) determination of the patient's ability to learn a new lifestyle and acquire new living skills.

DETOXIFICATION

The patient who prior to pregnancy has been maintained on a relatively high dose of methadone (>35 mg) or the patient who in the hospital setting has needed a large amount of methadone for control of withdrawal symptoms may require a slow detoxification during the course of the pregnancy. Although it has been debated as to whether lowering the maternal dose has any beneficial effect on the pregnancy, some studies have shown that the degree of neonatal withdrawal may be correlated with the maternal methadone dose in the last trimester of pregnancy.[29] If detoxification is elected, it should be performed slowly, preferably decreasing the dose by 5 mg every 2 weeks. Detoxification is not advised prior to 14 weeks' gestation because of a potential risk of inducing abortion and should not be performed after the 32nd week of pregnancy because of possible withdrawal-induced fetal stress. Zuspan et al.,[30] studying the effects of detoxification during the last half of pregnancy, found that a program lowering methadone levels could induce a marked fetal response of the adrenal gland with amniotic fluid levels of epinephrine and a response of the other sympathetic nervous system components manifested by increasing amniotic fluid levels of norepinephrine. This response was blunted if the methadone dose was increased. He concluded that detoxification late in pregnancy should not be recommended unless the fetus can be biochemically monitored for stress.

ABSTINENCE

Unfortunately, the course of abstinence in heroin addicts during pregnancy is not smooth. Pregnant women recently detoxified from narcotics have the same high rate of recidivism as non-pregnant addicts and thus become re-subjected to all of the attendant complications of illicit heroin use. The return to illicit heroin injection exposes the fetus to the risk of varying narcotic levels, which may well result in transient periods of fetal depression alternating with abstinence.[8,22,30-33] Uterine contractions during maternal withdrawal cause an intermittent obstruction to placental perfusion resulting in intermittent fetal hypoxia.

The multiple medical and pharmacologic complications during parenteral heroin abuse must be considered before rejecting methadone maintenance treatment or recommending detoxification from methadone during pregnancy. Also, polydrug or alcohol abuse may become an increasing problem if maintenance treatment is denied, if a dose reduction of methadone is carried out too rapidly, or if selected maintenance doses of methadone are too low to prevent supplementation with heroin. Many patients in these circumstances will use either illicitly obtained methadone or heroin. Others may turn to chronic abuse of tranquilizers, sedatives, barbiturates, or alcohol. Unfortunately, many well-meaning but poorly informed physicians may prescribe drugs such as diazepam for pregnant patients to blunt abstinence symptoms during methadone withdrawal. The use of such drugs not only may substitute another type of dependency, but also may be quite hazardous to the fetus.

It is recommended in most cases that heroin addicted women in an outpatient situation be given methadone maintenance utilizing the lowest possible dose that still maintains the woman in a comfortable state. With this therapy, injection of heroin is usually infrequent. It must be emphasized that informed consent for the use of methadone must be obtained, with all of the possible effects of methadone on both mother and baby being explained fully by the treating physician prior to initiating methadone therapy. Risks attendant to refusing treatment must also be fully explained.

METHADONE MAINTENANCE

Methadone maintenance services multiple purposes. Primarily, it attempts to remove the drug-addicted woman from the drug seeking environment, eliminates the necessary illicit behavior, and prevents the peaks and valleys in the maternal drug level that may occur throughout the day. Maternal nutrition is usually improved. The patients are more amenable to prenatal care and social and psychologic rehabilitation. Since the drug-seeking behavior is eliminated, the women are more able to prepare for the birth of the children and begin homemaking.

Drug-dependent women on methadone programs prior to pregnancy are maintained on their pre-pregnancy dosage, while women who are using street drugs are admitted to the hospital for intensive medical and psychologic evaluation and determination of an adequate methadone dosage. The heroin-addicted patient is initially evaluated for signs and symptoms of withdrawal, which include lacrimation, irritability, rhinorrhea, nausea, vomiting, abdominal cramping, uterine irritability, increased fetal activity, or rarely, hypotension. If evidence of withdrawal is present, 10 mg of methadone is given. Additional 5 mg doses are given every 4 to 6 hours if withdrawal symptoms are present. On the next day, the previous day's total dosage is given as the maintenance dose. The patient is evaluated for withdrawal, as previously, and supplemental doses given as needed. Most patients are able to be well-controlled on a dose of between 20 and 35 mg daily.

The pharmacology of methadone in the pregnant patient has been fairly well evaluated. It is widely distributed throughout the body after oral ingestion with extensive nonspecific tissue binding creating reservoirs that release unchanged methadone back into the blood, thus contributing to its long duration of action.[34] After ingestion of a maintenance dose of methadone, peak plasma levels occur between 2 and 6 hours, with less than 6% of the ingested dose in the total blood volume at this time.[35–37] Lower sustained plasma concentrations are present during the remainder of the 24-hour period. Methadone is metabolized primarily by the liver and excreted in the urine and feces both as unchanged methadone and a variety of metabolites.[35–38] Studies of methadone in pregnant women show a marked intra- and inter-individual variation, with plasma levels somewhat lower after a given dose during pregnancy than following delivery. This decrease in available methadone can be accounted for by an increased fluid space, a larger tissue reservoir for storing methadone, and drug metabolism by both the placenta and fetus.[39] Methadone-maintained women frequently complain of increasing withdrawal as pregnancy progresses and not infrequently need elevations of their oral dose in order to maintain the same plasma level and remain withdrawal free.

Methadone readily crosses the placenta and has been identified and measured in amniotic fluid, cord blood, and neonatal urine.[39–43] In the second trimester, both unchanged methadone and the two major N-demethylated metabolites have been identified in amniotic fluid, while the cord blood levels were below the lower limits of detection. At delivery, the mean ratio of amniotic fluid methadone to maternal plasma methadone was approximately 0.73 and the ratio of cord blood to maternal plasma levels approximately 0.5.[44,45]

NARCOTIC OVERDOSE

Narcotic overdose may occur from a variety of factors: the pregnant heroin addict may inject more heroin than intended; the pregnant methadone-maintained patient may accidentally ingest an overdose of methadone; pregnant sporadic drug abusers may self-administer a dose of narcotic beyond their degree of tolerance; a small child may accidentally ingest a treatment dose of methadone of a parent, a relative, or family friend. In each of these cases, a narcotic overdose syndrome may ensue. When an overdose is due to an intravenous injection of heroin or a similar rapid-acting narcotic, symptoms may occur within seconds. When excess methadone is accidentally or purposefully taken orally, symptoms may not appear for 1 to 3 hours and may progress over a 3 to 6 hour period with effects lasting for over 24 hours. Narcotic overdose may result in respiratory depression, apnea, obtundation, pulmonary edema, and coma.

After establishing an airway and supporting respiration, an intravenous line is placed and naloxone (Narcan), the pharmacologic treatment of choice for any narcotic overdose, is used. Naloxone is a pure narcotic antagonist with no agonist activity and no central nervous system depressant effects. It is safe to use in the treatment of narcotic overdose even if the diagnosis is not definitely established. Naloxone should be administered intravenously at a dose of 0.01 mg/kg body weight; this dose can be readministered at short intervals (e.g. every 5 minutes) until the patient regains consciousness. Naloxone has a maximum duration of action of only 2 to 3 hours, whereas most short-acting narcotics have a 6- to 8-hour duration of action, and methadone a 12- to 48-hour duration of action. Thus, once a patient has regained consciousness and the respiratory rate has returned toward normal, continued close observation is essential. Due to the duration of drug action, symptoms of overdose may be expected to recur within 3 hours and should be retreated as needed with naloxone given intravenously or intramuscularly.

Special care must be taken when it is necessary to give naloxone to methadone maintenance patients or physiologically dependent heroin addicts as severe acute narcotic withdrawal symptoms will be precipitated. In the pregnant addict, these may be hazardous for the fetus. Doses of naloxone should be titrated against clinical symptoms in this setting and a short-acting narcotic should be available for use to reverse acute symptoms of withdrawal.

Gastric lavage may be helpful when an oral drug has been ingested within 1 to 3 hours prior to institution of treatment. If lavage is necessary for treating a comatose patient, tracheal intubaton should be carried out first. Hemodialysis or peritoneal dialysis are not helpful since only small proportions of narcotic are free in plasma or serum. Most narcotics in the bloodstream are extensively bound to plasma proteins. Central nervous system stimulants are ineffective against the depressive action of narcotics and should not be used.

PSYCHOLOGIC CARE DURING GESTATION

The psychologic status of pregnant drug-dependent women must be evaluated as part of the ongoing care of these patients. An evaluation of drug-dependent women by such scales as the Profile of Mood States and the Beck Depression Inventory has found that these women have high levels of confusion and depression which may reflect their illicit drug use or may result from their generally chaotic social environments. Social and psychic intervention are warranted as early in pregnancy as possible. In addition, many factors have been shown to be associated with the occurrence of child abuse that include parental drug and/or alcohol abuse, extreme poverty, chaotic lifestyle, abuse experienced by the parents when they were children and violence between the parents. Drug dependent women have been found to have experienced an increased incidence of abuse, childhood rape, and sexual molestation. This violence, both sexual and non-sexual, coupled with depression, is seen in high incidence in drug dependent women. The potential for adversely affecting the quality of the attachment in the neonatal period as well as a long-term parent/child relationship exists. Evidence that abuse tends to be intergenerationally transmitted underscores the need for early and effective intervention.[46–48]

One of the most difficult challenges facing the primary care physician is the provision of prenatal care for the pregnant addict. Usually the patient does not like doctors and avoids the health care delivery system. These negative feelings are all too frequently reciprocated by the physician. How, then, can these polarized forces be brought together?

Most successful programs to care for pregnant addicts have adapted both prenatal and postnatal clinics to meet two needs.[5,8,9,31] First, the character of the pregnant addict must be taken into account, necessitating adaptation of the physician to the behaviors described below, rather than trying to force the patient to behave in a conforming manner. Secondly, the physicians (internist, obstetrician, and pediatrician) and other health care professionals require support in dealing with patients whose behavior may range from mystifying to infuriating.

In essence, the provision of adequate prenatal and postnatal care, including pediatric services, requires a setting which is non-judgmental and non-punitive. The mother, her children, her spouse, and other family members should feel welcome and comfortable in the clinic. Although appointments are made for many purposes, the clinic should be open at regular times every week. Service should not be denied because appointment schedules are not kept. In addition, the physician must realize that treatment for the mother's addiction is essential in order to obtain a positive response to medical treatment of both mother and infant. This will usually mean a specialized program with both professional and paraprofessional staff who are skilled in working with addicts. The staff of the addiction treatment program, by managing the disturbing aspects of the pregnant addict's behavior, can provide valuable support to the physician providing prenatal and postnatal care to both mother and infant.

CHARACTER OF THE PREGNANT ADDICT

Beneath a facade which appears to be uncaring and indifferent, the pregnant addict has conflicting emotions.[49,50] She usually experiences anxiety that is based on expectations, assumptions, and past experience. There is an expectation of criticism and rejection from the clinical staff. The woman expects that the physician will punitively order her to discontinue taking all drugs, under the guise of concern for the developing baby's welfare. A common underlying assumption is that the clinical staff will be either incapable of or disinterested in understanding her situation or problems. Her worst fears will be confirmed if the physician decides on the medications and doses to be used in treatment without consulting her. All too often past experience of her own or that of a friend has provided a strong basis for these expectations and assumptions.

Guilt and shame, coupled with low self-esteem, are also common emotions. There may be good reason for these feelings based on the addicted woman's perception of the effects of her behavior on herself, her children, her family, and the community in which she lives. These unpleasant feelings are usually denied and must be inferred from the woman's behavior. Staff comments that are designed to make the pregnant addict feel guilty or ashamed are not well tolerated. The usual result is a loss of willing contact with the staff and destruction of a positive therapeutic relationship, which is the cornerstone of adequate obstetric and pediatric care.

Awareness of the above and other emotions make the behavior of the pregnant addict easier to comprehend. The following behavior problems are frequently encountered:[51]

1. *Lateness or missed appointments:* The patient may appear at the end of a scheduled appointment or at some other time.
2. *Continued use of illicit drugs:* Frequent urine monitoring and close clinical observation will help bring this problem into the open.
3. *Intoxication:* Usually this will be from CNS depressants such as alcohol,

barbiturates, benzodiazepines, or other psychoactive agents, some of which may have been obtained from other physicians. A breathalyzer in the clinic can provide useful information and avoid angry confrontations. Stimulant intoxication from amphetamines, cocaine, or methylphenidate is less common and less easy to detect clinically.

4. *Illicit activity:* A variety of illegal behaviors used to support drug addiction may continue. This may result in arrests, but prenatal care is rarely terminated, since most judges are reluctant to incarcerate pregnant women. Negative emotional reactions of physicians, nurses, and other staff may then present a problem.

5. *Irritability:* Anger, often stemming from past or present hurts, may spill over onto people in contact with the pregnant addict. Children may be abused or neglected. Her spouse and/or other supporting family members may withdraw or leave. The result may be social isolation except from other active drug users. Health care professionals often have great difficulty with this behavior and may be tempted to respond in kind.

6. *Impulsive, demanding, provocative behavior:* Clinic rules may be broken in ways that alienate health care professionals and invite termination from treatment.

No one welcomes or easily tolerates these behaviors. The burden, however, can become manageable by sharing it with others. A structured program which includes paraprofessionals with "street" experience is usually most effective in controlling these behaviors in the clinic setting. Paraprofessionals are much less likely to be offended or to respond punitively. They are, therefore, of value in absorbing stress that disturbs other health care professionals. In this way, they may help preserve an effective therapeutic relationship.

The clinical staff should remember that the intolerable behavior of the pregnant addict reflects low self-esteem and devaluation of herself as a person. Abrupt termination from treatment is not a satisfactory solution. Through experience, it has been found that the woman terminated from care is at increased risk of suicide from drug overdose or some similar act, and further that the woman who discontinues prenatal care also places her fetus in jeopardy.

THE ROLE OF THE PHYSICIAN

The physician's role includes more than the provision of medical care. The pregnant addict is often in crisis and at a turning point in her life. Skilled handling may have an impact not only on her, but on other members of the family as well.

The first prenatal visit is particularly important. The pregnant addict is much less likely to return for a second visit than her non-addict counterpart. The likelihood of return depends much more on her subjective reaction to the first visit. A suggested format for the physician's activities during that visit is as follows:[52]

1. *Be supportive:* Emotional support for the woman does not mean support for her drug use or the aforementioned behaviors. The physician and other staff can strongly support the woman's participation in prenatal care and the implied intention of taking good care of herself and her developing baby.

2. *Explore treatment for addiction*: If the woman is in treatment, the physician needs to know where and with whom. If she is not, the importance of that treatment as an essential complement to prenatal care needs to be stressed. This issue should be raised early in the session so that the physician can call in a counselor from a known program to begin working with the woman on treatment for addiction. Personal contact is a far more effective method of referral for treatment than giving the woman an address or phone number. A review of the effects of drugs on the developing fetus may be beneficial at this time, especially if chemotherapy, such as methadone support, is to be used during the pregnancy. The addict may have an extensive knowledge of street pharmacology, but often has serious misconceptions about how damaging heroin and illicit methadone (because of unknown dose) are to the baby. On the other hand, she may minimize or be unaware of the more toxic effects of central nervous system depressants, such as alcohol. The physician can stress the fact that while abstinence is ideal, it may prove to be realistically impossible. In that case, the lesser of two evils is a known drug used under medical supervision and control. Street drugs or self-prescribed drugs of unknown quality and quantity, often laced with potentially infective and/or toxic impurities, are much more dangerous.

3. *Get baseline data:* A good history and physical examination (Table 16-2), as described earlier, provide essential data for management of the pregnancy and delivery. These activities also aid in establishing a positive relationship between physician and patient. Warm hands and instruments facilitate the development of this relationship. To ensure accurate data, the physician should refrain in a self-disciplined way from any negative judgmental emotional comments or reactions. Furthermore, this is not a good time to try to educate the patient. It can be viewed as a time when the patient educates the physician about her use of drugs, her lifestyle, and her state of mind and body.

4. *Initiate treatment:* The physician should resist impulses to detoxify every patient. If the woman herself wishes to attempt detoxification and there are no medical contraindications such as imminent delivery or potential fetal distress (first and third trimesters), then it can be cautiously attempted. It is wise to avoid multiple medications. If analgesics, hypnotics, and tranquilizers or antidepressants are needed to control withdrawal symptoms, then it is preferable to use a single substitute for the drug of abuse e.g. methadone for heroin. Treatment of infections and nutritional, metabolic, or other problems should be started. Assignment of medical and nursing staff who can follow the woman throughout her pregnancy should be made in view of the importance of stable, positive relationships in the treatment of the pregnant addict.

5. *Begin patient education:* A good beginning is with the medical findings, which are familiar ground for the physician and readily accepted by the patient. Chemotherapy and the patient's drug use, including alcohol and nicotine, can be reviewed including expression of the physician's concerns. It is at this point that the physician's own values may be expressed and a decision made about whether a working relationship can be established for the remainder of the pregnancy. The need for long-term treatment of the ad-

diction is an important concept to be emphasized. This will lead into the importance of long-term followup to assess the overall impact of the mother's drug use on her baby and to assure the child's best chance for long-term health without later drug abuse problems. The possibilities of a normal outcome for the pregnancy ought to be stressed by the physician. The expectant mother may be anticipating an abnormal outcome; she needs whatever hope can be offered without making false promises. Emphasis on the positive role the woman can play in her own prenatal care and later as an effective mother may also help increase her self-esteem.

6. *Explore sensitive areas*: Issues such as abortion, family planning, and adoption should be brought up at the end of the visit. Several purposes are served by raising these issues in a non-threatening, non-judgmental way. The woman may be relieved to find that she can consider options in what had been personally or culturally taboo areas. Possibilities may be raised of which she had been ignorant, or had never considered possible for herself. Through this process, the patient learns that emotionally loaded issues can be discussed confidentially and dispassionately with her physician. Perhaps most importantly, respect is communicated for the woman as a person who can make responsible decisions and who will benefit by any information the physician can provide.

Involvement of the family, including spouse, parents, children, or other close relatives living with the woman, should be considered by the physician. Although not essential to adequate prenatal care, family involvement is extremely important in treatment of the addiction and in positively influencing the environment in which the new baby will be raised.

The physician's language can be an important factor in determining the woman's response to treatment. Pejorative words relating to drug use should be avoided. Patients react negatively to terms such as "junkie," "wino," "lush," "druggy," or even "addict." The terms "addict,", "addicted," or "the littlest junkie" should never be applied to the infant, for it is not only inaccurate, but also arouses strong guilt feelings and resentment in the mother. The physician's language, therefore, impacts on the mother-child bond as well as on the physician-patient relationship.

MANAGEMENT OF OBSTETRICAL PROBLEMS DURING PREGNANCY

The management of most obstetrical problems in the drug-addicted patient is the same as in the non-addicted woman. However, the problems related to low birth weight are of such importance that a few points of special emphasis are necessary.

Identification of intrauterine fetal growth retardation must be emphasized. Studies have shown that a clinical impression of fetal growth failure, even in a high risk population, is correct only 50% of the time. To improve the accuracy, most drug-addicted women should have baseline ultrasound studies performed as early in pregnancy as possible and the growth evaluated by a second study at 32 to 36 weeks.

When the fetus is identified as manifesting growth failure, difficulty in evaluating fetal well-being exists. Fortunately estriol excretion is no longer used as a primary tool to evaluate fetal health. Estriol excretion in narcotic-addicted pregnant women during the last trimester does not truly reflect fetal welfare because the 24-hour production of estriol is generally below normal levels.[53] However, during the periods of withdrawal, the urinary estriol concentration rapidly increases, frequently exceeding expected values. This withdrawal-induced elevation is likely secondary to fetal adrenal stimulation, leading to increased production of estriol precursors. The non-stress and contraction stress tests have not been well evaluated in a drug-addicted population. In our unit, there is an increased incidence of non-reactive non-stress tests, when performed shortly after methadone was taken, but no increased incidence of falsely positive contraction stress tests. The increased incidence of fetal non-reactivity is not unexpected since narcotics have often been described as causing poor beat-to-beat variability.

Heat-stable alkaline phosphatase (HSAP) has been suggested as a means of following high risk pregnancies. Harper and colleagues[54] studied this enzyme in methadone-maintained pregnancies. They found high concentrations of HSAP in 80% of addicted women who were maintained on greater than 60 mg of methadone, while only 20% of women maintained on less than this had high concentrations. The higher levels of HSAP in women receiving large doses of methadone suggest that the drug may affect the maternal-placental-fetal unit in more subtle ways than previously considered. In practice, fetuses suspected of having intrauterine growth retardation should be followed by the standard biochemical and biophysical parameters.

The management of premature labor in the opiate-addicted woman includes bed rest, hydration, the use of tocolytics, and evaluation of pulmonary lung maturity. The initial evaluation should include an ultrasound examination for assessment of gestational age. Since these women have inaccurate reporting of their last menstrual period, what first may appear to be premature labor may simply be a term pregnancy. After determination of gestational age, a search should be made for an etiology.

Initially, it was thought that hyaline membrane disease almost never occurred in the infant of a heroin-addicted mother. This impression came from the work of Glass et al.[55] who evaluated 33 premature infants born to heroin-addicted women in whom no cases of hyaline membrane disease were identified. Since then, hyaline membrane disease has been seen in heroin-exposed infants. Studies have revealed that lung maturation in fetuses of narcotic-addicted mothers may occur at a point in gestation earlier than would be expected in the non-addicted infant.[56,57] Because of this early maturation and lack of reliability of the reported gestational age, an amniocentesis may aid in determining appropriate treatment of suspected premature labor.

MANAGEMENT OF LABOR, DELIVERY, AND THE POSTPARTUM PERIOD

Medical Management

The management of drug-dependent women during labor and delivery is similar to that for non-drug dependent women. There are, however, certain points that must be considered. Since the drug-addicted woman may confuse the early signs of labor with the signs of withdrawal, she may attempt to medicate herself and present in labor with a high blood level of narcotics. Accordingly, at the time of admission of all drug-abusing women, a urine drug screening should be obtained to identify drugs taken. This information will be of help not only to the obstetrician, but also to the pediatrician who will be treating the neonatal abstinence syndrome. If the patient is maintained on methadone, her usual dose should be given as soon after admission as possible in order to avoid withdrawal during labor which could lead to increased maternal and fetal oxygen consumption, uterine hyperirritability, and fetal distress. If the patient is un-registered and appears to be withdrawing, a dose of 10 to 20 mg of methadone is given intramuscularly.[58]

Most drug-abusing women have sclerotic veins making an intravenous in-sertion difficult. An intravenous line must be started prophylactically, however, to avoid serious delays in treatment if the need for medications or blood products arise. Therefore, many patients will need a subclavian intravenous line.[58]

Analgesia and Anesthesia

The choice of analgesia and anesthesia for the drug-dependent woman during labor is determined as in any non-addicted woman. Methadone is used only to prevent withdrawal and does not serve as adequate analgesia. Narcotics may be used in their regular dosage in addition to the patient's methadone. Both the mother and fetus are already physically dependent on narcotics and are therefore less sensitive than non-tolerant individuals to both the central nervous system and respiratory depressant effects. Regional anesthesia such as epidural, saddle block, or pudendal may be used. The amide group of local anesthetics require protein binding to prevent a large dose of drug from crossing into the fetus. Therefore, if the patient has marked malnutrition, is debilitated, or has a de-creased serum protein level, doses of these agents should be kept to a minimum. The use of ester type agents will eliminate this problem. If general anesthesia is necessary, it is administered in the same manner as for a non-drug dependent woman. It must be remembered, however, that a large percentage of drug-dependent women have liver dysfunction, and drugs utilizing this route for metabolism or those potentially toxic to the liver should be avoided.[58]

The use of narcotic antagonists such as naloxone is contraindicated for either the mother or the infant. These agents may cause severe withdrawal and should only be used in life-saving situations.[58]

Psychologic Management

Labor and delivery represent a period of high stress for the pregnant addict. Pain is a physiologic antidote to narcotics and also diminishes the effect of other drugs upon which the woman may be dependent. As a result, she may be admitted in a state of intoxication, having anxiously taken additional drugs to compensate for the real or anticipated stress. If not, she may be in a state of withdrawal even though taking the same amount of drugs which suppressed withdrawal symptoms before labor began.

The physician may find it useful to expect that the woman will have taken extra drugs. Then, if she has, he will not be surprised or react in an angry or punitive way. If she has not taken anything, the physician can then be genuinely pleased, supportive of the woman's courage, and less reluctant to use adequate doses of analgesic medication to ensure the highest possible level of cooperation from her during labor and delivery.

Active participation by the woman during labor and delivery may be beneficial for her and gratifying for the physician. This represents a change from her usual pattern of avoidance or passive withdrawal from stressful situations.

Participation by the spouse or mate and other primary family members offers additional benefits.[59] Encouragement by the physician will be necessary because the sexism of street lifestyles tends to preclude male involvement in many aspects of child rearing and other "women's" activities, including childbearing.[50]

Immediate parental contact with the newborn infant in the delivery room is desirable, if the mother intends to keep the baby.[60] There is some evidence that allowing the infant and parents to remain together for 45 to 60 minutes immediately following delivery enhances the quality of parent-child bonding and increases the likelihood that the child will thrive. At this time, either the physician or a nurse can assist the new parents to develop skill in tender, careful handling of their infant. This handling is characterized by full palmar rather than fingertip contact. It is skin to skin, warm, unhurried, and provides close physical contact. Support is provided, especially for the infant's head, encouraging an "en face" position between baby and parent. Responsive adjustments are made to the infant's movement without removing protective support. In addition to facilitating parent-child bonding, tender careful handling provides the parents with a real-life example of responding to feedback and stimulation from the child, thus setting the stage for two-way communication between parent and child during the next few years.

If a decision has been made to give up the child for adoption, it should be removed from the delivery room as soon as possible. This is an extremely stressful time for the mother, regardless of her calm appearance. The physician and other staff can help during this period of crisis by supporting her decision and facilitating contact with positive family members and staff from the woman's treatment program.

Postpartum Period

The postpartum course is monitored as in any other pregnancy. The necessity for continued methadone maintenance is obvious. The length of stay in the hospital depends upon whether there are obstetric problems. Close observation must occur for the potential of postpartum hemorrhage in these women. If there has been a normal labor and delivery, the patient is usually discharged on the second postpartum day. The infant, however, may stay longer, especially if withdrawal symptoms occur.[61,62]

A number of drug-dependent women express a desire to breast-feed their infants. Since narcotics are secreted in breast milk, it usually has been the practice to advise against this. Recently, information elucidating advantages to breast-fed infants, including the benefit from maternal-infant bonding, has led to a reconsideration of breastfeeding in more drug-dependent women. If the mother is abusing multiple drugs which would expose the infant to diverse agents in varying levels, then breastfeeding must still be considered contraindicated. However, if the mother has been maintained on methadone and is known to be free of other drug use, and has not shared needles for more than 4 years, then breastfeeding may be considered an option.[58] Breastfeeding is contraindicated if the mother is HIV positive.

FAMILY PLANNING

Beginning in the prenatal period, education for birth control and family planning should be provided and emphasized. The idea of spacing pregnancies should be introduced with reinforcement that there can be control over becoming pregnant and that there are many factors to consider when making the decision to have another child, i.e., the number of children born, the number wanted, the ability to care for the children present and future, and the drug-dependent status. The woman should be encouraged to feel satisfaction about controlling this aspect of her life.

Several routine methods of birth control are not optimal in the drug-dependent population, and evaluation on an individual basis is essential. Oral estrogen, preferably low dose, should be prescribed with care, as many of these women have vascular disease secondary to prolonged drug abuse, and they may not be conscientious in taking prescribed medication. Intrauterine devices (IUDs) may be considered if the patient's past history does not include pelvic infections; however, an additional complication with IUDs is the possibility of exposure to venereal disease. The barrier-type methods, which are the safest medically, are not the most effective and require consistent use.

The injectable, long-acting progestins (e.g. medroxy-progesterone acetate) have not as yet been approved by the FDA as contraceptives, but may be of potential value in the drug-dependent population. The safety of these agents and their use in women with specific medical disorders remains to be determined. Permanent sterilization can be introduced as a possibility, especially if the patient is extremely high risk. The procedure can be completed before discharge postpartum.

The need for appropriate family planning must be stressed because an unwanted pregnancy may only add unnecessary anxiety to an already precarious situation. Counseling should be readily available and should involve both parents whenever possible.

Professionals involved in the care of these women must also be aware that certain trends and changes in treatment programs with drug-dependent women have occurred over the last 5 to 8 years. In evaluating nearly 500 patients in Philadelphia over the last 8 years, it was noted that there were shifts in racial composition with an equal distribution in black and white women, an increased incidence of prematurity and maternal age, and a decrease in prenatal care. These changes were attributable to a shift in drug use from heroin and other drugs to predominantly cocaine, heroin, and depressants. Therefore, clinicians must realize that treatment modalities for drug-dependent women must be reassessed and restructured to reflect a changing population of women as well as their needs.[63]

REFERENCES

1. Cushman, P., and Kreek, M.J.: Some endocrinologic observations in narcotic addicts. In Narcotics and the Hypothalamus, Zimmerman, E. and George, R. (eds.), New York, Raven Press, 1974.
2. Gaulden, E.C., Littlefield, D.C., Putoff, O.E., et al.: Menstrual abnormalities associated with heroin addiction. Am. J. Obstet. Gynecol. *90*:155, 1964.

3. Santen, R.J., Sofsky, J., Bilic, N., et al.: Mechanism of action of narcotics in the production of menstrual dysfunction in women. Fertil. Steril., 26:538, 1975.
4. Stoffer, S.S.: A gynecologic study of drug addicts. Am. J. Obstet. Gynecol., 101: 779, 1968.
5. Blinick, G., Jerez, E., and Wallach, R.C.: Methadone maintenance, pregnancy, and progeny. JAMA, 225:477, 1973.
6. Horowitz, C.A., Maslansky, R., Waldinger, R., et al.: The effect of methadone on pregnancy tests: An analysis of 506 specimens with four currently available immunoassays. In Proceedings of the Fourth National Conference on Methadone Treatment. New York, NAPAN, 1972, pp.111–116.
7. Kreek, M.J.: Medical safety and side effects of methadone in tolerant individuals. JAMA, 223:665, 1974.
8. Wallach, R.C., Jerez, E., and Blinick, G.: Pregnancy and menstrual function in narcotic addicts treated with methadone. Am. J. Obstet. Gynecol., 105:1226, 1969.
9. Blinick, G., Wallach, R.C., and Jerez, E.: Pregnancy in narcotic addicts treated by medical withdrawal. Am. J. Obstet. Gynecol. 105:997, 1969.
10. Hatcher, R.A., Stewart, G.K., Guest, F., et al. (eds): Contraceptive Technology 1976–1977, New York, Irvington Publishers, 1976, pp.24–28.
11. Hutzel Hospital Laboratory, Detroit, Michigan: Unpublished data. (Dr. E. Booth, pathologist in charge).
12. Steel, W.B., and Taylor, K.J.W.: Grey scale ultrasonography in obstetrics, In Ultrasound in Medicine, Vol. I, White, D. (ed). New York, Plenum Press, 1975, p.415.
13. Wapner, R.J., Ross, R.D., FitzSimmons, J.M., et al.: Fetal growth in drug dependent women: quantitative assessments. Pediatr. Res., 15:1222, 1981.
14. Leifer, E.D., and Finnegan, L.P.: Application of toxicology reports to the management of pregnant methadone maintained women and their infants. Pediatr. Res., 17:387, 1983.
15. Livesay, S., Ehrlich, S., and Finnegan, L.P.: Cocaine and pregnancy: maternal and infant outcome. Pediatr. Res., 21:387, 1987.
16. Cherubin, C.E.: Infectious disease problems of narcotic addicts. Arch. Intern. Med., 128:309, 1971.
17. Cherubin, C.E., Kane, S., Weinberger, D.R., et al: Persistence of transaminase abnormalities in former drug addicts. Ann. Intern. Med., 76:385, 1972.
18. Cherubin, C.E., and Millian, S.J.: Serological investigations in narcotic addicts. I. Syphilis, lymphogranuloma venereum, herpes simplex and Q fever. Ann. Intern. Med., 69:739, 1968.
19. Cherubin, C.E., Rosenthal, W.S., Stenger, R.E., et al.: Chronic liver disease in asymptomatic narcotic addicts. Ann. Intern. Med., 76:391, 1972.
20. Cherubin, C.E., Schaefer, R.A., Rosenthal, W.S. et al.: The natural history of liver disease in former drug users. Am. J. Med. Sci., 272:244, 1976.
21. Cushman, P., and Grieco, M.H.: Hyperimmunoglobulinemia associated with narcotic addiction: effects of methadone maintenance treatment. Am. J. Med., 54:320, 1973.
22. Guttmacher, A.F., and Rovinsky, V.V.: Medical, Surgical, and Gynecological Complications of Pregnancy, Baltimore, Williams & Wilkins, 1965.
23. Naeye, R.L., Blane, W., Coblanc, W., et al.: Fetal complications of maternal heroin addiction: abnormal growth, infections, and episodes of stress. J. Pediatr., 83:1055, 1973.
24. Rogers, M.M.: Aids in children: a review on the clinical aphodemiologic and public health aspects. Pediatr. Infect. Dis., 4:230, 1985.
25. Stimmel, B., Vernace, S., and Tobias, H.: Hepatic dysfunction in heroin addicts: the role of alcohol. JAMA, 222:811, 1972.
26. Kreek, M.J., Dodes, L., Kane, S., et al.: Long-term methadone maintenance therapy. Effects on liver function. Ann. Intern. Med., 77:598, 1972.
27. Dosik, H., and Jhaveri, R.: Prevention of neonatal hepatitis B infection with high-dose hepatitis B immunoglobulin. N. Engl. J. Med., 298:602, 1978.
28. Connaughton, J.F., Reeser, D., and Finnegan, L.P.: Pregnancy complicated by drug addiction. In Perinatal Medicine, Bolognese, R., and Schwartz, R. (eds.), Baltimore, Williams & Wilkins, 1977.
29. Harper, R., Solish, G., Feingold, E., et al.: Maternal ingested methadone, body fluid methadone, and the neonatal withdrawal syndrome. Am. J. Obstet. Gynecol., 129:417, 1977.
30. Zuspan, F.P., Gumpel, J.A., Mejia-Zelaya, A., et al.: Fetal stress from methadone withdrawal. Am. J. Obstet. Gynecol., 122:43, 1975.
31. Davis, R.C., and Chappel, J.N.: Pregnancy in the context of narcotic addiction and methadone maintenance. In Proceedings of the National Conference on Methadone Treatment 2:1146, 1973.
32. Pelosi, M.A., Frattarola, M., Apuzzio, J., et al.: Pregnancy complicated by heroin addiction. Obstet. Gynecol., 45:512, 1975.
33. Strauss, M.E., Andresko, M., Stryker, J.C., et al.: Relationship of neonatal withdrawal to maternal methadone dose. Am J Drug Alcohol Abuse, 3:339, 1976.

34. Dole, V.P., and Kreek, M.J.: Methadone plasma level: sustained by a reservoir of drug in tissue. Proc. Natl. Acad. Sci., *70*:10, 1973.

35. Inturrisi, C.E., and Verebely, K.: A gas liquid chromatographic method for the quantitative determination of methadone in human plasma and urine. J. Chromatogr., *65*:361, 1972.

36. Kreek, M.J.: Plasma and urine levels of methadone. N.Y. State J. Med., *23*:2773, 1973.

37. Sullivan, H.R., and Blake, D.A.: Quantitative determination of methadone concentration in human blood, plasma, and urine by gas chromatography. Res. Commun. Chem. Pathol. Pharmacol., *3*:467, 1972.

38. Kreek, M.H., Dodes, L., Bowen, D.V. et al.: Fecal excretion of methadone and its metabolites: a major pathway of elmination in man. Proceedings of the Third National Drug Abuse Conference, San Francisco, May, 1977.

39. Kreek, M.J., Schecter, A., Gutjahr, C.L., et al.: Analyses of methadone and other drugs in maternal and neonatal body fluids: use in evaluation of symptoms in a neonate of mother maintained on methadone. Am. J. Drug Alcohol Abuse, *1*:409, 1974.

40. Peters, M.A., Turnbow, M., and Buchenauer, D.: The distribution of methadone in the non-pregnant, pregnant, and fetal rate after acute methadone treatment. J. Pharmacol. Exp. Ther., *181*:273, 1972.

41. Sanner, J.H., and Woods, L.A.: Comparative distribution of tritium labelled dihydromorphine between maternal and fetal rats. J. Pharmacol. Exp. Ther. *148*:176, 1965.

42. Yeh, Sy., and Woods, L.A.: Maternal and fetal distribution of H^3 dihydromorphine in the tolerant and non-tolerant rat. J. Pharmacol. Exp. Ther., *174*:9, 1970.

43. Blinick, G., Inturrisi, C.E., Jerez, E., et al.: Amniotic fluid methadone in women maintained on methadone. Mt. Sinai J. Med. N.Y., *41*:254, 1974.

44. Blinick, G., Inturrisi, C.E., Jerez, E., et al.: Methadone assays in pregnant women and progeny. Am. J. Obstet. Gynecol., *121*:617, 1975.

45. Rosen, T.S., and Pippenger, C.E.: Disposition of methadone and its relationship to severity of withdrawal in the newborn. Addict. Dis. *2*:169, 1975.

46. Regan, D.O., Leifer, B., and Finnegan, L.P.: Generations at risk: violence in the lives of pregnant drug abusing women. Pediatr. Res., *16*:77, 1982.

47. Regan, D.O., Tunish, S., and Finnegan, L.P.: Psychological status of pregnant drug dependent women: evaluation by the profile of mood states (POMS). Pediatr. Res. *17*:93, 1983.

48. Regan, D.O. Rudrauff, M.E., and Finnegan, L.P.: Parenting abilities in drug dependent women: the negative effect of depression. Pediatr. Res., *15*:90, 1981.

49. Coppolillo, H.P.: Drug impediments to mothering behavior.In Perinatal Addiction. Harbison, R.D. (ed.), New York, Spectrum Publications, 1975.

50. Eldred, C.A., and Washington, M.N.: Female heroin addicts in a city treatment program: the forgotten minority. Psychiatry, *38*:75, 1975.

51. Densen-Gerber, J., Wiener, M., and Hochstedler, R.: Sexual behavior, abortion, and birth control in heroin addicts: legal and psychiatric considerations. Contemp. Drug Probl., *1*:783, 1972.

52. Finnegan, L.P. (ed.): Drug dependence in pregnancy: clinical management of mother and child. A manual for medical professions and paraprofessionals prepared for the National Institute on Drug Abuse, Services Research Branch, Rockville, Maryland, 1978. U.S. Government Printing Office, Washington, D.C.

53. Northrop, G., Ditzler, J., Ryan, W.C., et al.: Estriol excretion profiles in narcotic-addicted women. Am. J. Obstet. Gynecol, *112*:704, 1972.

54. Harper, R.G., Solish, G.I., Purow, H.M., et al.: The effect of a methadone treatment program upon pregnant heroin addicts and their newborn infants. Pediatr. *54*:300, 1974.

55. Glass, L., Rajegowda, B.K., and Evans, H.F.: Absence of respiratory distress syndrome in premature infants of heroin-addicted mothers. Lancet, *2*:685, 1971.

56. Taeusch, H.W. Jr., Carson, S.H., Wang, N.S., et al.: Heroin induction of lung maturation and growth retardation in fetal rabbits. J. Pediatr., *82*:869, 1973.

57. Gluck, R., and Kulovich, M.V.: Lecithin/sphingomyelin ratios in amniotic fluid in normal and abnormal pregnancy. Am. J. Obstet. Gynecol., *115*:539, 1973.

58. Wapner, R.J., and Finnegan, L.P.: Perinatal aspects of psychotropic drug abuse. InPerinatal Medicine, 2nd Ed. Bolognese, R.J., Schwartz, R.H., and Schneider, J. (eds.), Baltimore, Williams & Wilkins, 1981, pp.384– 417.

59. Silver, F.C., Panepinto, W.C., Arnon, D, et al.: A family approach in treating the pregnant addict. *In* Development in the Field of Drug Abuse. Senay, E.C., Shorty, V., and Alksne, H. (eds.). Cambridge, Schenkman Publishing, 1975, p.401.

60. Klaus, M.H., and Kennell, J.H.: Maternal-infant Bonding. St. Louis, C.V. Mosby Co., 1976.

61. Finnegan, L.P., and MacNew, B.A.: Care of the addicted infant. Am. J. Nurs. *74*:685, 1974.

62. Finnegan, L.P.: Neonatal abstinence. InCurrent Therapy in Neonatal-Perinatal Medicine, Nelson, N. (ed.), Ontario, Canada, B.C. Decker, Inc., Publisher, 1984.

63. Ehrlich, S., and Finnegan, L.P.: Trends and changes in a treatment program for drug-dependent pregnant woman: an 8 year study. Pediatr. Res., *21*:1324, 1987.

Chapter 17

Marijuana and Cocaine Use During Pregnancy*

Ernest L. Abel and Robert J. Sokol

About 25% of the adult American population uses marijuana to some degree[1] and cocaine use in America has risen sharply since the 1970s to the point where about 10 million Americans have used cocaine at least once and 5 million are reported to be regular users.[2] However, the possibility and extent of birth defects related to either of these substances will continue to be difficult to assess adequately because of some of the same problems relating in general to drug abuse in pregnancy.[3] Among these problems are (1) cocaine use is illegal and marijuana use is still illegal in many states so that patients may be unwilling to admit to such usage, (2) heavy marijuana or cocaine users may not seek prenatal care, and (3) use of other drugs simultaneously with marijuana and/or cocaine is common.

Despite such problems, there is a growing body of information concerning marijuana's effects on pregnancy and the conceptus and some reports are beginning to appear concerning cocaine use during pregnancy.

In this review, we will summarize current information concerning the use of these two drugs during pregnancy and will offer some suggestions for managing pregnant patients who use these drugs.

MARIJUANA

Marijuana is a crude drug preparation made from the plant *Cannabis sativa*. The principal psychoactive ingredient in marijuana is delta-9-tetrahydrocannabinol (delta-9-THC), also called delta-1-tetrahydrocannabinol. Hashish is another crude *Cannabis* preparation and differs from marijuana in that only the tops of the plant are used and therefore the delta-9-THC concentration tends to be about twice as high. There are about 60 other cannabinoids present in marijuana, but few have known psychoactive properties, although they may affect the actions of delta-9-THC.

Marijuana is generally taken by inhalation of a hand-rolled cigarette ("joint"). The smoker inhales deeply and the breath is held for several seconds to increase maximal exposure of lung tissue and therefore maximal absorption.

The concentration of delta-9-THC is about 8% in the marijuana generally used in North America, which is considerably increased from concentrations encountered a decade ago.

*Supported by Grant DA 04148-02 from the National Institute on Drug Abuse to E. Abel and NIAAA AA06334-1 to R. Sokol.

A typical "joint" usually contains about 2.5 to 5.0 mg delta-9-THC. Average peak plasma levels after smoking one marijuana cigarette containing about 5 mg delta-9-THC are in the range of 50 ng/ml and decline to about 5 ng/ml within an hour.[4] Although the psychoactive effect ("high") lasts for only 2 to 3 hours, delta-9-THC has a half-life of 24 hours and accumulation of delta-9-THC in the body is likely for daily marijuana users.[4]

Use During Pregnancy

About 14% of all pregnant women use marijuana to some degree (Table 17–1). Since delta-9-THC is able to cross the placenta,[5,6] there is the potential for damage to the conceptus. However, the placenta in some species of rodents appears to provide a barrier to complete transplacental passage.[7,8] A recent study by Blackard and Tennes[9] suggests that in humans, the placenta may also provide a similar barrier. These authors reported that levels of delta-9-THC in maternal blood at time of delivery were about 2.5 times higher than in cord blood. Likewise, Greenland et al.[10] noted positive serum delta-9-THC levels in 7 mothers at time of delivery but none of their infants had positive cord blood levels. Thus, a placental barrier may account in part for the fact that no serious birth defects have as yet been noted in connection with maternal use of marijuana during pregnancy. Early reports of malformations in children born to marijuana users[11,12] were inconclusive because the mothers of these children used many other drugs as well.

Effects on Pregnancy, Labor and Delivery

Marijuana has been used for centuries to hasten delivery.[13] In the 19th century, hashish was reported to stimulate uterine activity during labor.[14] More recent studies have supported these earlier observations.

Length of Gestation

Several studies have found that marijuana use during pregnancy is associated with a shortened gestation. In a prospective study involving 583 women, gestational duration was shortened by 0.8 weeks in heavy marijuana users (more than 5 "joints" per week) after adjustment for use of other drugs (e.g. alcohol, smoking) and prepregnancy weight.[15] Among heavy marijuana users, the amount of marijuana used was dose-related to shortened gestation.

An even stronger relation between marijuana use and length of gestation was reported by Gibson and co-workers.[16] In this prospective study of 7,301 births

Table 17–1. Extent of Reported Marijuana Use Among Pregnant Women

Study Site	%	N	Reference
Boston	14	1690	Hingson et al., 1982[24]
Boston	10	12424	Linn et al., 1983[17]
Boston	14	1630	Weiner et al., 1983[42]
Ottawa	14	583	Fried, et al., 1984[15]
Australia	5.4	7301	Gibson, et al., 1983[16]
Los Angeles	13	Not Stated	Greenland et al., 1984[10]
Ann Arbor	13	245	Rayburn et al., 1982[43]

in Australia, marijuana users had a significantly higher incidence of premature births (<37 weeks) than nonusers after controlling for maternal age, parity, and alcohol and tobacco use.

In another large scale prospective study involving 12,424 women, Linn et al.[17] likewise found that marijuana users had a significantly higher incidence of premature labor, but this was no longer significant after controlling for maternal factors such as medical history, age, parity, race, alcohol and tobacco use.

These results suggest that marijuana use during pregnancy is associated with a shortened length of gestation.

Effects on Labor

Greenland et al.[10] compared 35 marijuana users (using at least once a month) with 36 age, race, and parity-matched nonuser controls in a prospective study. Marijuana users who used other drugs were excluded from participation. A significantly higher incidence of precipitate labor (<3 hours) occurred among marijuana users compared to nonusers (29% vs 3% respectively). Infants born to marijuana users also had a higher incidence of meconium passage (57% vs 25%). Data were adjusted for various labor and neonatal differences and presumably for birth weight as well as other factors. After such adjustment, the authors concluded that marijuana use added 32% to the risk for meconium passage.

In a second study by this same group,[18] marijuana users again were found to have higher incidences of precipitate labor and meconium passage, but differences were not statistically significant. A major difference between these two studies was that women in the second group participated in a low-risk home-delivery program, whereas those in the first study were hospital-delivered.

Linn and her co-workers[17] found a significant increase in abruptio placentae among marijuana users and in a case study of 5 heavy marijuana users, Qazi et al.[19] reported that 2 out of the 5 women had gestation periods of less than 37 weeks.

In contrast to these studies, no effect on duration of labor was noted by Fried[20] in his prospective study of 420 women, 14 of whom were heavy marijuana users (6 to >100 "joints" per week).

Other complications of pregnancy have not generally been noted in connection with maternal marijuana use. In a prospective study of 1120 pregnancies, we did not observe a significant effect of marijuana use or the combination of marijuana and alcohol on spontaneous abortion rate,[21] although animal studies had suggested the occurrence of such an effect.[22] Since detailed histories of marijuana use were not conducted for women in our study, the failure to corroborate the observation in animals may have been related to relatively light marijuana use during pregnancy.

Birth Weight and Other Neonatal Outcomes

Several investigators[15–17,23] have reported that birth weights of childen born to marijuana users are decreased but when corrected for gestational duration, these decreases are not signficant. An exception to this general finding is found in the report by Hingson et al.[24] These investigators found that infants born to marijuana smokers weighed 105 g less than those born to nonusers and the effect on birth weight was related to frequency of use. However, the effect on birth weight was primarily due to shortened gestational age.

In a clinical case study, Qazi and co-workers[19] also reported decreased birth weights in children born to heavy marijuana smokers. Although there was no correction made for confounding factors, gestational ages do not appear to be able to account for this effect. These case reports are also of interest because they represent outcomes in women smoking considerably more marijuana than those studied in prospective studies.

In animals, in utero exposure to cannabinoids reliably produces intrauterine growth retardation.[25,26] However, administration of cannabinoids to pregnant animals causes decreased weight gain during pregnancy,[25] therefore, this confounding factor must be taken into account. Fortunately, control procedures are available for this drug-related effect. Even when maternal weight gain is taken into account, animals prenatally exposed to cannabinoids are growth retarded at birth.[25,27] Interestingly, supplementation of regular diet with protein has been shown to attenuate some of marijuana's effects on birth weight in rats.[28]

Studies in animals have also shown that the effects of cannabinoids on birth weight are related to period of exposure. In utero exposure to cannabinoids during the first or second trimesters of pregnancy in the rat has minimal effects on birth weight, whereas exposure during the last trimester of pregnancy significantly decreases birth weight and increases postnatal mortality.[27]

Animals stuides have also shown that prenatal cannabinoid exposure can affect body composition at birth, decreasing calcium and lipid content and increasing sodium content.[29]

Congenital Anomalies

As previously noted, marijuana use during pregnancy has not been found to be associated with a higher incidence of congenital anomalies in several prospective studies.[15,16] Nonetheless, Linn et al.[17] found that children born to marijuana users were more likely to have one or more major malformations, but no specific malformation. The increased risk was calculated as 1.36 times higher, but when other risk factors were taken into account, the association was no longer significant.

Hingson et al.[24] and Qazi et al.[19] reported that women who smoked marijuana delivered children with features compatible with fetal alcohol syndrome (FAS). Since such features are nonspecific and can include decreased birth weight and relatively mild effects, e.g. hirsutism, hemangiomas, decreased length, small head, epicanthic folds, posteriorly rotated ears, long philtrum and abnormal palmar creases, this outcome is difficult to assess.

Studies of teratogenic effects of cannabinoids have been reviewed by Abel.[30] In general, cannabinoids are not teratogenic to animals. An exception is the mouse, which seems more sensitive to cannabinoids than other species. However, this increased sensitivity mainly occurs when the drug is administered intraperitoneally.

Neurobehavioral Effects

Most of the postnatal evaluations of children born to marijuana smokers have been reported by Fried in his ongoing prospective study in Ottawa.[20,31]

In his first study,[31] infants were evaluated using the Brazelton Neonatal Assessment Scale. Children born to heavy marijuana smokers were less responsive (in terms of a startle response) to light and of those that did, 2 out of 4 did not habituate. Infants of heavy marijuana users also were less able to self-quiet themselves and they also had a higher incidence of tremors and startles. A higher incidence of cri-du-chat syndrome in marijuana-exposed infants was also noted but observations of this effect were not recorded systematically.

In a subsequent study[20] involving additional women (n = 420), infants prenatally exposed to marijuana again had a higher likelihood of not responding to light or habituating. The previously observed failure to self-quiet, however, was not corroborated. Tremors and startles again occurred with a higher frequency among marijuana-exposed infants. Cri-du-chat syndrome was noted among one-third of the marijuana-exposed infants, but did not occur among any of the control infants.

Fried administered the Prechtl neurologic examination to 6 infants of heavy marijuana users and infants of women who reduced marijuana use during pregnancy at 9 and 30 days of age. Infants of heavy marijuana users continued to have a diminished startle response to light at 9 days but by 30 days, they no longer differed from controls. No interpretation has as yet been offered for this difference in response to light. Tremors were also still evident at 9 but not 30 days. Infants did not differ on Bayley Scales at 12 months of age.

STUDIES IN ANIMALS

There have been several studies of the behavioral consequences of prenatal cannabinoid exposure, but results have been inconsistent.[13] Exceptions to this general conclusion are studies showing decreased sexual responsiveness in male mice prenatally exposed to cannabinoids.[26,32,34]

Another interesting behavioral effect observed in monkeys exposed to delta-9-THC during pregnancy and nursing is similar to effects reported by Fried in his studies of children born to mothers who used marijuana during pregnancy. In these studies, monkeys were given a test of visual attention at 1 year of age which involved looking at a slide of an unfamiliar scene and a blank slide of equal light intensity. The cannabinoid-exposed monkeys spent more time than controls viewing both slides, suggesting less habituation or a greater effect of novelty. When animals were 2 years of age, they were given a similar test. The complexity of the slide did not affect attention but novelty did prolong viewing time for cannabinoid-exposed monkeys.[35,36]

In summary, decreased habituation associated with prenatal marijuana exposure has been noted in both human infants and monkeys. This is possibly indicative of immature nervous system development. Studies in animals have unfortunately not been able to offer suggestions as to possible effects in humans to be evaluated.

COCAINE

Cocaine hydrochloride is a white, odorless, crystalline, water soluble powder made from the leaves of the coca bush, *Erythroxylon coca*. "Free base" is pure cocaine. Cocaine is a CNS stimulant and has local anesthetic effects and marked vasoconstrictive effects.

Cocaine is usually taken by sniffing ("snorting") or by injection. In general, "social" users sniff about 5 to 20 mg at a time and may repeat such exposures 2 or 3 times an hour for several hours. Heavy users may use about 10 g per day.

Cocaine and Pregnancy

A major problem in evaluating the effects of cocaine in pregnant women is that many cocaine users are also users of other drugs.[37,38] As a result, it is difficult to determine if any adverse effects seen in children born to cocaine users are due to cocaine or to the other drugs taken by the cocaine user. Currently, there are only two clinical studies of infants born to cocaine users.[37,38] Consequently, conclusions regarding the effects of prenatal cocaine use are still quite tentative.

Complications of Pregnancy

Acker et al.[39] reported uterine contractions, and vaginal bleeding and abruptio placentae occurred in 2 women shortly after cocaine use. Abruptio placentae was also noted in 4 out of 23 cocaine users in Chasnoff's study, but did not occur in controls or women using drugs other than cocaine.[37] As in Acker's study, the onset of effects occurred shortly after intravenous administration.

In isolated human placenta, cocaine causes vasoconstriction and potentiates bradykinin-induced pressor response.[40] Cocaine also causes initial placental vasoconstriction in mice followed by marked vasodilation.[40] The implications of these observations on the placenta are that cocaine may produce episodes of decreased blood flow to the fetus resulting in episodic periods of hypoxia. In addition, there is the possibility of increased fetal exposure to agents normally innocuous but rendered noxious due to rebound vasodilation. This should especially be of concern because of polydrug use by cocaine users.

Duration of Pregnancy

All pregnant cocaine users studied by Chasnoff et al.[37] delivered at term. One of the 8 infants studied by Madden et al.[38] was premature at 33 weeks of gestation. There was no indication that this prematurity was related to cocaine use.

Birth Weight and Congenital Malformations

There are no unequivocal published reports of cocaine use during pregnancy and congenital malformations or growth retardation in offspring. None of the 8 infants born to the cocaine users studied by Madden et al.[38] had any malformations or any common facial features, but 2 were considered small-for-gestational age.

One of the cocaine users in Chasnoff's study[37] gave birth to an infant with multiple congenital anomalies. Women in this group were users of alcohol and marijuana and some of the anomalies have been noted in conjunction with fetal alcohol exposure e.g. hydronephrosis and cryptorchidism. By 1 month of age, 2 of the cocaine infants died, 1 due to sudden infant death syndrome, and the other from meningitis.

Surprisingly, few studies of cocaine's effects on the conceptus have been reported in animals. Mahalik et al.[40] reported that a single injection of cocaine to pregnant mice during the period of organogenesis (equivalent to first trimester in women) produced an increased incidence of soft tissue anomalies (e.g. hydronephrosis, cryptorchidism, anophthalmia) and skeletal defects (delayed ossification of skull and paws, extra ribs, malformed sternebrae). In contrast to these results, Fantel and Macphail[41] did not observe a significant increase in anomalies in rats or mice prenatally exposed to cocaine, but did note significant decreases in birth weight for such animals.

Neurobehavioral Effects

Chasnoff et al.[37] reported that infants prenatally exposed to cocaine had a greater degree of tremulousness and startle response than methadone-exposed or control infants.

RECOMMENDATIONS FOR MANAGEMENT OF MARIJUANA AND COCAINE USE

The main problem for the obstetrician/gynecologist and perinatologist in connection with marijuana is the possibility of shortened gestation and an associated decrease in birth weight. Marijuana does not produce congenital anomalies but nervous system development may be delayed. Chronic marijuana users are also prone to use other drugs as well, and the physician should be alert to this possibility.

Cocaine use during pregnancy appears to be a risk factor for abruption and reduced placental perfusion. There is not enough information yet available to determine if cocaine is a teratogen or has postnatal effects on behavior. As in the case of marijuana, or perhaps even more so, cocaine users are likely to be polydrug users.

The most reasonable clinical approach at this time is to advise patients concerning the risks associated with marijuana or cocaine use during pregnancy and to offer support and encouragement to those willing to reduce their use of these drugs. The neonatologist should be alerted to the prenatal drug histories of these infants so that special attention may be paid to them.

REFERENCES

1. U.S. Department of Health, Education, and Welfare, Public Health Service, Marijuana and Health. Eighth Annual Report to the Congress from the Secretary of Health, Education and Welfare, 1980, DHEW Pub. No. (ADM) 80-945. Washington, D.C.: U.S. Govt. Print. Off., 1980.
2. Fishburne, PM: National Survey on Drug Abuse: Main Findings: 1979. National Institute on Drug Abuse, Rockville, Maryland, 1980.
3. Judge, N.E. and Sokol, R.J.: Drug abuse in pregnancy. *In* Quilligan, EJ (ed) Current Therapy in Obstetrics and Gynecology. Philadelphia, W.B. Saunders Co., 1983, pp.74–77.
4. Agurell, S., Gillespir, H., Halldin, M., et al.: A review of recent studies on the pharmacokinetics and metabolism of delta-1-tetrahydrocannabinol, cannabidiol, and cannabinol in man. *In* Harvey, D.J. (ed) Marihuana '84, Oxford, England, IRL Press, pp.49–62.
5. Idanpaan-Heikkila, J., Fritchie, G.E., Englert, L.F., et al.: Placental transfer of tritiated 1-delta-9-tetrahydrocannabinol. N Engl J Med, *281*:330, 1969.
6. Ryrfeldt, A., Ramsay, C.H., Agurell, S., et al.: Whole-body autoradiographic studies on the distribution of delta-1 (6)-tetrahydrocannabinol (THC) in mice after intravenous administration. Act Pharmaceut Suec *8*:704, 1971.
7. Harbison, R.D., and Mantilla-Plata, B.: Prenatal toxicity, maternal distribution and placental transfer of tetrahydrocannabinol. J. Pharm. Exp. Ther., *180*:446, 1972.
8. Vardaris, R.M., Weisz, D.J., Faze, A., et al.: Chronic administration of delta-9-tetrahydrocannabinol to pregnant rats: studies of pup behavior and placental transfer. Pharm Biochem Behav, *4*:249, 1976.
9. Blackard, C. and Tennes, K.: Human placental transfer of cannabinoids. N Engl J Med, *311*: 1984.
10. Greenland, S., Staisch, K.J., Brown, N., et al.: The effects of marijuana use during pregnancy. I. A preliminary epidemiology study. Am J Obstet Gynecol, *150*:23, 1984.
11. Hecht, F., Beals, R., Lees, M., et al.: Lysergic-acid diethylamide and cannabis as possible teratogens in man. Lancet, 2:1087, 1968.

12. Carakushansky, G., Neu, R.L., and Gardner, L.I.: Lysergide and cannabis as possible teratogens in man. Lancet, *1*:150, 1969.
13. Abel, E.L.:Prenatal exposure to cannabis: A critical review of effect on growth, development and behavior. Behav Neurol Biol, *29*:137, 1980.
14. Grigor, J.: Hashish in childbirth. J Pharm Chim, *3*:386, 1853.
15. Fried, P.A., Watkinson, B., and William A.: Marijuana use during pregnancy and decreased length of gestation. Am J Obstet Gynecol, *150*:23, 1984.
16. Gibson, G.T., Baghurst, P.A., and Colley, D.P.: Maternal alcohol, tobacco and cannabis consumption and the outcome of pregnancy. Aust NZ J Obstet Gynecol, *23*:15, 1983.
17. Linn, S., Schoenbaum, S.C., Monson, R.R., et al.: The association of marijuana with outcome of pregnancy. Am J Pub Health 73:1161, 1983.
18. Greenland, S., Richwald, G., and Honda, G: The effects of marijuana use during pregnancy. II. A study in a low-risk home-delivery population. Drug Alcohol Dep, 1983.
19. Qazi, Q.H., Mariano, E., Milman, D.H., et al.: Abnormalities in offspring associated with prenatal marihuana exposure. Dev Pharm Ther, *8*:141, 1985.
20. Fried, P.A.: Marihuana use by pregnant women and effects on offspring: An update. Neurobehav Toxicol Teratol, *4*:451, 1982.
21. Sokol, R.J., Martier, S., Ager, J., et al.: Human pregnancy loss and prenatal alcohol-marijuana exposure; no synergism detected. Alcohol Clin Exp Res, *10*:101, 1986.
22. Abel, E.L.: Alcohol-enchancement of marihuana-induced feto toxicity. Teratol, *31*:35, 1985.
23. Tennes, K., and Blackard, C.: Maternal alcohol consumption, birth weight, and minor physical anomalies. Am J Obstet Gynecol, *138*:774, 1980.
24. Hingson, R., Alpert, J., Day, N., et al.: Effects of maternal drinking and marijuana use on fetal growth and development. Pediatr, *70*:539, 1982.
25. Abel, E.L., Dintcheff, B.A., and Day, N.: Effects of marijuana on pregnant rats and their offspring. Psychopharm, *71*:71, 1980.
26. Fried, P.A. and Charlebois, A.T.: Cannabis administered during pregnancy: first-and second-generation effects in rats. Physiol Psychol, *7*:307, 1979.
27. Abel, E.L., Bush, R., Dintcheff, B.A., et al: Critical periods for marihuana-induced intrauterine growth retardation in the rat. Neurobehav Toxicol Teratol, *3*:351, 1981.
28. Charlebois, A.T. and Fried, P.A.: Interactive effects of nutrition and cannabis upon rat perinatal development. Devel Psychobiol, *13*:591, 1980.
29. Greizerstein, H.B. and Abel, E.L.: In utero exposure to marihuana extract: changes in neonate rat body composition. Neurobehav Toxicol Teratol, *3*:53, 1981.
30. Abel, E.L.: Marihuana. The First Twelve Thousand Years. New York, Plenum Press, 1980.
31. Fried, P.A.: Marihuana use by pregnant women: neurobehavioral effects in neonates. Drug Alcohol Depend, *6*:415 1980.
32. Dalterio, S. and Bartke, A.: Perinatal exposure to cannabinoids alters male reproductive function in mice. Science, *205*:1420, 1979.
33. Dalterio, S.: Perinatal or adult exposure to cannabinoids alters male reproductive functions in mice. Pharm Biochem Behav, *12*:143, 1980.
34. Hatoum, N.S., Davis, W.M., Elsohly, M.A., et al.: Perinatal exposure to cannabichromene and delta-9-tetrahydrocannabinol: separate and combined effects on viability of pups and on male reproductive system at maturity. Toxicol Letter, *8*:141, 1981.
35. Golub, M.S., Sassenrath, E.N. and Chapman, L.F.: Regulation of visual attention in offspring of female monkeys treated chronically with delta-9-tetrahydrocannabinol. Devel Psychol, *14*:507, 1981.
36. Golub, M.S., Sassenrath, N., and Chapman, L.F.: An analysis of altered attention in monkeys exposed to delta-9-tetrahydrocannabinol during development. Neurobehav Toxicol Teratol, *4*:469, 1982.
37. Chasnoff, I.J., Burns, W.J., Schnoll, S.H., et al.: Cocaine use in pregnancy. N Engl J Med *313*:666, 1985.
38. Madden, J.D., Payne, T.F. and Miller, S.: Maternal cocaine abuse and effect on the newborn. Pediatr *77*:209, 1976.
39. Acker, D., Sachs, B.P., Tracey, K.J., et al.: Abruptio placentae associated with cocaine use. Am J Obstet Gynecol, *146*:220, 1983.
40. Mahalik, M.P., Gautieri, R.E., and Mann, D.E.: Teratogenic potential of cocaine hydrochloride in CF-1 mice. J Pharmaceut Sci, *69*:703, 1980.
41. Fantel, A.G. and Macphail, B.J.: The teratogenicity of cocaine. Teratol, *26*:17, 1982.
42. Weiner, L., Rosett, H.L., Edelin, K.C., et al.: Alcohol consumption by pregnant women. Obstet Gynecol, *61*:6, 1983.
43. Rayburn, W., Wible-Kant, E.J. and Bledsoe, P.: Changing trends in drug use during pregnancy. J Reprod Med, *27*:569, 1982.

Chapter 18

Caffeine in Pregnancy

Timothy R.B. Johnson and Jennifer R. Niebyl

Caffeine is a naturally occurring xanthine derivative which structurally resembles metabolically important purines and other xanthines such as theophylline and theobromine. The stimulant properties of caffeine have led to its extraction from coffee, tea, cocoa and kola plants, and its widespread popular consumption. The approximate caffeine content of commonly used beverages is shown in Table 18–1. Depending on methods of brewing, as much as 300 mg of caffeine can be extracted in a cup of coffee. Caffeine is also a common additive in a large number of over-the-counter preparations, mostly mild analgesics,[1] which generally contain 100 to 200 mg.

Biologically, caffeine is rapidly absorbed, metabolized, and excreted primarily in urine. It passes readily to the fetus, but it is believed that the fetus is not able to metabolize caffeine.[2] The elimination half-life of caffeine is 3.5 hours in the adult, but approximately 4 days in newborn infants.[3]

In sheep, after a maternal intravenous infusion of 3.5 mg/kg of caffeine, maternal blood pressure rose and uterine blood flow decreased by 10%[4] At 10 times that dose, maternal and fetal tachycardia resulted. Fetal blood levels of caffeine were 82% of maternal levels.

In human pregnancy, maternal ingestion of 2 cups of coffee resulted in significant elevations of epinephrine concentrations after 30 minutes,[5] and the intervillous placental blood flow decreased.

Although there is a body of data implicating caffeine as a teratogen in animals, there is no convincing scientific evidence that caffeine is teratogenic in humans.[6–8] In their prospective study, Heinonen et al.[9] showed no increased incidence of congenital defects in 5773 women taking caffeine in pregnancy, usually in a fixed dose analgesic medication. Nelson and Forfar[10] found no statistical increase in congenital abnormalities associated with caffeine use in a retrospective case-control study of 458 women with anomalous infants. Le Chat et al.[11] showed a

Table 18–1. Approximate Caffeine Content of 1 cup (8 oz) of Beverage

Beverage	Caffeine, mg
coffee-brewed	75–150
coffee-instant	30–80
tea	40–60
cola	30–60
cocoa	2–40

small risk of heavy coffee use in a small population (202) and are themselves cautious in drawing definitive conclusions.

There is some evidence to suggest that heavy ingestion of caffeine is associated with increased pregnancy complications. In a prospective study, Mau and Netter[12] found an increased incidence of low birth weight infants in women using coffee, but they stressed that confounding variables might be more important than any direct effect of caffeine. Van den Berg[13] showed a similar increase in low birth weight neonates born to mothers using more than 7 cups of coffee per day. She recognized that tobacco, and probably also alcohol consumption seem to be higher in this group of women making interpretation difficult, and socioeconomic variables may also be critically important. In a retrospective study, Weathersbee found that 15 of 16 women who apparently used more than 600 mg caffeine per day (about 8 cups of coffee) suffered increased miscarriages, prematurity and stillbirths, and found a similar risk in wives of men using such high levels of caffeine.[2]

Linn et al.[14] showed no association between coffee consumption and adverse outcomes of pregnancy in 12,205 women. Low birth weight and prematurity occurred more often among offspring of women who drank 4 or more cups of coffee a day and more often among the offspring of smokers. After controlling for smoking and other habits, demographic characteristics and medical history, they found no relationship between coffee consumption and any adverse outcome. Also, there was no excess of malformations among coffee drinkers. Kurppa et al.[15] also found no increeased risk of birth defects in women who drank at least 6 cups of coffee per day.

Srisuphan et al.[16] found that moderate-to-heavy caffeine users (>151 mg caffeine daily) were more likely to experience late first or second trimester spontaneous abortions than non-users or light users (<150 mg).

It is unlikely that low exposure to caffeine is a significant teratogenic risk to humans. Heavy caffeine use may be a signal of risk in pregnancy, and when such a history is elicited during the nutritional interview, other questions should be directed to elicit other known contributors to poor pregnancy outcome. Appropriate counseling can begin there. For the present, the Food and Drug Administration suggests that "prudence dictates that pregnant women and those who may become pregnant avoid caffeine-containing products or use them sparingly."[17]

REFERENCES

1. Graham, D.M.: Caffeine: its identity, dietary sources, intake and biological effects. Nutr Rev, *36*:97, 1978.
2. Weathersbee, P.S., Olsen, L.K. and Lodge, J.R.: Caffeine and pregnancy: a retrospective study. Postgrad Med, *62*:64, 1977.
3. Aldridge, A., Aranda, J.V., and Neims, A.H.: Caffeine metabolism in the developing human infant. Pharmacol, *20*:263, 1978.
4. Wilson, S.J., Ayromlooi, J., and Errick, J.K.: Pharmacokinetic and hemodynamic effects of caffeine in the pregnant sheep. Obstet Gynecol, *61*:486, 1983.
5. Kirkinen, P., Jouppila, P., Koivula, A., et al.: The effect of caffeine on placental and fetal blood flow in human pregnancy. Am J Obstet Gynecol, *147*:939, 1983.
6. Mulvihill, J.J.: Caffeine as a teratogen and mutagen. Teratol, *8*:69, 1973.
7. Weathersbee, P.S. and Lodge, J.R.: Caffeine: its direct influence on reproduction. J Reprod Med, *19*:55, 1977.
8. "Soda Water; Amendment to Standard." Federal Register, *45*:69816, 1980.
9. Heinonen, O.P., Slone, D. and Shapiro, S.: Caffeine and other xanthine derivatives, in Birth

Defects and Drugs in Pregnancy, Littleton, Mass. Publishing Services Group, Inc., 1977, pp.366–370.

10. Nelson, M.M. and Forfar, J.O.: Associations between drugs administered during pregnancy and congenital abnormalities of the fetus. Br Med J, *1*:523, 1971.

11. Le Chat, M.F., Borlee, I., Bouckaert, A., et al.: "Caffeine Study" (letter) Science, *207*:1296, 1980.

12. Mau, G., and Netter, P.: Kaffee-und alkoholkonsum—risikofaktoren in der schhwangerschaft? Geburtsh U Frauenheilk, *34*:1018, 1974.

13. Van den Berg, B.J.: Epidemiologic observations of prematurity; effects of tobacco, coffee and alcohol in The Epidemiology of Prematurity, ed. Reed D.M. and Stanley, F.J. Baltimore, Urban and Schwartzenberg, 1977.

14. Linn, S., Schoenbaum, S.C., Monson, R.R., et al.: No association between coffee consumption and adverse outcomes of pregnancy. N Engl J Med, *306*:141, 1982.

15. Kurppa, K., Holmberg, P.C., Kuosma, E., et al.: Coffee consumption during pregnancy. N Engl J Med, *306*:1548, 1982.

16. Srisuphan, W., and Bracken, M.B.: Caffeine consumption during pregnancy and association with late spontaneous abortion. Am J Obstet Gynecol, *154*:14, 1986.

17. Caffeine and Pregnancy, FDA Drug Bulletin, *10*:19, 1980.

Chapter 19

Treatment of the Common Cold in Pregnancy

Jennifer R. Niebyl and John T. Repke

Pregnant women seem particularly susceptible to the common cold and often have several colds during pregnancy. They should be reassured that this is normal as their resistance is down in the pregnant state. They should also be reassured that the viruses that cause the common cold have not been shown to be teratogenic.

First, non-pharmacologic remedies should be encouraged such as increased rest and fluid intake. The use of a humidifier can be helpful in soothing a dry throat.

As far as medications are concerned, it should be explained to the patient that over-the-counter symptomatic treatments are not therapeutic. Many patients have the misconception that some of these preparations act like an antibiotic to the etiologic agent. Many of the over-the-counter preparations contain several agents including antihistamines, decongestants, expectorants, and analgesics (Table 19–1). A history should be taken to elicit from the patient the symptom that is bothering her the most and then the most appropriate specific drug therapy rather than combination therapy can be used. This will minimize fetal exposure to drugs which are not indicated.

Antihistamines

If the patient has an allergy, an antihistamine may be all that is necessary. The most commonly used antihistamine is chlorpheniramine (Chlortrimeton) (Table 19–1). Most antihistamines are not associated with any known teratogenic risk.[1] Of 1070 first trimester exposures to chlorpheniramine in the Collaborative Perinatal Project,[1] and 175 exposures in another study,[2] no association with birth defects was noted. However, in the Collaborative Perinatal Project, in 65 exposures in the first trimester to brompheniramine (in Dimetane, Dimetapp), the relative risk for birth defects was increased three-fold which was statistically significant. In this study, triprolidine alone, the antihistamine in Actifed, was only evaluated in 16 patients with no obvious teratogenic risk.[1] Triprolidine plus pseudoephedrine (Actifed) was not found to be associated with any risk of birth defects in 244 exposures.[2] Antihistamines have been further discussed in Chapter 2.

Decongestants

In the Collaborative Perinatal Project, there was a statistically significant association of increased birth defects with use of sympathomimetic drugs in the

235

Table 19–1. Over-The-Counter Cold Preparations

	Antihistamines						Decongestants			Expectorants		Acetaminophen	Alcohol % (Liquid Forms)
	pyrilamine	chlorpheniramine	doxylamine succinate	triprolidine	brompheniramine	dexbrompheniramine	pseudoephedrine	phenylpropanolamine	phenylephrine	dextromethorphan	guaifenesin		
Actifed				X			X						0
Allerest		X						X				±	—
ARM		X						X					—
Chlortrimeton		X											
Chlortrimeton decongestant		X					X						7
Contac		X						X				±	—
Coricidin		X										X	
Coricidin decongestant		X					X	X					<0.5
Cotylenol		X					X			X		X	7
Dimetane					X								3
Dimetane decongestant					X				X				2.3
Dimetapp					X			X					2.3
Dristan		X							X			X	—
Drixoral						X	X						0
4 Way		X						X					
Robitussin											X		3.5
Robitussin night relief	X								X	X		X	25
Sinarest		X						X				X	—
Sinutab		X					X					X	
Sudafed							X						2.4
Sudafed Plus		X					X						0
Vicks 44										X			10–20
Vicks Nyquil			X				X			X		X	25

(—) = Not available in liquid form.

first trimester, and these were usually taken for upper respiratory symptoms.[3] Significant associations were noted for epinephrine and phenylpropanolamine.[3] Less risk is associated with phenylephrine,[2,3] and no increased risk of birth defects has been reported in 460 exposures to pseudoephedrine.[2,3] Phenylpropanolamine is present in several cold preparations, including Allerest, ARM, Contac, Coricidin decongestant, Dimetapp, and Sinarest, and should be avoided in the first trimester.

If a decongestant is necessary alone, pseudoephedrine (Sudafed) is recommended. For combinations with an antihistamine, pseudoephedrine plus triprolidine (Actifed), or pseudoephedrine plus chlorpheniramine (Chlortrimeton decongestant or Sudafed Plus) are recommended.

The occurrence of viral illness was not noted in the Collaborative Study and so the possibility remains that a viral agent contributed to the defects as well as the drugs to treat the symptoms. However, there is no association between cough medicines or most antihistamines and malformations suggesting that indeed, the sympathomimetic drugs themselves may have contributed to the problem.

Topical Nasal Decongestants

Sometimes saline nose drops will give relief. If the patient needs a decongestant, topical administration will result in a lower blood level than will oral administration, where the same blood level of the drug is delivered to the uterus as to the patient's nose. Chronic use of topical decongestants should be avoided, however, because of the problem of rebound nasal congestion. If a long-acting topical decongestant is used at night, usually none is necessary during the daytime if the patient can tolerate some rhinorrhea in order to minimize fetal exposure.

Phenylephrine is the most frequently used short-acting and oxymetazoline the most commonly used long-acting topical decongestant (Table 19–2). Among topical decongestants, no increased risk of birth defects was found with 155 first trimester exposures to oxymetazoline[2] (Afrin, Coricidin, Dristan Long-Acting, Duration, 4 way Long-Acting, NTZ, Nostril Long Acting, Vicks Sinex Long Acting), 207 exposures to xylometazoline (Otrivin),[2] 373 exposures to ephedrine (Vicks Vatronol),[3] or 550 exposures to phenylephrine (Dristan, 4 Way Fast Acting, Neo-Synephrine, Nostril, Vicks Sinex).[2,3] No information is available about use in pregnancy of prophylhexedrine (Benzedrex) naphazoline (Privine) or desoxyephedrine (Vicks inhaler).

Cough Medicines

The major cough medicine to be avoided in pregnancy is saturated solution of potassium iodide. This can cross to the fetus and cause significant goiter, on occasion enough to cause respiratory obstruction in the newborn.[4]

Other expectorants have not been shown to be of any risk. Of 300 infants exposed to dextromethorphan in the first trimester in the Collaborative Perinatal Project, there was no increased risk of birth defects. Of 197 exposed to guaifenesin (glyceryl guaiacolate; Robitussin) in the perinatal projects and 241 exposures in another study,[2] no association with birth defects was found. Of 292 exposures to cetylpyridinium chloride (Cepacol), no increased risk was noted.[2]

Some liquid cold preparations do have a significant alcohol content. Of the

Table 19–2.   Topical Nasal Decongestants

	oxymetazoline	phenylephrine	xylometazoline	prophylhexedrine	naphazoline	desoxyephedrine	ephedrine	pheniramine
Afrin	X							
Benzedrex				X				
Coricidin	X							
Dristan		X						X
Dristan LA	X							
Duration	X							
4 Way Fast Acting		X						
4 Way Long Acting	X							
NTZ	X							
Neo-Synephrine		X						
Nostril		X						
Nostril LA	X							
Otrivin			X					
Privine					X			
Vicks Inhaler						X		
Vicks Sinex		X						
Vicks Sinex LA	X							
Vicks Vatronol							X	

formulas listed, Vicks Nyquil and Robitussin Night Relief had the highest alcohol content by volume (25%). If the maximum recommended daily dosage is used (1 ounce every 6 hours), this would be the equivalent of 1 ounce of absolute alcohol. One report described a woman who abused cough syrup consuming 480 to 840 ml per day of a mixture containing 9.5% alcohol. The infant had features of fetal alcohol syndrome.[6] Preparations with low or no alcohol content should be recommended for use in pregnancy (Table 19–1). Also, the alcohol and sugar content of liquid preparations should be kept in mind for women who are diabetic or on special diets.

Patients should be educated that over-the counter cold preparations provide purely symptomatic relief and have no influence on the course of the disease. The use of these drugs for trivial indications should be discouraged as long term effects are unknown.

REFERENCES

1. Heinonen, O.P., Slone, D., and Shapiro, S.: Birth Defects and Drugs in Pregnancy. Littleton, Mass., Publishing Sciences Group, Inc., 1977, p. 322.
2. Aselton, P., Jick, H., and Milunsky, A., et al.: First-trimester drug use and congenital disorders. Obstet Gynecol, 65:451, 1985.
3. Heinonen, O.P., Slone, D., and Shapiro, S.: Birth Defects and Drugs in Pregnancy. Littleton, Mass., Publishing Sciences Group, Inc., 1977, p. 348.
4. Senior, B. and Chernoff, H.L.: Iodide goiter in the newborn. Pediatrics, 47:510, 1971.
5. Heinonen, O.P., Slone, D., and Shapiro, S.: Birth Defects and Drugs in Pregnancy. Littleton, Mass., Publishing Sciences Group, Inc., 1977, p. 383.
6. Chasnoff, I.J., Diggs, G., and Schnoll, S.H.: Fetal alcohol effects and maternal cough syrup abuse. Am J Dis Child, 135:968, 1981.

INDEX

Page numbers in *Italics* indicate figures; page numbers followed by "t" indicate tables.